T024890

KT-491-917

Research Methods for Health and Social Care

WB25
10/09

Also by the editor:

Neale, J. (2002) *Drug Users in Society* (Basingstoke: Palgrave – now Palgrave Macmillan)

Research Methods for Health and Social Care

Edited by
Joanne Neale

palgrave
macmillan

First published 2009 by
PALGRAVE MACMILLAN

Palgrave Macmillan in the UK is an imprint of Macmillan Publishers Limited,
registered in England, company number 785998, of Houndmills, Basingstoke,
Hampshire RG21 6XS.

Palgrave Macmillan in the US is a division of St Martin's Press LLC,
175 Fifth Avenue, New York, NY 10010.

Palgrave Macmillan is the global academic imprint of the above companies
and has companies and representatives throughout the world.

Palgrave® and Macmillan® are registered trademarks in the United States,
the United Kingdom, Europe and other countries.

ISBN-13: 978–0–230–50078–5
ISBN-10: 0–230–50078–1

This book is printed on paper suitable for recycling and made from fully
managed and sustained forest sources. Logging, pulping and manufacturing
processes are expected to conform to the environmental regulations of the
country of origin.

A catalogue record for this book is available from the British Library.

10 9 8 7 6 5 4 3 2 1
18 17 16 15 14 13 12 11 10 09

Printed and bound in China

In memory of Jo Campling

Contents

PART 4
Qualitative Research 195

List of Figures, Tables and Boxes

Figures

Tables

Boxes

Contributors

Dr Hamed A. Adetunji (B.Sc., M.Sc., MPH, Ph.D., Dip. Epid., PGCHE, FRIPH) is Course Leader for the M.Sc. in Public Health at Oxford Brookes University. He has worked in public health practice, teaching and research for more than two decades and his current research interests include internationalising the curriculum, occupational health risks from exposure to nano-particulates, and students' health behaviours and well-being.

Dr Debby Allen (B.Sc. Hons, M.Sc., Ph.D., PG Dip. HE, RGN, DN Dip.) is a Senior Lecturer and Research Associate in the School of Health and Social Care at Oxford Brookes University. Debby's research focuses on substance use/misuse, particularly in relation to young people.

Dr Jane V. Appleton (BA Hons, M.Sc., Ph.D., RGN, RHV, PGCEA) is Reader in Primary and Community Care at Oxford Brookes University. Jane's research focuses on health visiting, children in need, and safeguarding children. She is a nurse member of Warwickshire Research Ethics Committee, professional editor for *Community Practitioner* and co-editor of *Child Abuse Review*.

Dr Helen Aveyard (B.Sc., MA, Ph.D., RGN, PDCE) is Senior Lecturer in the School of Health and Social Care, Oxford Brookes University, and is involved in the teaching and development of research education. Helen's recent publications include *Doing a Literature Review in Health and Social Care,* which was published by Open University Press in 2007.

Professor Mary Boulton (BA, Ph.D., Hon MFPH) is Professor of Health Sociology and Director of Research in the School of Health and Social Care, Oxford Brookes University. Her academic interests are in the social aspects of health and healthcare and her teaching and research have been concerned largely with primary care, children with disabilities, and families and health. Mary is also interested in research ethics and informed consent. Her current research is on the role of primary care in supporting individuals and families living with cancer.

Lindsey Coombes (BA Hons, MA, RMN, RGN, PGCEA) is Senior Lecturer in Mental Health Nursing and a Research Fellow at Oxford Brookes University. For the past 20 years, he has taught a variety of healthcare modules at diploma, undergraduate and postgraduate level. Since January 2000, Lindsey has conducted research relating to mental health promotion, community nursing, substance misuse, young people, and children's services.

Dr Jill Dawson (BA Hons, M.Sc., D.Phil.) is Senior Research Scientist at the University of Oxford and Visiting Professor at Oxford Brookes University. She has been a full-time researcher since 1987 and has focused on the measurement of health status and outcomes for most of that time. Jill is currently researching outcomes following shoulder rotator cuff surgery and outcomes and satisfaction related to foot and ankle surgery.

Dr Annette K. Dearmun (B.Sc. Hons, Ph.D., RSCN, RGN, DN, DNE, RNT, ITEC) is Associate Lecturer at Oxford Brookes University. She has been teaching in the field of child health since 1986 and is currently Chief Nurse at the Oxford Children's Hospital, Oxford Radcliffe Hospitals NHS Trust.

Lorraine Dixon (Dip. HE Palliative Care, PGDip.Ed., M.Sc.) is Palliative Care Services Manager at Leckhampton Court Hospice, Sue Ryder Care, and until recently was Field Chair Cancer and Palliative Care/Senior Lecturer at Oxford Brookes University. Lorraine is currently researching carer involvement within professional education.

Julia Foster-Turner (MBA, PGCert.Ed., DMS, Dip.COT) is Senior Lecturer/Senior Consultant at the London Centre for Leadership in Learning at the Institute of Education. She was a manager within the NHS for 20 years and has worked in higher education, teaching on a variety of topics in the field of management and leadership for the past eight years. Her practice specialism is in developmental relationships, such as coaching and mentoring, and in the crafting and utilisation of intra- and inter-organisational learning networks.

Professor David R. Foxcroft (B.Sc. Hons, Ph.D., CPsychol) is Professor of Health Care at Oxford Brookes University. He has been teaching health psychology and research methods for over ten years. David is currently researching the effectiveness of alcohol and drug misuse prevention programmes.

Professor John Hall (BA, M.Sc., Ph.D., FBPsS) is Visiting Professor of Mental Health at Oxford Brookes University and Director of Research at the Health and Social Care Advisory Service in London. As a clinical psychologist, John has been involved in research relating to severe mental health problems, and is currently working on a number of projects to improve the quality of mental health services.

Professor Sarah Harper (MA Cantab, D.Phil. Oxon) is Professor of Gerontology at the University of Oxford and Director of the Oxford Institute of Ageing. An ethnographer by training, Sarah's research focuses on the implications of population ageing, with particular focus on work and the family.

Deborah Humphrey (BA Hons, M.Sc., RMN) is a Nurse Consultant in older people's mental health at Oxfordshire and Buckinghamshire Mental Health Partnership Trust. She has been working in older people's healthcare practice and education for about 20 years. Deborah is currently researching the types of knowledge that contribute to nursing in older people's services.

Dr Michelle Jackson (BA Hons, M.Sc., D.Phil.) is Research Fellow in the Centre for Research Methods in the Social Sciences (Department of Politics and

International Relations) at Nuffield College, Oxford. She is a sociologist with research interests in the sociology of education, social stratification and mobility. She currently holds an ESRC Research Fellowship within the Understanding Population Trends and Processes research programme.

Professor Peter A. Kemp (B.Sc. Hons, M.Phil., D.Phil.) is Barnett Professor of Social Policy at the University of Oxford and Fellow of St Cross College. His current teaching is mainly in the field of comparative social policy. Peter's recent publications include *Private Renting in Transition* (2004), *Cash and Care: Policy Challenges in the Welfare State* (2006), *Sick Societies? Trends in Disability Benefits in Post-industrial Welfare States* (2006) and *Housing Allowances in Comparative Perspective* (2007).

Jenny La Fontaine (MA, RMN, DPSN, Cert. Ed. FAHE, PG Cert) is Research Officer at the Oxford Institute of Ageing, University of Oxford. She has worked with people with dementia and their families for over 20 years, and taught health and social care professionals in this speciality. Jenny is currently engaged in an ethnographic study exploring the impact of dementia upon grandparent and grandchild relationships.

Martin Leach (BA Hons, M.Sc.) is Senior Lecturer in Health Care at Oxford Brookes University, where he specialises in healthcare research methods. He has more than ten years' experience of research into the genetic epidemiology of rheumatic disease.

Professor Joanne Neale (BA Hons, MA, D.Phil., CQSW) is Professor of Public Health in the School of Health and Social Care at Oxford Brookes University. She has been researching illicit drug use since 1996 and has undertaken both qualitative and quantitative studies, exploring topics such as non-fatal drug overdose, drug driving, drug users' views and experiences of treatment services, homelessness among drug users, and drug users' everyday lives and recovery processes.

Debora Osborne (BA Hons, Grad. Dip. Ed., RN) currently studies and teaches part-time at Griffith University, Brisbane, Australia. Her research is focused on constructions of female sexuality and her chosen methodology is Foucauldian Discourse Analysis.

Dr Charlotte Ritchie (BA Hons, M.Sc., D.Phil., DipSW) is Senior Lecturer in Social Work at Oxford Brookes University and Deputy Director of the Oxford Centre for Research into Parenting and Children. Prior to moving to Oxford Brookes, Charlotte carried out research at the University of Oxford, specialising in policy, parenting and children.

Professor Terence J. Ryan (DM, FRCP) is Emeritus Professor at the University of Oxford and Oxford Brookes University. His early career focused on blood supply and lymphatic drainage of the skin while heading the Oxford Hospital's Dermatology Department. Over the past two decades, Terence has taken skin care into the developing world through contracts with international organisations, such as the World Health Organization; the United Nations Educational, Scientific and Cultural Organization; and the International Society of Dermatology.

Dr Lesley Smith (BA Hons, Ph.D.) is Principal Lecturer in Quantitative Research Methods, School of Health and Social Care, Oxford Brookes University. She has been active in teaching healthcare professionals and students for the past 12 years, with a particular emphasis on evidence-based medicine. Her current research includes an evaluation of diagnostic screening tools for alcohol use in primary care, alcohol consumption in pregnancy, and methodological issues of meta-analysis for determining drug safety.

Bridget Taylor (BA Hons, M.Sc., RGN, Cert. Ed.) is Senior Lecturer at Oxford Brookes University. She has been teaching in the field of sexual health for the past 15 years. Bridget is currently researching the experiences of patients and partners of patients with life-limiting conditions in relation to sexuality and intimacy.

Dr Sharon Vitali qualified as a Social Worker in Canada and began her career as a child protection worker specialising in sexual abuse. She is currently Senior Lecturer at Oxford Brookes University, where she teaches across a wide variety of modules and disciplines. Sharon has a special interest in distance and blended learning and the psychosocial impact of chronic illness on patients, marriages, children and caregivers. Her recent research has explored the acquisition of professional competency in educational programmes.

Professor Robert Walker (BSocSci, MA, M.Sc., Ph.D., FRSA) is Professor of Social Policy and Fellow of Green Templeton College at the University of Oxford where he directs the M.Sc. programme in Comparative Social Policy. Robert's research interests are eclectic but include poverty, family dynamics, and policy evaluation; embrace quantitative and qualitative methodologies; and are increasingly applied across the old global East–West and North–South divides.

Dr Marion Watson (B.Sc. Hons, Ph.D., ARCS, PGCM, PGCTHE) is Senior Research Support Associate at the University of Oxford, with particular interests in clinical trials and gene therapy. Previously, she spent 15 years in pharmaceutical research and also worked at Oxford Brookes University, where she taught research methods and undertook primary care-centred research studies.

Neil Wheeler (EdD, MBA) is Principal Lecturer at Oxford Brookes University. Following a career in NHS senior management, he has been teaching public sector management and research methods for 15 years. Neil's research is in the area of management education.

Acknowledgements

My first acknowledgement goes to Professor Griffith Edwards of the National Addiction Centre, London, UK. In 2004, Griffith asked me to write an article for the journal *Addiction*. The aim was to provide an overview of qualitative research, highlighting its strengths and weaknesses and outlining some of the important principles and processes involved in its undertaking. The article was published as Neale, J., Allen, D. and Coombes, L. (2005) 'Qualitative research methods within the addictions', *Addiction,* **100**, 1584–93. While working on this paper, it occurred to me that Griffith's vision of a short, balanced overview of what qualitative research is and how to do it could, with a bit of reworking, be applied to a wide range of study designs. And so the idea for a health and social care research methods textbook was born. I would like to thank Griffith for unwittingly starting this volume on its journey.

Relatively soon thereafter, I mentioned my tentative thoughts for a book to Professor Peter Kemp (then at the University of York and now at the University of Oxford), Dr Amanda Root (then at Oxford Brookes University), and Professor David Foxcroft (then, and still, at Oxford Brookes University). These three individuals were all positive and encouraging and I am very grateful for that. Over the months that followed, Peter has continued to listen, discuss and debate ideas relating to the book. He has also provided unfailing wise counsel and contributed to one of the chapters. Amanda was involved in the early stages of writing the book proposal and helped to identify contributors. Life, however, diverted her down a different route and she left Oxford Brookes early in 2007. David has been around throughout the project and also co-authored one of the chapters.

Turning an idea for a book into a reality obviously requires the support of a publisher. For this, as in the past, I turned to Jo Campling. Jo, a freelance publishing consultant, visited the School of Health and Social Care at Oxford Brookes University in the summer of 2005 and gave us one of her fascinating talks on the publishing process. She also read our book proposal, provided invaluable feedback and promised to help us find a publisher. It is through her efforts that we obtained a contract with Palgrave Macmillan. Jo very sadly died in 2006. She is irreplaceable and sorely missed. I am very sorry that I cannot thank her again in person, but I hope that we have done justice to her faith in us and that she would have been pleased with the final product.

Wise as ever, Jo left us in the very capable hands of Lynda Thompson at Palgrave. Over the past year and a half, Lynda has provided me with a perfect combination of support, advice, patience, distance, good humour and plan Bs. This has helped to make the writing and editing process much easier and (on occasions) even good fun. I would like to acknowledge Lynda for her invaluable input as the book slowly came together. Then, as the final stages of drafting and redrafting began (the point where the end was in sight, but the mind and body were weary), my colleague Professor Mary Boulton, Director of Research in the School of Health and Social Care at Oxford Brookes University, did a wonderful job of nudging me and the book towards and over the finishing line.

Finally, of course, I must thank all the contributors – particularly for their willingness to accommodate my interventionist editorial style. With a book of this size, it is inevitable that jobs change, illnesses occur, babies are born, and other life events happen. To my amazement, we finished with the twenty chapters we promised at the outset. This is testimony to the commitment of my colleagues both at Oxford Brookes University and the University of Oxford. Having volunteered to become involved, they stuck faithfully to their words and delivered. I promise that I am now going to stop emailing, phoning and generally interfering, so allowing them all well-earned peace, quiet and time to get on with other things.

JOANNE NEALE
Oxford Brookes University

The publishers are grateful for permission to reproduce Table 13.1. Reproduced with permission and copyright © of the British Editorial Society of *Bone and Joint Surgery*, Dawson, J., Fitzpatrick, R. and Carr, A. (1996) Questionnaire on the perceptions of patients about shoulder surgery. *Journal of Bone and Joint Surgery* [Br], **78-B**: 593–600. (Table 1).

Every effort has been made to acknowledge copyright. The publisher apologises should there have been any accidental infringements, and would welcome any information to redress this situation.

Abbreviations

ADL	activities of daily living
AIMS	Arthritis Impact Measurement Scales
ANOVA	analysis of variance
AUDIT	alcohol use disorders identification test
AWHONN	Association of Women's Health, Obstetric and Neonatal Nurses
BCS70	1970 British Cohort Study
BMI	body mass index
BMJ	*British Medical Journal*
CBA	cost–benefit analysis
CEA	cost-effectiveness analysis
CENTRAL	Cochrane Central Register of Controlled Trials
CI	confidence interval
CIOMS	Council for International Organizations of Medical Sciences
CIT	critical incident technique
CMA	cost-minimisation analysis
CONSORT	consolidated standards of reporting trials
CRD	Centre for Reviews and Dissemination
CSCI	Commission for Social Care Inspection
CUA	cost–utility analysis
DTCA	direct-to-consumer advertisements
DSM-IV	*Diagnostic and Statistical Manual of Mental Disorders-IV*
DWP	Department for Work and Pensions
EPPI-Centre	Evidence for Policy and Practice Information Co-ordinating Centre
ER	emergency room
ESRC	Economic and Social Research Council
FBI	Federal Bureau of Investigation
FCC	Federal Communications Commission
GMG	Glasgow Media Group
GP	general practitioner
HAQ	Stanford Health Assessment Questionnaire
HRT	hormone replacement therapy
HuGENeT	Human Genome Epidemiology Network
ICER	incremental cost-effectiveness ratio
IEC	institutional ethics committee
IMRAD	introduction, methods, results and discussion

IRB	institutional review board
IQOLA	international quality of life assessment
ITT	intention-to-treat
JMMR	*Journal of Mixed Methods Research*
MIDIRS	Midwives' Information and Resource Service
MRC	Medical Research Council
NCDS	National Child Development Study
NHS	National Health Service
NICE	The National Institute for Health and Clinical Excellence
NRES	National Research Ethics Service
OSS	Oxford Shoulder Score
PROMS	patient-reported outcome measures
QALY	quality adjusted life year
QOF	quality and outcomes framework
QRI	Queensland Radium Institute
R&D	research and development
RCT	randomised controlled trial
REB	research ethics board
REC	research ethics committee
SCIE	Social Care Institute for Excellence
SD	standard deviation
SE	standard error
SF-36	Short-Form 36
SOGC	Society of Obstetricians and Gynaecologists of Canada
SPSS	statistical package for the Social Sciences
SSCI	Social Science Citation Index
SSI	Social Services Inspectorate
UK	United Kingdom
US	United States
USA	United States of America
USSR	Union of Soviet Socialist Republics
VAS	visual analogue scale
WHO	World Health Organization
WHOQOL	World Health Organization Quality of Life Assessment

Part 1

Research Preliminaries

Why Research?

CHARLOTTE RITCHIE AND SHARON VITALI

The Importance of Research

In today's information-driven society, almost all policy and practice decisions demand consideration and evaluation of the evidence base. Thus, health and social care practitioners can no longer rely solely on the theoretical knowledge acquired from 'clever' lecturers and professors while taking an academic degree, nor the practice wisdom of mentors, borne of their many years of experience. The ability to comprehend and master research is required of both undergraduate and postgraduate students of health and social care, and this is reflected in the growth of modules such as *research methods*, *critical appraisal* and *evidence-based practice*, as well as the ubiquitous *research dissertation*. Meanwhile, qualified nurses, midwives, physiotherapists, social workers, occupational therapists, paramedics and others are increasingly utilising research findings and undertaking studies themselves in order to inform their practice.

The holy grail of conclusive evidence regarding 'what works, when, how, why and with whom' can, however, seem difficult to locate – particularly for the new researcher confronting multiple and often conflicting presentations of fact and opinion in books, academic and professional journals, reports, web pages and more popular media. Most frustratingly, the key details of a study are frequently obscured within the mysterious language and rituals of the world of researchers. For many students and practitioners, the mere mention of research methods, data analysis and publication can be enough to induce panic and cognitive freezing. Yet, research is an exciting activity that can be personally and professionally rewarding, as well as leading to wider benefits for services and their users. It is therefore important that today's health and social care students and professionals understand how studies are undertaken and what research findings mean. Crucially, this means being able to:

- Understand and critically appraise research papers and reports

- Conduct literature searches in order to determine the current knowledge and evidence base regarding a health or social problem and potential interventions

- Lead on and/or participate in studies which evaluate policy, practice and programme-based initiatives

● Lead on and/or participate in studies which improve understanding of the experiences, needs and behaviours of those using and working within health and social care services

● Collect, collate, appraise and present research evidence in a confident and cognisant manner.

This book is written for those of you – students, professionals and even lecturers – who are looking for a user-friendly interpretation of the essential, but sometimes apparently impenetrable, world of research. Without confusing you with unnecessary jargon, the book will clarify the role of research within health and social care and help you to identify which methods and research designs are most suited to particular types of research question. Using examples from the field, it will also guide you through the various stages of conducting a study – from identifying a topic to disseminating your findings – and highlight the strengths and weaknesses of different methods, thus providing balanced accounts that will enable you to reflect critically on the wide range of possible approaches.

Our primary goal is to help you to develop your research knowledge and skills so that you will feel confident in your ability to use research effectively. This should liberate you from reliance on, and fear of, the 'research expert'. In keeping with that philosophy, the book has been designed so that you can consume it in its entirety or move quickly to the chapter(s) dealing with the method(s) that most interest you – either as an introduction or as a refresher session. The rest of this chapter will help to set the scene. To this end, we reflect on the contested meaning of scientific knowledge, explore the role that patronage and funding have played in research, and acknowledge the limitations of evidence-based practice. We also argue that the future of health and social care research is bright, and conclude with a brief overview of the chapters that are to follow.

The Contested Nature of Scientific Knowledge

There is no absolute knowledge.
And those who claim it,
whether they are scientists or dogmatists,
open the door to tragedy.
All information is imperfect.
We have to treat it with humility. (Bronowski, 1953: 353)

How do we know that anything we measure or observe is accurate? The early discoverers soon learned that challenging a pre-existing theory required fortitude, but also a methodology that could be verified by their contemporaries. Units of measurement, for example, had to be recognisable, if not universal, and calculations and observations had to be open to the inspection of others – their peers. Today, whenever a study is published in an academic journal, it will have been reviewed first by at least two other academics familiar with the subject, a process known as peer review. But this still leaves many questions unanswered and key amongst them is 'how true are research findings?'

To begin to answer this question, it is important to contemplate the relationship between research and truth and the strengths and limitations of both natural and social science methods. This is particularly important for health and social care researchers who routinely engage with studies from both traditions.[1] Essentially, natural science claims to be a rational approach to studying the objective 'real' world, which, like chemical reactions or the fusion of particles, is governed by rules or laws of natural origin. In contrast, social science is concerned with exploring human behaviour and society, phenomena which are difficult to measure or define since they are socially, culturally and historically specific, as well as underpinned by individual agency, choice and free will.

By way of illustration, we can take a natural world problem and juxtapose it with one from the social world. Let us suppose that water has found its way to the edge of a sharp drop and that nothing stands in the way of it tipping over the edge. We know from past experience that it will flow over and down the hillside. This is driven by the laws of nature. As Karl Popper[2] might have argued, unless or until we see water travelling unaided uphill, we know that the hypothesis that water, unhindered, flows downhill will always be true. This is a natural science problem, but the same is not true of human subjects, whose behaviour is governed not on the whole by scientific laws and inevitability, but by personal choices made within the structures and contexts of their broader life circumstances (see also Giddens, 1995).

For example, a very hungry person who is offered food will usually make a rational decision to eat it. However, we cannot assume that this will always be so. They may have rational reasons for not eating it – they may not like its taste or smell or they may be on a diet, religious fast or hunger strike. They may also have seemingly irrational 'reasons' for not eating it. They might simply be in a bad mood or a 'fussy' eater. The logic of whether they eat or not might even be a matter for professional medical or psychiatric debate. So, someone who has an eating disorder and does not eat despite being very hungry might be described as behaving rationally within the constraints of their illness or irrationally if they are risking their health and even life.

At first sight then, it may seem that the natural sciences and the social sciences are dealing with two entirely different worlds: the first objective, inevitable and capable of measurement; and the second lacking objectivity, contingent and unable to demonstrate causality. Yet, this is an unhelpful distinction. Over the years, social scientists have valiantly sought to prove that their work – like the work of natural scientists – is objective, verifiable and therefore true. The origins of this crusade date back to the eighteenth century when philosophers and intellectuals – such as John Locke (1602–1704), Isaac Newton (1642–1727) and David Hume (1711–1776) – introduced the concept of empiricism. This was the principle that knowledge should always be based on observations of the real world, rather than on mere reasoning or conjecture.

Subsequently, Auguste Comte (1798–1857) argued that all science should not only involve observation, but also procedures for verification (that is, methods for checking the accuracy of its claims). Moreover, science should be value-free (not make judgements about worth, utility or importance) and measurable (able to quantify what has been done and found). Additionally, science should discard any theory which could not be verified or proved true. Comte is generally regarded as the first Western sociologist and his writings – along with those of others, such as Jeremy Bentham (1748–1832), John Stuart Mill (1806–1873), Durkheim (1858–1917), Marx (1818–1883) and Weber (1864–1920) – helped to establish positivism within social science. The philosophy of positivism maintains that knowledge can only come from positive affirmation of theories through strict scientific method, involving observation and experience.

More recently, social scientists have drawn back from positivism, instead arguing that science can never be truly objective and verifiable since all knowledge is socially constructed (Berger and Luckmann, 1966; Latour and Woolgar, 1979; Lyotard, 1984). Research hypotheses and theories always involve questions of meaning, definition and value, and are therefore by their very nature contingent. For example, we may hypothesise that intervention A will solve problem B. Yet, to test this, we need to be certain of what exactly both A and B are. Problematically, we cannot be sure that everyone will necessarily agree on what – or how important – A is, or on how B should be implemented. Furthermore, the impact of A on B cannot be divorced from the subjective experiences of those affected. For example, being diagnosed with a particular illness can have very different meanings for individuals depending on their personal, social, cultural and economic circumstances.[3]

It is also not possible to assume that science (natural or social) can explain everything. We cannot conclude that something does not exist, just because we have not observed or measured it. Maybe we were simply looking in the wrong place or at the wrong time. Nor can we be certain that our experimental observations (however carefully controlled) have not missed some crucial explanatory factor or causal process – perhaps one that we did not consider or one that simply could not be factored into the research. In practice, natural science researchers cannot conclusively predict which individuals will develop a particular condition and how it will develop. Similarly, social scientists cannot foretell with any absolute certainty which children will be abused or treated badly by their parents or which young people will grow up to engage in a life of drugs or crime.

In short, the quest for truth founded on neutral and objective scientific knowledge appears to be an ephemeral goal. Knowledge is rather contingent and contested and this becomes even more evident when we consider not only what researchers do, but how they are enabled (or not) to do it – crucially, how their work is funded.

The Role of Patronage and Funding

In the days of the Renaissance,[4] wealthy princes and others sponsored scientists, mathematicians and artists in order to glorify their own name and self-image

(Pumfrey and Dawbarn, 2004). However, this patronage also stimulated innovation in scientific thinking. Whilst the sixteenth- and seventeenth-century universities maintained rigorous disciplinary divides between cosmology and mathematical astronomy, the courts of princes provided an opportunity for more groundbreaking and innovative ideas. Thus, the Renaissance led to an exponential increase in scientific discoveries which would not have occurred without the support and funding of some of society's wealthiest and most powerful families and institutions. However, this patronage did not always come without a cost.

Galileo, for example, found financial support from the court of the Medicis in Italy and deftly named the satellites of Jupiter after the Grand Duke's four sons. In time, he worked his way up to the papal court at the Vatican, the most powerful court in a largely Catholic Europe. At that point, Pope Urban VIII asked Galileo to give arguments for and against the Copernican theory that the planets revolved around the sun. Galileo's work concurred with the Copernican theory and this angered the Vatican because the Church, taking a literal interpretation of the Old Testament, held that the earth was static.[5] As a result, Galileo was summoned before the Inquisition, placed under house arrest, and his publications and all future works were banned.

During the middle years of the twentieth century, the power of ruling ideologies in accepting or dismissing new knowledge and theories became increasingly evident. For example, there were calls for Einstein's work on relativity to be banned in the Union of Soviet Socialist Republics (USSR) because his theories resonated with bourgeois decadence. In America, meanwhile, he was investigated by the Federal Bureau of Investigation (FBI) as a 'dangerous' liberal and freethinker. The development of nuclear weapons during and after the Second World War further confirmed that science was anything but value-free. Even the lunar landings of the 1960s were enabled by Nazi rocket technology, powered by the Cold War between the USSR and America, and motivated by potential military applications.

So, academic work has often needed the endorsement of a powerful institution or patron. Yet, in order to benefit, its findings have generally had to fit – at least for the moment – within the ideas and priorities set by those offering their support. An important benefit of this is that paradigms and patronage have often focused academic thought and led to innovation. Additionally, understanding has developed incrementally with a degree of coherence and logical structure as new theories have been added to old. Despite this, the paradigms and patronage of the privileged can become all-powerful, making innovation more difficult. Equally, those whose scientific interests have lacked economic or social viability, or not fitted within prevailing belief structures, have often found that the door to discovery was firmly closed.

Today, funding opportunities for health and social care research come from many different sources: government departments; international bodies; the National Health Service (NHS); research councils; charities; trusts; industry; commerce; and private donors. Each of these sources will inevitably have its own priorities and commitments. Equally, these will change and evolve over time. When assessing the objectivity of any research findings, the source of funding for a study has to be considered. It is naive to assume that the interests of those financing research do not directly or indirectly lead to pressure to investigate/or not investigate a particular topic or to publish/or not publish in a certain area. This is, of course, even more pertinent when the researchers are themselves employees of those providing the funding, such as researchers working for campaigning organisations, political parties or lobbying groups.

In recent years, such bias has been particularly evident within the pharmaceutical industry where the pressure to market pharmaceutical products appears to have resulted in companies being reluctant fully to report research findings on the safety of particular drugs (Wise, 1997; Melzer, 1998). This apparent lack of integrity not only adulterates the available body of knowledge, but also puts health and welfare at risk. Meanwhile, bias can be more covertly present in the research funding priorities of governments, which tend to favour topical issues high on the political agenda, and even charitable organisations, which often have limited budgets and therefore award numerous small stipends for relatively superficial studies in the hope that this will produce immediate results at relatively little cost.

The Limitations of Evidence-based Practice

As indicated at the start of this chapter, there has lately been a groundswell of enthusiasm for evidence-based practice. The roots of this 'movement' can be found in medicine during the early 1990s and are closely associated with Archie Cochrane, a British medical researcher, who argued that limited healthcare resources should be used to provide services that have been shown to be effective (Cochrane, 1972). To this end, Cochrane promoted the use of randomised controlled trials (RCTs) to evaluate treatment methods (see Chapter 11) and pioneered the use of systematic reviews and meta-analyses (see Chapter 5). His work also led to the emergence of the Cochrane Collaboration, an international network to support the development of evidence-based medicine.

Since then, evidence-based practice has spread into many other professional fields, including nursing, social work, probation, education and public health (Trinder, 2000). It is underpinned by the belief that practitioners should make rational decisions on the basis of structured critical appraisals of empirical evidence relating to what works in their field. Ideally, this empirical evidence should come from RCTs using large sample sizes, the random allocation of participants to comparison groups, high follow-up rates, and outcome measures of known or probable clinical importance. Better still, it will involve quantitative reviews of more than one RCT by meta-analysis. Advocates of this evidence-based approach maintain that this results in both the best practice possible and the optimal use of resources.

Despite widespread acclaim, the rise of evidence-based practice has not been universally welcomed. Those who are reluctant to embrace the concept do not tend to baulk at the idea of advancing knowledge or improving health and social care delivery. Their objections rather relate to the limitations they perceive in an approach that pitches undisputed fact against the more complex and messy reality of everyday life (Tobin, 2003). Such negativity will probably seem clearer now that we have reflected on the contingent nature of scientific knowledge. It does indeed seem difficult to be certain of what best practice is when we cannot guarantee that knowledge is objective or value-free and when science can never promise the truth of its conclusions (Popper, 1945; Kuhn, 1970).

Building upon this, many health and social care practitioners have argued that the causes of health and/or social problems are extremely complex, chaotic and ever-changing (Sheldon and Chilvers, 2000; Darlington and Scott, 2002). Yet the kinds of research which underpin evidence-based practice tend to oversimplify problems and attribute mistaken certainty to their findings. They also tend to be costly and time-consuming to undertake (Reid and Zettergren, 1999). Furthermore, evidence-based practice is based largely on studies conducted in experimental situations, the findings of which may not apply in real-world settings. Indeed, it can actually be difficult to implement evidence-based practice as the evidence available often lacks obvious relevance to everyday practice (Richardson et al., 1990; Darlington and Scott, 2002).

Such difficulties have been expressed in terms of the 'high, hard ground' of complex technical knowledge which may be of interest to a minority of experts in the field and the 'swampy lowlands' which are messy but preoccupy the majority of health and social care clients and professionals:

> In the varied topography of professional practice, there is a high, hard ground where practitioners can make effective use of research-based theory and technique, and there is a swampy lowland where situations are confusing 'messes' incapable of a technical solution. The difficulty is that the problems of the high ground, however great their technical interest, are often relatively unimportant to clients of the larger society while in the swamp are the problems of the greatest human concern. (Schon, 1983: 42–3)

It is often difficult to see how the findings of a narrowly specified RCT or systematic review will help the young person who struggles with myriad problems including depression, homelessness, poor family relationships and substance misuse or, indeed, the social worker working with them. In fact, some have argued that evidence-based practice actually impedes professionals since it erodes their autonomy in decision-making processes and effectively functions as a covert method of rationing resources (Trinder, 2000: 2).

The impenetrability of very complex health and social problems, along with the high costs of conducting studies long and large enough to produce reliable findings, have been addressed to some extent by the advent of meta-analysis (see Chapter 5). However, reviews of published work will inevitably repeat the gaps existing in the original research. There are few large scale RCTs of many health and social care interventions because of the difficulty of securing sufficient time and funding, the ethics of withholding potentially important treatment and services from some individuals, and the near impossibility of controlling for the full range of variables (personal, social, psychological, cultural and economic) that are likely to affect outcomes. This lack of a research base can threaten services which may well be effective, although not formally evidenced.

An overreliance on large RCTs has also meant that the findings of other types of study, particularly qualitative research, have often been marginalised or overlooked. Qualitative research seeks in-depth information from relatively small samples and this allows topics to be explored in a level, depth and detail that is not possible using more structured, quantitative formats. Indeed, a key strength of qualitative research is that it enables research participants to be open and reflective about their experiences (Stewart et al., 1995). Equally, it can provide the questioning professional with the opportunity to explore the reality of their practice as they encounter it. As we shall see in Part 4, qualitative research prioritises different forms of knowledge and values from quantitative research. However, it has provided many important insights into how people feel and behave within a wide range of health and social care settings and is thus crucial to health and social care research as well as to evidence-based practice.

Towards an Optimistic Research Future

Quantitative researchers have often argued that qualitative research is of minimal value except in the exploratory phase of a study. In contrast, qualitative researchers have claimed that the application of purely quantitative evaluation techniques distorts reality into overly simplistic data analysis (Susman and Evered, 1978; Macdonald et al., 1992; Gabor et al., 1998; Hart and Bond, 1998). Such diametrically opposed positions – with the proponents of quantitative and qualitative data each believing in the superiority of their own approaches – were well-documented in the 1970s when methodology paradigm wars monopolised the research literature (Hersen and Barlow, 1976).

During the 1980s, however, some of the rigid boundaries between quantitative and qualitative researchers began to relax. Qualitative methods (especially focus groups) crept into the previously quantitative realm of market research (see Chapter 15) and service user involvement – which emphasises the importance of involving those who use services in deciding what they want and need and potentially even delivering those services – became embedded in health and social care research and practice (Stewart et al., 1995). The availability of personal computers and software packages additionally accelerated the blurring of methodological boundaries by facilitating the transformation of qualitative data into quantitative data and vice versa (Bazeley, 1999). Gradually, the complementarity of qualitative and quantitative techniques has been recognised and mixed methods protocols have been accepted (see Chapter 19).

The plurality of funding sources available for health and social care research today also means that individual researchers are much less reliant on the patronage and interests of the wealthy and privileged than was the case in the past. The world of research is in principle now open to all who are appropriately trained and briefed, with projects varying in size from very small local studies to large international collaborations. Meanwhile, formalised ethical and research governance procedures provide better guidance and security to research participants and researchers (see Chapters 2 and 3), whilst peer review processes for deciding which studies should be funded and which research findings should be published help to ensure that methodological rigour is maintained.

Certainly, it is wise to retain a healthy degree of scepticism regarding academic processes of self-regulation – especially given all we have already said about research serving the interests of the powerful and privileged. Undoubtedly, those whose studies are not funded and those whose papers are rejected will sometimes claim that the system of peer review favours those who have professional allies, share a common perspective on a research question, or are established researchers in their field – and, on occasions, it is likely that they will be right. Yet, we cannot deny that the scrutiny of research protocols and findings by those who are knowledgeable of the topic and methodology has helped to ensure that more research than ever is being undertaken by reputable and proven scientists who will produce robust findings that they share to the good of all.

Finally, we should perhaps remain optimistic about the role that serendipity and inspiration can play in shaping knowledge and increasing understanding. The natural sciences are littered with remarkable discoveries that are, in effect, the result of accidents or of bold scientific imagination – for example, Newton's work on gravity, Harrison's work on longitude, Archimedes' discovery of the principle of buoyancy, and Fleming's work on penicillin. Such scientific breakthroughs were not necessarily recognised as such at the time – perhaps because the discoverers were not well-known or because the findings did not 'fit' the body of knowledge already held or were not in an area deemed to be of interest. Yet, over time they have resurfaced, been recognised and changed lives. Inquisitive open minds remain as important today as they were in the past to the broad scientific endeavour.

The Rest of the Book

Some of you may be commencing this book with a heavy heart: a necessary read for a module or an essay to write. Others will be reading with an air of excitement and anticipation as you prepare to undertake a research project of your own: a student dissertation or thesis, or maybe in hope of finding some answers to aspects of your practice that interest, concern or frustrate you. The history of research is littered with great lives: from Pythagoras to Bowlby; from Euclid to Marie Curie – men and women who have struggled to get their ideas and their research into the public domain. Your own research may add to an existing body of knowledge, or it may begin – alongside the work of others – to chip away at a prevailing set of beliefs and methods of practice.

This introductory chapter will have hopefully provided you with some realistic insights into what can and cannot be achieved within the constraints of a single study. The findings of any research project, however large or small, are but a drop in a much larger ocean of uncertainty. We cannot say that they will ever represent the absolute truth on any one subject, but as findings link together, the evidence becomes stronger. Research is rewarding and challenging. As we have seen, an astute mind may find a fault seam running through even an apparently strong body of knowledge built up over the years, and from there initiate change. Meanwhile, it is the constant search for truth, however ephemeral, that often inspires and drives researchers on.

Whether you are an aspiring researcher or a consumer of research literature, the skills that you will acquire from reading this book will help to inform and guide you on your investigative journey. In the remainder of Part 1, we consider other necessary preliminaries to undertaking research. These include designing and planning your study (Chapter 2) and research ethics (Chapter 3). Chapters 4 to 18 then each critically explore one method or design commonly used by health and social care researchers. Whilst we have sought to include a diverse and balanced range of approaches, we do not claim to have been exhaustive. For example, we are particularly conscious of the lack of a chapter on emancipatory and participatory research. However, we are reassured that there are other excellent texts to fill this void (c.f. Oliver, 1997; Ramcharan et al., 2004; Koch and Kralik, 2006). Moreover, those wishing to conduct emancipatory and participatory research should still find much that is useful within the methods and designs that are covered.

Chapters 4 to 18 each use the following standard format:

- *Introduction*: a short, clear definition of the method/design

- *Historical context*: a brief note on the origins and history of the method/design

- *Current use*: an overview of when, why and by whom the method/design is currently used

- *Strengths*: the main strengths of the method/design

- *Weaknesses*: the main weaknesses of the method/design

- *Conducting a study*: a brief account of how to undertake a study using the method/design

- *A published example*: an overview of one recent high-quality health or social care study using the method/design

- *Further reading*: a short list of suggested further reading with brief commentaries.

We hope that this structured approach will enable you to compare and contrast methods, but also provide you with balanced accounts that reveal how and when each approach is best used, as well as an understanding of its limitations. The sections on 'conducting a study' and 'a published example' aim to provide you with enough information to grasp what undertaking research using a particular method or design entails, whilst the further reading will point you in the right direction for developing your knowledge and skills further. One book chapter cannot possibly equip you with everything you need to know in order to undertake your own study. Thus, you will inevitably find yourself consulting other texts and discussing your work with colleagues and experts in the field. You are also likely to require specialist training in statistics and/or qualitative data analysis techniques. Nonetheless, each chapter should give you a good grounding in, and broad understanding of, the method or design which is featured.

With some niggling reservations, we have called Part 2 of the book 'Desk-based Research', Part 3 'Quantitative Research' and Part 4 'Qualitative Research'. Each method or design has been allocated to the part of the book with which it seemed most strongly connected (historically, philosophically and in practice). Yet, we recognise that this arrangement is not wholly satisfactory. The term 'desk-based research' tends to refer to methods that utilise existing data sources, particularly written documents. However, it is possible to analyse new empirical data using desk-based methods – for example, interview data can often be subject to a discourse or content analysis. Equally, as later chapters will illustrate, research designs which have generally been considered quantitative are increasingly being used by qualitative researchers and qualitative data can often be analysed quantitatively.

The world of research is complex and new approaches to data collection, analysis and interpretation are constantly evolving. This is a positive development and we do not wish to seem rooted in the past by unduly prioritising a qualitative versus quantitative divide or by resurrecting old methodology paradigm wars. Nonetheless, our decision to divide the fifteen methods chapters into three parts gives the book a structure and coherence which seems, for the most part, relevant and sensible. In Part 5, we then seek to 'bring it all together' with two concluding chapters. Chapter 19 explores the possibilities of using qualitative and quantitative research within a single study, whilst Chapter 20 reviews the various ways of ensuring that research findings reach an appropriate audience and thus have maximum impact.

Whether your intention is to read this book from cover to cover or to turn to the chapter(s) that most interest you, our advice is to be thoughtful, creative, critical, inquisitive, honest and transparent, but also to enjoy your research. Ultimately, these are the values that should predominate within your academic work as much as within your life as a committed health and social care practitioner. We hope that *Research Methods for Health and Social Care* will become a well-thumbed and comforting companion, as well as a useful resource, for many new researchers. We also hope that it will inspire and encourage rigorous studies that go on to generate valuable findings for future health and social care policy and practice.

References

Bazeley, P. (1999) 'The bricoleur with a computer: Piecing together qualitative and quantitative data', *Qualitative Health Research*, **9**, 279–87.

Berger, P.L. and Luckmann, T. (1966) *The Social Construction of Reality: A Treatise in the Sociology of Knowledge* (Garden City, NY: Anchor Books).

Bronowski, J. (1953) *The Common Sense of Science* (Cambridge, MA: Harvard University Press).

Cochrane, A. (1972) *Effectiveness and Efficiency: Random Reflections on Health Services* (Oxford: The Nuffield Provincial Hospitals Trust).

Darlington, Y. and Scott, D. (2002) *Qualitative Research in Practice: Stories from the Field* (Buckingham: Open University Press).

Gabor, P., Unrau, Y. and Grinnell, R. Jr. (1998) *Evaluation for Social Workers: A Quality Improvement Approach for the Social Sciences*, 2nd edn (Boston, MA: Allyn & Bacon).

Giddens, A. (1995) *Politics, Sociology and Social Theory: Encounters with Classical and Contemporary Social Thought* (Cambridge: Polity).

Hart, E. and Bond, E. (1998) *Action Research for Health and Social Care: A Guide to Practice* (Buckingham: Open University Press).

Hersen, M. and Barlow, D. (1976) *Single Case Experimental Designs: Strategies for Studying Behavior Change* (New York: Pergamon Press).

Koch, T. and Kralik, D. (2006) *Participatory Action Research in Healthcare* (Oxford: Blackwell).

Kuhn, T.S. (1970) *The Structure of Scientific Revolutions* (Chicago, IL: Chicago University Press).

Latour, B. and Woolgar, S. (1979) *Laboratory Life: The Social Construction of Scientific Facts* (Beverly Hills, LA: Sage).

Lyotard, J.F. (1984) *The Postmodern Condition: A Report on Knowledge,* Translated by Bennington, G. and Massumi, B. (Minneapolis, MN: University of Minnesota Press).

Macdonald, G., Sheldon, B. and Gillespie, J. (1992) 'Contemporary studies of the effectiveness of social work', *British Journal of Social Work*, **22**, 615–43.

Melzer, D. (1998) 'New drug treatment for Alzheimer's disease: Lessons for healthcare policy', *British Medical Journal*, **316**, 762–4.

Oliver, M. (1997) 'Emancipatory research: Realistic goal or impossible dream?' In Barnes, C. and Mercer, G. (eds), *Doing Disability Research* (Leeds: The Disability Press).

Popper, K. (1945) *The Open Society and Its Enemies* (Vols 1 and 2) (London: Routledge).

Pumfrey, S. and Dawbarn, F. (2004) 'Science and patronage in England, 1570–1625: A preliminary study', *History of Science*, **42**, 137–88.

Ramcharan, P., Grant, G. and Flynn, M. (2004) 'Participatory and emancipatory research: How far have we come?' In Emerson, E., Hatton, C., Thompson, T. and Parmenter, T. (eds), *International Handbook of Applied Research in Intellectual Disabilities* (London: Wiley).

Reid, W. and Zettergren, P. (1999) 'A perspective on empirical practice'. In Shaw, I. and Lishman, J. (eds), *Evaluation and Social Work Practice* (London: Sage).

Richardson, A., Jackson, C. and Sykes, W. (1990) *Taking Research Seriously: Means of Improving and Assessing the Use and Dissemination of Research* (London: HMSO).

Schon, D. (1983) *The Reflective Practitioner: How Professionals Think in Action* (London: Temple Smith).

Sheldon, B. and Chilvers, R. (2000) *Evidence-based Social Care: Study of Prospects and Problems* (Dorset: Russell House Publishing).

Stewart, M., Brown, J.B., Weston W.W., McWhinney I.R., McWilliam C.L. and Freeman T.R. (1995) *Patient Centred Medicine: Transforming the Clinical Method* (London: Sage).

Susman, G. and Evered, R. (1978) 'An Assessment of the Scientific Merits of Action Research', *Administrative Science Quarterly*, **23**, 582–603.

Tobin, M. (2003) 'The role of a journal in scientific controversy', *American Journal of Respiratory and Critical Care Medicine*, **168**, 511–15.

Trinder L. (2000) 'Evidence-based practice in social work and probation'. In Trinder, L. and Reynolds, S. (eds), *Evidence-Based Practice: A Critical Appraisal* (Oxford: Blackwell Publishing).

Wise, J. (1997) 'Research suppressed for seven years by drug company', *British Medical Journal*, **314**, 1145.

Notes

1 Medicine, Biology and Anatomy, for example, are largely natural science disciplines, whilst Sociology, Social Work and Psychology are predominantly social science subjects.

2 Karl Popper was arguably one of the twentieth century's greatest philosophers of science. He queried whether firm scientific laws could be established through observation and experiment and argued that absolute truth was alien to the scientific method. His falsification principle suggests that a statement cannot be said to be 'true' unless it can be verified, which is perhaps impossible in an infinite and changing world. See, for example, Popper, K. (1945).

3 Such as their age, gender, family relationships, employment situation, social networks, material resources, and local health and social care facilities.

4 An economic and intellectual movement with its roots in the ancient Western civilisations of Rome and Greece.

5 Psalm 93:1, Psalm 96:10, and Chronicles 16:30 state that 'the world is firmly established, it cannot be moved.' Psalm 104:5 says, '[the LORD] set the earth on its foundations; it can never be moved.' Ecclesiastes 1:5 states that 'the sun rises and the sun sets and hurries back to where it rises.'

2 Starting a New Research Project

JANE V. APPLETON

Introduction

The prospect of starting a new research project can be quite daunting. It might be the first study that you have ever undertaken or you might be using a new method for the first time. The purpose of this chapter is to identify some of the common preliminary stages in undertaking research in order to help you focus on the skills and knowledge required and plan the work ahead. You will be encouraged to think about your particular areas of interest, why you are doing research, and your working habits and preferences. You will also be alerted to some of the key challenges and milestones that you are likely to face along the way. Being clear about these issues from the outset should help to ensure that your study has every chance of being a success.

Deciding on a Topic

The first stage in getting started in research is to identify a topic that really intrigues you and will sustain your interest and motivation. This is important for all types of research – regardless of whether you are planning to undertake empirical work, audit, a literature review or a theoretical study. A research topic is essentially a broad problem area or issue 'sometimes referred to as the focus of the research' (Polit and Hungler, 1999: 49). Within health and social care, research topics can be extremely diverse. For example, they might include: adolescent substance misuse; wound care management; child protection; care of the elderly; obesity; or patient/professional communications.

Research topics can be either internally generated by researchers themselves or externally driven by employers, research funding agencies, charitable organisations or government bodies that commission research in particular areas (Clifford, 1997). Whilst some health and social care practitioners are fairly clear about the topic they wish to investigate, others are much less certain (Walliman, 2001). For those who are struggling to think of a suitable topic, it may be helpful to consider some of the following.

Your own professional experience

Thinking about your own daily work can help research seem more meaningful and relevant. Often professionals have hunches about their day-to-day practice that they would like to explore in more depth. Equally, there may be questions that they routinely ask themselves – perhaps relating to patient care or why a particular treatment is working or not working. It can also be fruitful to think about challenging clients, conversations with colleagues, or organisational issues that are a concern. Attending professional conferences or meetings, where it is possible to network with peers, can be an additional way of generating ideas. Meanwhile, reading the professional literature can stimulate research ideas relating to current practice developments (Depoy and Gitlin, 2005).

Existing research evidence

There are a wealth of health and social care journals publishing peer-reviewed primary research and secondary evidence (such as literature reviews and systematic reviews). Reading academic papers will ensure that you are up-to-date with the latest research evidence. Moreover, many of these publications actually make suggestions for future research, based on the findings of the study that they are reporting. It can also be productive to think about who the key authors and researchers are in the field that interests you. Following the work of these individuals via their publications and websites and attending academic conferences where you might have the opportunity to hear them present and discuss their latest findings can also be very stimulating.

Social trends and policy developments

Interest in a particular research topic might additionally be generated by your knowledge of, and concern for, social or political issues. As Polit and Hungler note, a research idea might emerge from your 'familiarity with social concerns or controversial social problems' (Polit and Hungler, 1999: 52). For example, the children's rights movement has over the years raised important research questions about the impact of domestic violence on children's emotional health and well-being; it has also led to research on youth participatory rights. National and international development plans, consultation papers, strategies and policy documents can all be particularly good starting points for research ideas as they highlight key current and developing policy issues.

Practical activities to help generate research topics

If you are still struggling to identify a topic – or, conversely, feel overwhelmed by possibilities because you have so many different interests – you can always share your thoughts with work colleagues or engage in debate with friends or fellow students. Talking preliminary topics over with a supervisor or manager, or with other people who have research experience, can help you to shape and hone your thinking. Even the simple act of getting some initial thoughts written down can be very productive. To this end, you might brainstorm ideas on to a large sheet of plain paper or create a mind map or spider diagram.[1]

Arthur (2000: 7) also emphasises the need to 'write down the subject area(s) that have been nagging away at you for a while' and 'think about why they interest you and what was the trigger that made you interested in them in the first place'. He notes that 'elegant research projects start with vague ideas'. Walliman (2001), meanwhile, suggests keeping three questions in mind when searching for and clarifying a research topic. These are: What is motivating you to conduct the research?; What relevant practice interests, experience or expertise you bring to the subject?; and What is going to be your end product? Reflecting on these issues should help to ensure that your topic is something that genuinely interests and motivates you; that you have good background knowledge to help inform your study; and that you understand what your research might realistically achieve.

Formulating a Research Question

Once you have decided upon a broad topic area, you need to refine your thinking to produce a clear research problem and thereafter a focused research question. The process of moving from a general topic to a research problem can best be achieved by a period of further reading, reflection and discussion with colleagues and peers. As part of this process, it is important to ask oneself challenging questions, such as: What is going on here?; Why is this happening?; Under what circumstances does this phenomenon occur?; How common is this problem?; What factors contribute to this issue?; and Who is actually affected, and how?

Such reflections should enable you to state your research problem in one to two clear sentences. For example, you may be interested in the topic of adolescent substance misuse, but your research problem might relate to whether, and if so why, young people who are excluded or truant from school are more likely to misuse illicit drugs than young people who have a good record of school attendance. According to Walliman (2001), a good research problem will really interest you; be important; be clearly delineated; and be expressed clearly and concisely. You should also be confident that you are able to access the data or information necessary to draw some meaningful conclusions.

Having identified a research problem, the next stage is to undertake a more focused and thorough review of the literature in order to refine the problem into a manageable research question. People starting out on research for the first time are often over-ambitious and want to do too much. It is essential to be realistic about the scope of your study and the time available to you to complete your work (Walliman, 2004). It is also important to remember that new data do not always need to be collected. There may be existing literature that can be reviewed (see Chapters 4 and 5) or existing data sets that can be reanalysed (see for example, the UK data archive, http://www.data-archive.ac.uk).

In essence, a research question can be defined as 'the specific query the researcher wants to answer to address the research problem' (Polit and Hungler, 1999: 49). Most studies will have a primary research question and a number of secondary, or more specific, research questions (Cormack and Benton, 2000; Punch, 2006). These will provide a framework to guide the entire research process. As Stone (2002) argues, clearly identified research questions promote clarity of thought; generate the study protocol;[2] inform the choice of research methodology; guide data analysis; and increase the chances of publication.

Research questions are often classified as: descriptive, relational or causal (Meadows, 2003; Burns and Grove, 2005). *Descriptive* research questions seek to describe what is happening, for example: How is adolescent binge-drinking represented in the media? *Relational* research questions examine the relationships between variables and concepts, for example: What is the relationship between moderate depression and an increase in general practice attendance amongst older male patients? Meanwhile, *causal* questions examine the cause and effect interactions between variables, for example: Does a particular home-visiting intervention programme prevent childhood injury?

A good research question should be clearly worded and written in a single sentence. It needs to be unambiguous, specific, answerable, realistic and worthwhile (Robson, 2002; Punch, 2006). In some research designs, the research idea might be formulated in terms of a research *hypothesis* rather than a research question (Hancock, 2000; Walliman, 2004). A *hypothesis* is generally used in studies that seek to test out an idea or prediction statistically. For example a researcher might hypothesise that a new drug treatment is more effective than an existing drug treatment by undertaking a randomised controlled trial (see Chapter 11). In other research designs, particularly qualitative research, the research idea might be formulated in terms of a study aim (a general statement of intent about what the study will achieve, such as to explore the experience of parenthood amongst young teenage parents) and a series of more specific and measurable objectives (or research outcomes, such as to identify how teenagers adjust to parenthood and to explore differences between young fathers and young mothers) (Graham, 2007).

Choosing a Methodology and Appropriate Methods

Confusion sometimes exists around the terms *methodology* and *method*, compounded by the fact that the two are often used imprecisely and interchangeably. *Methodology* is concerned with the question 'How should the inquirer go about finding out knowledge?' (Guba, 1990: 18). It is the rationale and philosophy underpinning the study design and its execution, including a researcher's ontological or epistemological[3] perspectives. Examples of research methodology are: experimental methodologies; constructivism; and participatory inquiry. A *method*, conversely, is a specific data collection and analysis technique, such as systematic reviews (Chapter 5); surveys (Chapter 9); or focus groups (Chapter 15). Polit and Hungler (1999: 707) define research methods as 'the steps, procedures and strategies for gathering and analysing the data in a research investigation'.

Research methods are often described as being either quantitative or qualitative. Quantitative methods are primarily concerned with gathering numerical data and factual knowledge about the social world, often under controlled conditions. Quantitative research examines relationships and sometimes the strength of relationships between variables using statistical techniques. In contrast, qualitative methods explore people's subjective experiences and opinions in order better to understand and give meaning to social phenomena. Whilst quantitative research methods tend to be deductive in their approach (that is, they seek to test theory or ideas using previously established categories of data), qualitative research methods tend to be inductive (that is, they build insights or theory using categories generated from their own data).

Although Part 3 of this book focuses on quantitative research and Part 4 considers more qualitative techniques, the distinction between these two approaches is often blurred. Moreover, many questions in health and social care research benefit from adopting a mixed methods approach – combining both quantitative and qualitative techniques within one study (see Chapter 19 for a detailed discussion). A careful reading of Chapters 4–18 should help to ensure that you have the basic knowledge needed to choose an appropriate method for your particular research question, hypothesis or aim and objectives.

Planning the Study

Be clear about what the study will achieve

Reflecting on why exactly you want to do your research will help you to focus on what you hope your study will achieve (Potter, 2006). The end points of research are often expressed in terms of outputs and outcomes. Outputs are the tangible products of a study and might include a dissertation or thesis, a research report, a book, new practice guidelines, a journal article or a conference presentation. Outcomes refer to the impact of a study, such as the introduction of a new drug or a change in working practices. Generally speaking, good outputs are the key to ensuring good research outcomes. This is because a study needs to be taken seriously and disseminated widely to achieve maximum impact (see Chapter 20 for how to write up and present your research to a range of audiences).

Careful time management

Developing effective time management is an early skill to master when conduct-ing research. To this end, preparing a realistic timetable with manageable goals and milestones is essential. This can be done using a simple table produced in Microsoft Word, with dates in the first column and key activities in the second. Alternatively, many researchers use a Gantt chart.[4] Developed by Henry Gantt in 1917, this is a type of bar chart that visually illustrates a project's schedule and timescale, including start and completion dates. A Gantt chart allows the duration and ordering of tasks to be plotted against the progression of time which is very helpful in monitoring study progress.

Irrespective of whether a simple table or more sophisticated Gantt Chart is chosen, the timetable is probably most easily produced by listing all the steps in the intended study and estimating on a weekly basis the amount of time needed to complete each step (see Sharp et al. (2002) for a longer discus-sion). It is also crucial to build in some extra time for delays or scope creep. Scope creep refers to unanticipated changes in a study's extent, usually an increase in the amount of work needed for its successful completion. Both delays and scope creep should be avoided whenever possible and this is best achieved by careful planning. Nevertheless, it is not possible to predict every-thing that might go wrong with a study – such as problems in securing access to a study site or illness amongst key personnel – so some over-budgeting of time is sensible.

Effective working practices

How and when you work

As Phelps et al. (2007) recommend, it is worth taking time at the beginning of a study to examine your own personal working practices. Knowing yourself and the way that you work are important in terms of maximising the return on your effort invested. This will involve thinking about when you will have uninterrupted time, when you are able to write best and when you are able to do your most creative thinking: for example, when you are debating ideas with colleagues at work or when you are contemplating things alone in a relaxed atmosphere. 'Only you know how best you work, and only you know how organized you want to be and feel' (Phelps et al., 2007: 36). Walliman (2004) argues that self-motivation and self-discipline are the two key factors influencing successful research completion. For those with limited time avail-able, who are perhaps working in the evening when children are in bed, Oliver (2004: 44) suggests the concept of 'little and often' and recommends getting into the habit of trying to write about three hundred words every day to estab-lish continuity and a routine.

Workspace and working systems

Planning also involves thinking about where you are going to undertake most of your research and then organising your office, room or workspace to your liking. A good working environment needs to be conducive to reading, writing and thinking. This will require privacy and minimal distractions. In today's technology-dependent world, you will need a computer and (preferably high-speed) internet access. Equally, you should consider whether you require any training in database searching, referencing software (such as ENDNOTE[5]), or software data analysis packages (such as NViVo[6] or SPSS[7]).

From the moment you begin your research, it is crucial to establish an efficient system for managing your ideas, notes and to-do lists. Whilst it may be necessary to jot down a sudden flash of inspiration on the nearest scrap of paper, this must subsequently be recorded and filed in a systematic way so that it can easily be retrieved later. One useful strategy is to keep a research diary (in paper or electronic format). This should be maintained on a regular basis in order to log progress, such as literature search strategies, any contact with research sites, and dates of experiments or interviews. It can also be used to record pertinent thoughts, reflections and insights about the research process. The research diary can provide an audit trail justifying your actions in the study's development. Moreover, as Rossman and Ralliss (1998: 43) comment, 'documenting your intellectual and methodological journey is crucial for establishing the soundness of the study'.

Other research materials – such as, journal articles and other retrieved literature; letters, ethics and research governance documentation, consent forms and other formal paperwork; interview transcripts, returned questionnaires and fieldnotes; data files; and drafts of research findings and so on – also need to be kept in an accessible but secure location. A password-protected computer is essential for storing confidential electronic data and a lockable filing cabinet is needed for other confidential material. Boden et al. (2005: 54) recommend developing a good hard copy or computer filing system to enable you to locate all the material relating to your project; keep valuable things safe; maintain a complete history of your research; work efficiently; know what materials you have; and effectively manage the project. For lots of useful additional practical tips on managing and organising your research, see Phelps et al. (2007).

Researcher physical and emotional safety

One important, but often overlooked, issue in planning your study is researcher safety. Fieldwork may involve contact with strangers, travel to unfamiliar places, and being away at weekends or evenings. It may also be emotionally distressing, since it can involve discussing sensitive or upsetting topics with vulnerable people. Whilst it is not possible to prepare for every potential hazard, it is essential to consider ways of minimising risks as much as possible. For example, researchers out on fieldwork should always leave details of their whereabouts with a reliable third party and make regular phone calls back to them. In addition, it is sensible to identify someone (a peer, colleague, or supervisor) who is willing to provide a sympathetic listening ear as and when the need arises. The Social Research Association has produced a useful code of practice for the safety of social researchers (available at http://www.the-sra.org.uk/staying_safe.htm) and a report by Bloor et al. (2007) helpfully summarises a range of issues that can threaten the safety of qualitative researchers, as well as strategies that will help them to stay physically and emotionally safe.

Securing support

Financial support

Undertaking research can be a costly process and obtaining appropriate funding will often be the factor that determines whether or not a research idea can become a reality. Some postgraduate and research students are successful in securing a studentship, bursary or training fellowship from their employer, a university, a research funding body or even a charity. This is likely to cover their university fees, very basic living expenses, and even some of their fieldwork costs and conference attendance. Other health and social care students find themselves combining part-time research study with paid employment (and often family commitments as well). This can be extremely demanding. However, they may be able to negotiate a financial contribution or study leave from an employer, particularly if the research being undertaken is directly related to their paid work.

For those wishing to undertake research as part of their job (that is, not as a student project), there is a diverse range of local, national and international funding sources available. These include research councils,[8] government departments, statutory and voluntary health and social care providers, as well as charities. Although some organisations will consider funding research on any topic (via 'open calls' for proposals), most will have their own agendas and priorities (see Chapter 1). Funding organisations will often advertise research opportunities in the national or professional press and through websites and electronic mailing lists. They usually have their own guidelines and application procedures and it is important to become familiar with, and adhere to, these in order not to waste valuable time and energy submitting an application to an inappropriate source.

If you are applying for external financial support, you will need to prepare an itemised list of proposed expenses. These will commonly include:

- Staffing (researcher time and any necessary secretarial or administrative support)

- Equipment (computers, software, audio or video recorders, measuring instruments and so on)

- Books, reports and interlibrary loans

- Travel (to and from fieldwork sites and for meetings with any research collaborators)

- Subsistence (for the researcher and research participants)

- Expenses for research participants (it is often necessary to reimburse individuals for any out-of-pocket expenses and/or to give them a small payment for their time)

- Transcription costs or costs for data entry

- Job advertisement (if it is necessary to recruit anybody new to work on the study)

- Dissemination costs (to pay for the production of any reports, leaflets or web-based material to publicise the study findings)

- Conference/professional meeting attendance (to keep up-to-date with developments in the field and to disseminate one's own findings at the end of the study)

- Office costs (such as stationery, postage, printing and photocopying).

In addition, those working within universities will usually be expected to include a sum to cover indirect costs (a contribution to their institution's library costs, finance and personnel services and so on) and estate costs (a contribution to costs related to buildings and premises, such as maintenance, utility bills, cleaning and security). If you are a postgraduate student undertaking research, it is also worth scrutinising the above list since you will undoubtedly find yourself needing to cover at least some of these expenses.

Supervisor support

Those undertaking research as part of a university degree will be allocated an academic supervisor and possibly a small team of two or three supervisors. However, it is important to remember that the study belongs to the student and they must take ownership and responsibility for it. Postgraduate students might be in the lucky position of having some choice about who their supervisor will be – perhaps someone who has expertise in their research area or someone they perceive as having what Crofts (1999: 29) describes as 'super-vision'. Both Potter (2006) and Phillips and Pugh (1994) offer some very useful suggestions for establishing a good relationship with a supervisor and getting the most out of the supervisory process. University degree regulations commonly indicate the amount of supervision time a student can expect from their supervisors and it is sensible to clarify this from the outset.

Novice researchers undertaking research as part of their job are advised to seek the support of someone in their organisation who has responsibility for research or who themselves has research experience. This person may be available to act as a mentor or may be helpful in terms of facilitating access to research sites. Within a university setting, the best person to contact might be very obvious. Practitioners employed in health or social care settings might need to ask around or attend local research seminars or events to find out about relevant research networks. In the UK, for example, regional research and development (R&D) departments run courses and training programmes which are often very helpful for those beginning research in clinical settings. Individuals associated with these departments may also provide one-to-one advice to healthcare professionals on planning and conducting a specific study.

Seeking and Obtaining Approvals

In order to undertake empirical research or an audit study within a health, social care, voluntary or university setting, it is generally necessary to seek and obtain approval from a series of gatekeepers. These are likely to include the following:

The senior manager at the research site

This might be a local authority or voluntary sector service manager, a director of nursing in a hospital, or medical director of a hospice. Support from this individual is required to gain access to the specific service or services where the research will hopefully be conducted. Initial permission is usually best sought by writing to the senior manager, enclosing key information about the study or a copy of the research proposal. This will then need to be followed up with a phone call, and if possible a visit, to discuss the research in more detail.

Research and development (R&D) management and governance

Before any research or audit can be conducted in a UK healthcare setting, it must first be approved by R&D management and governance (Appleton and Caan, 2004; Appleton et al., 2007). This will ensure that the research proposal complies with the local arrangements in place for all research work in the organisation. For example, all UK NHS Trusts have systems in place to administer the management and research governance of proposals involving their Trust. This is the R&D management and governance function, which is tasked with ensuring that any proposed study is justifiable scientifically and organisationally. R&D management and governance will scrutinise such factors as the use of health service data; staff time and other resources; health and safety issues; financial project management and sponsorship arrangements; research ethics committee approval (see below); and intellectual property. Those planning to undertake research in a local authority setting will similarly need to have their proposal vetted by someone responsible for research in the organisation. In the voluntary sector, the management and governance aspects may be separated. Nevertheless, details of the agreed process must still be recorded by the researcher.

Research ethics committee

Any study involving human participants will usually need to be reviewed by a formal research ethics committee to ensure that the dignity, rights, safety, inclusivity and well-being of participants will not be negatively affected by their participation (for a more detailed discussion of research ethics and ethics committees see Chapter 3). Sometimes, it will be necessary to seek approval from more than one committee. For example, a postgraduate research student wishing to undertake research in a health or social care setting may find that they first need to seek approval from a university research ethics committee, after which they will need to apply for permission from an external research ethics committee. In the UK, all research involving NHS staff, patients, premises or records must be reviewed by the National Research Ethics Service (NRES) (http://www.nres.npsa.nhs.uk/). Each local authority and many charitable organisations have their own equivalent of a research ethics committee.

Writing a Proposal

Any study requires a research proposal. This is a written plan that outlines the problem and question that will be investigated and provides a detailed overview of the methods to be used. Burns and Grove (2005: 747) note that the research proposal is 'a formal way to communicate ideas about a proposed study to receive approval to conduct the study and to seek funding'. According to Locke et al. (2000: 3), it is a means of communication, a plan and a contract. Writing the proposal can, however, also be a useful way of refining and clarifying your research ideas and getting preliminary feedback from colleagues and peers.

The proposal is thus a central part of the research process and, when complete, should provide a clear rationale for why and how you are intending to undertake your study. Most funding bodies demand a proposal in order to determine whether a study is worth supporting. It is also a requirement of research management and governance and research ethics committees (see above). In addition, those wishing to undertake a Ph.D. will often be required to submit an outline proposal as part of any university application procedure. A potential supervisor will then use this to assess how realistic and feasible a project is likely to be and whether the topic fits their specialist interests. Meanwhile, a potential research student might send it to a range of institutions to help identify a supervisor with appropriate methodological and subject area knowledge.

Box 2.1 provides a suggested structure and some key headings to consider when writing a research proposal. This is only a broad guide since funding bodies, research ethics committees, university departments and so on will often have their own guidelines and application forms. Furthermore, the content of the proposal will vary depending on the methods being proposed (quantitative, qualitative or literature review). Both Locke et al. (2000) and Punch (2006) provide more detailed information on writing effective research proposals, including some helpful worked examples using different methodologies.

BOX 2.1

Suggested Structure for a Research Proposal

Title: be relevant, explicit and concise

Summary: provide a short overview of the background, aims, methods and anticipated outcomes

Introduction: explain succinctly what you want to do and why

Background literature: summarise key issues and limitations in the existing literature, including the theoretical or conceptual basis for your research and any key policy or relevant theory

Research question, hypothesis or study aim/objectives: be clear and concise, and ensure that the research question, hypothesis, aims/objectives are achievable

Research methodology: consider the appropriateness of your chosen methodology to answer your research question, hypothesis or study aim/objectives

Research methods: include an overview of the sample/population; access and recruitment; data collection methods; and data analysis methods. Also outline any proposed pilot work[9] and address issues of validity and reliability or rigour and credibility

Ethical considerations: discuss potential ethical issues, such as informed consent; confidentiality; anonymity; sensitivity issues; and risk of harm/safety. Also, describe plans for seeking ethical and governance approval

Limitations/potential problems: describe any potential study limitations/problems and how these might be overcome

Planned study outcomes: specify the planned benefits of the research and link these to current health and social care policy

Dissemination: explain what will happen to the research results (see also Chapter 20)

Timescale: include a timetable or Gantt chart outlining the study milestones and plan of work

Budget and resources: list all the resources required to complete the research

References: ensure that all references in the proposal are pertinent, up-to-date and accurate, and list these in a final reference list

Appendices: include, where relevant, letters of support; participant invitation letter; participant information sheet; consent form; interview schedule/questionnaire or data extraction tool and so on

Researcher curriculum vitae: include a brief curriculum vitae for each researcher outlining their relevant skills and experience including previous research grants held, notable awards and publications

When starting to write a proposal, it can be helpful to make notes using the headings outlined in Box 2.1. The aim is to be simple, clear and concise and to use language which is understandable to a lay person. It is important to avoid complicated terminology or jargon and the proposal should be written in the future tense. The finished research proposal is essentially a sales tool. Thus, it should be well laid out, word processed, without spelling or grammatical errors, correctly referenced, and neat and inviting in its presentation.

Conclusion

This chapter has identified the key steps that need to be considered when getting started on a study. Getting started on research is never straightforward and the chapter has offered a number of strategies and practical suggestions to help you on your way. It has explored six critical stages in the research process. These were: topic identification; question formulation; selecting an appropriate methodology and methods; planning; seeking and obtaining approval for the research; and designing a research proposal. Perseverance, self-motivation and a willingness to learn are the key to success in research at any level. By following the steps outlined in this chapter, you should be in a good position to start confidently on the research journey that lies ahead of you.

 ## References

Appleton, J.V. and Caan, W. (2004) 'Guidance on research governance', *Community Practitioner*, **77**, 303–5.

Appleton, J.V., Caan, W., Cowley S. and Kendall S. (2007) 'Busting the bureaucracy: Lessons from research governance in primary care', *Community Practitioner*, **80**, 29–32.

Arthur, A.J. (2000) 'Starting a research project and applying for funding'. In Saks, M., Williams, M. and Hancock, B. (eds), *Developing Research in Primary Care* (Oxford: Radcliffe Medical Press).

Bloor, M., Sampson, H. and Fincham, B. (2007) *Qualiti (NCRM) Commissioned Inquiry into the Risk to Well-being of Researchers in Qualitative Research* (Cardiff: Qualiti).

Boden, R., Kenway, J. and Epstein, D. (2005) *Getting Started on Research* (London: Sage Publications Ltd).

Burns, B. and Grove, S.K. (2005) *The Practice of Nursing Research: Conduct, Critique and Utilization,* 5th edn (St Louis, MO: Elsevier/Saunders).

Clifford, C. (1997) *Nursing and Health Care Research. A Skills-based Introduction,* 2nd edn (London: Prentice Hall).

Cormack, D.F.S. and Benton, D.C. (2000) 'Asking the research question'. In Cormack, D.F.S. (ed.), *The Research Process in Nursing,* 4th edn (Oxford: Blackwell Science).

Crofts, L. (1999) 'Research in the raw: Research supervision in a busy trust', *Nurse Researcher,* **6**, 29–39.

Depoy, E. and Gitlin, L.N. (2005) *Introduction to Research: Understanding and Applying Multiple Strategies,* 3rd edn (St Louis, MO: Elsevier Mosby).

Graham, M. (2007) 'The youngest parents: Teenage mothers' and fathers' accounts of their early experiences of becoming a parent'. Conference Paper. *Shaping the Future.* CPHVA Annual Professional Conference, Torquay, Friday 2 November.

Guba, E.G. (1990) *The Paradigm Dialog* (London: Sage Publications).

Hancock, B. (2000) 'An introduction to research methodology'. In Wilson, A., Williams, M. and Hancock, B. (eds), *Research Approaches in Primary Care* (Oxford: Racliffe Medical Press).

Locke, L.F, Spirduso, W.W. and Silverman, S.J. (2000) *Proposals that Work: A Guide for Planning Dissertations and Grant Proposals,* 4th edn (London: Sage Publications).

Meadows, K. (2003) 'So you want to do research? 2: Developing the research question', *British Journal of Community Nursing,* **8**, 397–403.

Oliver, P. (2004) *Writing Your Thesis* (London: Sage Publications).

Phelps, R., Fisher, R. and Ellis, A. (2007) *Organizing and Managing Your Research: A Practical Guide for Postgraduates* (London: Sage Publications).

Phillips, E.M. and Pugh, D.S. (1994) *How to Get a PhD: A Handbook for Students and Their Supervisors* (Buckingham: Open University Press).

Polit, D.F. and Hungler, B.P. (1999) *Nursing Research Principles and Methods*, 6th edn (London: Lippincott).

Potter, S. (2006) *Doing Postgraduate Research*, 2nd edn (London: Sage Publications and The Open University).

Punch, K.F. (2006) *Developing Effective Research Proposals*, 2nd edn (London: Sage Publications).

Robson, C. (2002) *Real World Research: A Resource for Social Scientists and Practitioner-researchers* (Oxford: Blackwell).

Rossman, G.B. and Ralliss, S.F. (1998) *Learning in the Field: An Introduction to Qualitative Research* (London: Sage Publications).

Sharp, J.A, Peters, J. and Howard, K. (2002) *The Management of a Student Research Project* (Aldershot: Gower Publishing).

Stone, P. (2002) 'Deciding upon and refining a research question', *Palliative Medicine,* **16**, 265–7.

Walliman, N. (2001) *Your Research Project. A Step-by-step Guide for the First Time Researcher* (London: Sage Publications).

Walliman, N. (2004) *Your Undergraduate Dissertation. The Essential Guide for Success* (London: Sage Publications).

Notes

1   Mind maps and spider diagrams are very easy ways of developing and organising your thinking visually in relation to a central idea or topic. This is done by noting related concepts and adding these around the central topic to generate further ideas.

2   The terms 'study protocol' or 'research protocol' are often used interchangeably with 'research proposal'.

3 Ontology is the study of being or existence; epistemology is the study of knowledge and what can be known.

4 This can be produced with a range of software including Microsoft EXCEL.

5 http://www.endnote.com/

6 http://www.qsrinternational.com/

7 http://www.spss.com/

8 Such as the Medical Research Council (MRC) and Economic and Social Research Council (ESRC) in the UK.

9 Any research should begin with a pilot study. This is essentially a trial run of the main study to ensure that there are no unforeseen problems.

Research Ethics

3

MARY BOULTON

Introduction

Ethics is 'a generic term for various ways of understanding and examining the moral life' (Beauchamp and Childress, 2001: 1). Research ethics is its application to the conduct of research. In designing, carrying out and disseminating their studies, researchers must consider the ways in which their activities could impact on those involved. Knowing how to act in a morally right way is not as straightforward as it may sound, and researchers often face difficult ethical decisions in the course of their work. At the same time, public and professional concern about the consequences of research that goes wrong has led to progressively tighter regulation of the ethics of research and, more recently, to the regulation of a broader range of issues in the form of research governance (see Chapter 2).

This chapter will describe the historical development of research ethics; the main theories, principles and codes of practice or research conduct intended to help researchers in making ethical decisions; and the mechanisms and procedures that have been established to regulate and monitor the way research is conducted. The aim is to provide an overview of research ethics and some practical guidance on how health and social care researchers might respond to a range of common ethical issues.

Historical Development of Research Ethics

Modern research ethics has developed since the Second World War, driven largely from within biomedicine where the need to protect the dignity and well-being of research subjects has been most acutely felt (Israel and Hay, 2006). Its progress has been marked by the publication of four key documents: the *Nuremberg Code;*[1] the *Declaration of Helsinki;*[2] the *Belmont Report*[3] and the *International Ethical Guidelines for Biomedical Research Involving Human Subjects.*[4]

The *Nuremberg Code* is commonly regarded as marking the point at which the ethics of research became a major concern in its own right. It was published at the end of the Nuremberg Trials in 1947, in response to the atrocities of Nazi experiments on humans and out of concern for the loss of public trust in doctors and researchers which it was feared would follow. The *Code* makes clear that the welfare of individual research participants must be prioritised over any potential benefits to humankind that might result from the research, and sets out ten standards for human experimentation. These standards identify circumstances in which human experimentation is unacceptable and emphasise voluntary and informed consent (discussed more fully below) and the right of subjects to withdraw from a study.

The guidance provided by the *Nuremberg Code* was subsequently amended and extended by the World Medical Association in its *Declaration of Helsinki*, first adopted in 1964 and revised for the fifth time in 2000/02. The *Declaration of Helsinki* has come to be regarded as the 'fundamental document' on the ethics of biomedical research and has influenced national legislation and international codes of conduct ever since. It attempts to ensure protection for research subjects by requiring: that research conforms to scientific principles and is conducted by an expert; that strong, independent justification is provided before individuals are exposed to substantial risk of harm; and that research protocols are reviewed by an independent research ethics committee. It also elaborates on the require-ments for informed consent and addresses the position of subjects legally incompetent or incapable of giving consent (Israel and Hay, 2006).

Despite wide acceptance of these documents, it soon became clear that research continued to be conducted without regard for the welfare of partici-pants. In the 1960s, Pappworth (1967) in the UK and Beecher (1966) in the USA published high-profile accounts of many years of harmful experiments conducted by doctors on vulnerable people without their consent. In the 1970s, a series of well-publicised research 'scandals'[5] provided further fuel for those who argued that closer attention should be paid to ethical matters. In this context, the US government established a National Commission for the Protection of Human Subjects of Biomedical and Behavioral Research and, in 1979, this Commission published the *Belmont Report: Ethical Principles and Guidelines for the Protection of Human Subjects of Research*. The *Belmont Report* set out three basic principles to guide research involving human subjects (described below) and examined the main requirements which arise from the applications of these principles to the conduct of research. In 1991, they were converted into regulations for all research funded by the American federal government and its agencies with the publication of a Federal policy known as the Common Rule.[6]

In 1982, the Council for International Organizations of Medical Sciences (CIOMS) moved the focus away from Western societies and onto issues raised by research involving developing countries. The social, cultural and legal traditions of developing countries can be very different from those of industrialised nations and adverse economic conditions can leave them vulnerable to exploitation by multi- or transnational corporations. CIOMS published the *International Ethical Guidelines for Biomedical Research Involving Human Subjects*, a document which 'grapples with the application of "universal" ethical principles in a diverse and multicultural world' (Israel and Hay, 2006: 37). Particular attention is given to informed consent, research with vulnerable groups and women, and the mechanisms and procedures for ethical and scientific review of research protocols. The document also provides an extended discussion of unacceptable practices that abuse or exploit vulnerable countries and the responsibilities of researchers to leave such countries better, rather than worse, off when a study ends.

Theories of Ethics

While researchers may wish to act in a way that is morally right and respectful of the well-being of others, it is not always evident what this would entail. Theories of ethics provide *general perspectives* from which to consider ethical issues. Consequentialism, deontology (non-consequentialism), and virtue ethics represent the major strands of Western normative ethics, and the ethics of care is a more recent attempt at a form of ethical reasoning based on feminist principles. Each of these theories provides a distinctive way of looking at ethical issues and attempting to resolve them (Ridley, 1998; Beauchamp and Childress, 2001).

Consequentialism

According to consequentialism, an action should be judged by its consequences. The morally right action is, therefore, the one which produces the greatest balance of benefit over harm. Utilitarianism is the best-known form of consequentialism and is closely allied with the work of John Stuart Mill (1806–1873) and Jeremy Bentham (1748–1832). Critics of consequentialism point to the difficulties of knowing what is good or beneficial and what is evil or harmful, and of foreseeing what the consequences of actions might be for all those involved. Focusing solely on the consequences of actions also means that intentions are not considered and at the extreme may be taken as arguing that 'the ends justify the means'.

Deontology

Deontology (or non-consequentialism) takes the view that an action should be judged in relation to certain fundamental moral rules (for example honesty) and the duties and obligations which flow from them. The morally right action is therefore the one which accords with duties and obligations and the morally wrong action is the one which violates an obligation or duty. The challenge for a deontologist facing an ethical issue is to determine which duties or obligations are relevant in any particular case. Deontology is most closely associated with the work of Immanuel Kant (1724–1804), who argued that we should treat ourselves and others in ways consistent with human dignity and worth – as 'an end in themselves and not as a means to an end'. In more recent years, deontology has provided a basis for the increasingly common argument that people's 'rights' should be respected in considering ethical issues (Williamson, 2007).

Critics of deontology point to the difficulties of identifying an ultimate justifica-tion for duties and obligations and to the potential conflict between different sets of duties and obligations. Focusing exclusively on duties and obligations also means that the consequences of actions count for nothing and, at an extreme, may be seen as arguing for a moral absolutism.

Virtue ethics

Virtue ethics, taking inspiration from the work of the Greek philosopher Aristotle (384BC–322BC), shifts attention from the moral quality of an action to that of the *actor* and her/his motives and intentions. It takes the view that a virtuous person will act in a virtuous way and seeks to describe the features of a virtuous or morally upstanding character. It thus provides the basis for the argument that the best protection participants in a study can have is a researcher with high personal integrity and a good grounding in research ethics. Critics of this theory note both the difficulties of agreeing on what constitutes a 'virtue' (as these change over time and between communities) and its essentially conservative stance (because of its focus on established ways of being and doing) (Israel and Hay, 2006).

Ethics of care

The ethics of care is associated with the work of Gilligan (1982) and Noddings (2003), who argue that theories which emphasise rights, autonomy and abstract reasoning (ethics of justice) represent an approach to ethical deliberation that is used by men. Women, by contrast, more usually use an approach which emphasises interdependence, nurturing relationships and the importance of context. From this perspective, the morally right action must take account of responsibilities and relationships, rather than rules and rights, and be grounded in practical knowledge and attention to specificity and contextual detail (Edwards and Mauthner, 2002). Critics argue that the ethics of care has no central moral principle and that its applications to research are poorly developed. Nevertheless, the ethics of care is important in challenging established orthodoxies and high-lighting the broad range of relationships in which researchers are embedded and which are often overlooked.

BOX 3.1

A Case Example

To illustrate differences between the various theories of ethics discussed, we can consider the example of a researcher who is designing an observational study to explore social exclusion amongst older people in a nursing home:

- From a **consequentialist** perspective, the researcher might argue that better insights could be obtained if the research were conducted 'undercover' (so that 'real' rather than 'socially desirable' behaviour could be observed) and that doing so would not harm those involved. Covert research would therefore be the most appropriate study design.

- From a **deontological** perspective, the researcher might argue that he/she has an obligation to treat the others involved in the study (older people, the nurses and the managers of the nursing home) with respect. Doing so requires openness and honesty about what he/she, as researcher, is doing and acceptance of others' decisions regarding participation, regardless of the difficulties this might create for robust observations and insights.

- From the perspective of **virtue ethics**, the researcher might assert his/her moral character and argue that, over the course of the study, he/she will draw on his/her interpersonal skills and experience and show sensitivity to those involved in the study, so navigating a course through silence and disclosure which respects the values and concerns of the community.

- From the perspective of the **ethics of care**, the researcher might propose to gain an understanding of daily life in the nursing home, relationships amongst residents, the circumstances of individual residents, and the relationships of residents with staff and their own family members. Having achieved this, she would then decide what to disclose about the research, to whom, when and in what manner, always recognising the potential impact of the research on others.

Ethical Principles

Ethical principles are more specific than ethical theories, providing more *prescriptive guidelines* for ethical reasoning. Competing ethical theories nonetheless acknowledge a shared set of ethical principles (Ridley, 1998), of which the most important for health and social care research are those set out in the *Belmont Report*, elaborated by Beauchamp and Childress (2001) in the USA and extended by Gillon (1994) in the UK. These principles are: *beneficence*; *non-maleficence*; *respect for persons* (autonomy); and *justice*. They are regarded as binding principles; that is, each must be respected unless they conflict, in which case a choice must be made between them.

Beneficence is the principle that one should attempt to do good and to benefit others. In relation to research, this means that the aims of a study should have social and/or scientific value and its design and conduct should ensure valid or trustworthy findings. *Non-maleficence* was subsequently distinguished from beneficence as an independent principle that one should avoid doing harm. This means that risks to participants should be minimised and in proportion to the anticipated benefits. *Respect for persons* states that one should treat individuals as autonomous agents, giving due weight to their goals, preferences and interests, and that those with diminished autonomy should be protected from the risk of harm. This means, for example, allowing individuals to decide for themselves whether they wish to take part in a study and protecting the privacy of those who do. The principles of beneficence and respect for persons may conflict with each other, in which case one must be given precedence over the other: a choice which favours beneficence over respect for autonomy is *paternalistic*; a choice which favours respect for autonomy over beneficence is *libertarian*.

Justice is the principle that like cases should be treated alike and that differences in the way cases are treated should be justified by reference to relevant differences between them. The main implication for research is that participants should be selected in a fair and equitable way: that is, that vulnerable or dependent groups (such as those in institutions or low-resource countries) should not be targeted for research which involves higher risks and that individuals or groups of individuals (such as women or older people) should not be excluded from research without a good scientific reason. Justice is a more general principle than the other three. It cannot be determined by examining any particular case, but requires a comparison between cases in the way they are treated (Ridley, 1998).

Codes of Practice or Research Conduct

Codes of professional practice and/or research conduct interpret ethical principles in relation to the circumstances of their own profession or research focus. In so doing, they provide *practical advice* on the conduct of research which reflects the norms, values and experience of their members. Most professional and academic organisations have their own codes (see Box 3.2) to protect the welfare of patients, clients and research participants. Although they vary in their focus, emphasis and detail, they generally provide a set of guidelines in relation to such issues as informed consent, respect for privacy and confidentiality, and the balance of risks and benefits. Some also address the researcher's responsibilities towards other stakeholders including colleagues, employers and society.

BOX 3.2

Examples of Codes of Practice and Research Conduct

Professional codes of practice

- American Occupational Therapy Association:
  http://www.aota.org/general/docs/ethicscode05.pdf

- Nursing & Midwifery Council:
  http://www.nmc-uk.org/aArticle.aspx?ArticleID=3057

- British Association of Social Workers:
  http://www.basw.co.uk/Default.aspx?tabid=64

- The Chartered Society of Physiotherapy:
  http://www.csp.org.uk/uploads/documents/csp_effecprac_res07.pdf

- National Association of Social Workers:
  http://www.socialworkers.org/pubs/code/code.asp

Academic codes of research conduct

- American Anthropological Association:
  http://dev.aaanet.org/committees/ethics/ethrpt.htm

- British Psychological Society:
  http://www.bps.org.uk/downloadfile.cfm?file_uuid=6D0645CC-7E96-C67F-D75E2648E5580115&ext=pdf

- British Sociological Association:
  http://www.sociology.org.uk/as4bsoce.pdf

- Economic and Social Research Council:
  http://www.esrcsocietytoday.ac.uk/ESRCInfoCentre/Images/ESRC_Re_Ethics_Frame_tcm6-11291.pdf

- RESPECT:
  http://www.respectproject.org/code/index.php

- Social Research Association:
  http://www.the-sra.org.uk/ethical.htm

Informed consent

Informed consent refers to the way participants are included in a study: that is, on the basis of a decision by the participant, which has been made *voluntarily*[7] and with an understanding of *all the information likely to be relevant* to their decision. Informed consent is commonly regarded as fundamental to ethical research and the main means for protecting the rights, dignity and well-being of research participants (Boulton and Parker, 2007). All codes of practice or research conduct indicate that researchers should obtain the informed consent of participants before they begin, although many also recognise that there are circumstances (see below) in which this might not be possible or required.

'Valid consent' is a broader concept than informed consent and specifies that the person who gives consent should be competent to do so. If individuals are legally or medically not competent to give consent (perhaps because they are too young or too ill), proxy consent from their parent or guardian may be required. However, this should not preclude seeking the participants' agreement as well, and no study should proceed against the will of those actually involved (Bartlett and Martin, 2001; Alderson and Morrow, 2004).

In order to meet the requirements of valid or informed consent, information about the research should be provided to participants in a way that they can understand. This should usually be both in writing (in the form of an *information sheet*) and verbally; keeping sentences simple, translating information into other languages or providing it in Braille or audio format as necessary. Box 3.3 indicates the main headings that should be used in an information sheet. Participants should be given such a document well in advance of being asked to agree to take part in a study so that they have time to read, consider and talk about it with others. Equally, they should be given an opportunity to discuss it with the researcher.

BOX 3.3

Main Headings to be Included in an Information Sheet

- Study title

- Invitation to take part in a study

- What is the purpose of the study?

- Why have I been chosen?

- Do I have to take part? Do I have to carry on until the end if I start to take part?

- What will taking part involve for me? What will happen to me if I take part?/If I don't take part?

- What are the possible disadvantages or risks of taking part?

- What are the possible benefits of taking part?

- What if there is a problem?

- Will my taking part in the study be kept confidential?

- What will happen to the results of the study?

- Who is organising and funding the study?

- Who has reviewed the study?

- Further information and contact details

Adapted from the National Research Ethics Service (2007) *Information Sheets and Consent Forms: Guidance for Researchers and Reviewers*. Version 3.2 May 2007: http://www.nres.npsa.nhs.uk/rec-community/guidance/#InformedConsent

Securing consent also requires the researcher to ensure that individuals are not subject to manipulation, coercion or undue pressure to take part in the study. For this reason, special measures must be taken in research which involves those who are in a dependent relationship with the researcher (for example as a patient, client, student or employee) or who may feel an obligation to them (for example as a user of the services they represent) (Berglund, 1998; Scullion, 1999). Such measures may include protecting the identities of those who have been invited to take part from those providing care or keeping researchers quite separate from care providers, lecturers or employers. Incentives/inducements or payments for taking part may constitute undue pressure and researchers are generally advised to keep these to a level proportionate to the time participants give to the study and/or the disruption they experience as a result.

Researchers are commonly expected to document informed consent or proxy consent by obtaining a signed *consent form*. The consent form should ask the participant to confirm that they have seen and had time to read and digest the information sheet and that they understand and agree to each of the various elements of the study to which they are being asked to give consent (to take part in the study; to have the interview audio-recorded; to have verbatim quotes used in publications and so on) (Tarling, 2002; Boynton, 2005).

While a signed consent form is essential in any study which involves an intrusive clinical intervention, health and social care researchers conducting other types of studies have argued that it may be impossible or undesirable to ask a participant to sign a consent form. This is commonly the case where participants are engaged in illegal or stigmatising behaviour (for example illicit drug use or self-harm) or feel vulnerable to discrimination (for example those using mental health services or people diagnosed with HIV/AIDS). Signed consent forms are also seen as legalistic and hence as inconsistent with the development of a relationship of collaboration and trust (for example in ethno-graphic research – see Chapter 17) and with the notion of consent as an on-going process (Ramcharan and Cutcliffe, 2001; Kent et al., 2002; Murphy and Dingwall, 2007).

Covert research and research involving deception violate the principle of respect for autonomy and the requirement for informed consent. They may be justified, however, when the research question is of significant social or scientific value and a more open approach would distort the investigation. Wherever possible, participants should be debriefed at the end of such a study and informed consent obtained *post hoc*. Observational studies in public places may also take place without the knowledge or consent of those involved if it is not practically possible to obtain it. In these circumstances, care should be taken not to infringe the privacy or 'private space' of an individual or group. Epidemiological research involving anonymised patient records and the second-ary analysis of some data sets may also be exempt from the requirement for informed consent.

Respect for privacy and confidentiality

Respect for privacy and confidentiality is particularly important in health and social care research which is likely to involve the collection of sensitive information on personal beliefs, behaviours and experiences or on intimate bodily structures and functions. Researchers should attempt to minimise any distress to participants by keeping the collection of intrusive information to a minimum and by collecting it in a sensitive way.

A number of techniques are commonly used to protect participants' identity and to preserve their confidentiality (Oliver, 2003). These include not recording names or identifying data (collecting anonymous data); removing names and identifying details from data at the earliest possible time and storing them in separate places (de-identifying data); and using pseudonyms and disguising people, places and events in reports and publications. In quantitative research, various statistical methods can be used to conceal individual identities, such as combining categories of individuals below a certain size into larger categories when presenting data. Recordings, transcripts and data sets should also be stored and disposed of in ways that conform to relevant data protection legislation – for example, they should be kept in locked drawers or on password-protected computers and then shredded or electronically wiped.

As with informed consent, some codes of practice or research conduct provide for *exceptions* to the protection of confidentiality. Thus, many codes acknowledge that it is not necessary to offer confidentiality to those in public office who are speaking about their public work and recognise that information given to a researcher may need to be shared with a supervisor or other members of a research team. However, in both cases, this should be made clear to participants before the study begins. In addition, some codes of research conduct now make provision for researchers to deposit their data – suitably consented to, fully anonymised and properly documented – in a data archive where they may be made available to other researchers for secondary analysis. Many codes also require that confidential information is disclosed when it is in the public interest to do so; for example, where there is evidence of child or elder abuse or serious risk of harm to the participant or other identifiable individuals.

The balance of harms and benefits

All research entails some risk of harm as well as potential benefits, not least within the research process itself (Kent et al., 2002: 5.13). In much health and social care research, risks may be limited to relatively minor 'costs', such as demands on time, disruption to normal activities, fatigue or boredom. However, it is important not to underestimate the significance of these 'costs' to participants, nor to overlook the risk of more enduring harms; for example, the risk of significant discomfort or physical damage where research involves some form of therapeutic intervention (Seale and Barnard, 1999, Burgess 2007). In addition, research in health and social care commonly involves sensitive topics or vulnerable individuals and here the risk of social and psychological harm can be very high (Renzetti and Lee, 1993).

Strategies to minimise the risk of harm include adopting the research design which entails least risks, ensuring that researchers have appropriate knowledge and skills to carry out the research, actively monitoring participants over the course of a study, and providing a safety net of professional support for those who become distressed or suffer ill effects. Incorporating participants or members of their community in designing and monitoring the study may be a useful way of anticipating and avoiding potential risks and responding to those which do occur in a timely and appropriate manner.

Research participants are not generally regarded as the main beneficiaries of research. Nonetheless, they may benefit indirectly from access to treatments not otherwise available, the attention and support of the researcher, or the satisfaction of helping others. In addition, researchers are increasingly arguing for research designs which benefit participants directly (for example by providing better services for those whom they are studying or by engaging in advocacy on their behalf) or which maximise the benefits to the community as a whole (for example by increasing the skills and confidence of the community). Health and social care researchers who work regularly with disadvantaged groups are also increasingly adopting methodologies which involve participants directly in researching and improving their circumstances (Truman, 2003).

Responsibilities towards other stakeholders

While codes of research conduct generally emphasise responsibilities towards research participants, they may also set out the researcher's responsibilities towards other stakeholders in the research process. Responsibilities to other *members of the research team* include clarifying their work responsibilities, access to data and rights regarding publication and co-authorship, as well as attending to their safety and well-being over the course of the study. Responsibilities to *colleagues and the discipline* more generally include avoiding actions that would make it difficult for future researchers to work in the area or would adversely affect the reputation of the discipline. With regard to *employers and/or funders*, researchers' responsibilities include being honest and open about their own expertise and any factors which could affect the satisfactory completion of the study. Finally, researchers have a responsibility to *society* to consider the likely (negative) consequences of their work for those not directly involved in the research and to communicate their findings for the benefit of all (see Chapter 20 for further discussion on the importance of communicating research findings).

Research Ethics Review

While codes of practice or research conduct are important in providing guidance to researchers in the way they plan and conduct their research, many countries now also require that research involving human participants be reviewed and approved by an independent committee before it can begin. These are known as research ethics committees (RECs) in the UK, institutional review boards (IRBs) in the USA, research ethics boards (REBs) in Canada and institutional ethics committees (IECs) in Australia.[8] As a consequence, most universities, hospitals, social care departments and other institutions which conduct or commission research have established their own committees, and these generally comprise a Chair, Secretary, several members with subject and methodological expertise and lay members drawn from relevant communities. Collectively, their role is to protect the dignity, rights and well-being of participants by scrutinising research proposals and the way studies are to be conducted (Parker, 1994).

Applying to an ethics committee can be time-consuming and researchers should allow two to four months for final approval (Tarling, 2002; Boynton, 2005; Haigh, 2007). The first step for the researcher is to identify the appropriate committee, obtain its application form and establish the dates that it meets and the deadlines for submitting paperwork. In some cases, approval by several different committees may be required. This may occur if a university or research institution requires a protocol to be approved by an internal committee before it is submitted to an external hospital or social care committee, or if the research is to be conducted in a number of different areas or countries. Application forms are likely to vary between committees, but most will cover aims, objectives and background to the study; research design and methods of data collection and analysis; identification, selection and recruitment of participants (including inducements, coercion, deception and consent); potential benefits and risks to participants; handling, storage and disposal of data; and funding. As well as the completed form, the committee is likely to require copies of the research protocol; the principal investigator's curriculum vitae; the participant invitation letter, information sheet and consent form; indemnity arrangements; interview schedules, questionnaires and topic guides; and advertisements for the study (see also Chapter 2).

Research ethics committees meet regularly and review a limited number of applications at each meeting. Box 3.4 provides a summary of the key issues RECs consider and about which they must be adequately reassured before they give a 'favourable opinion' of an application. Applicants may be invited to the meeting to answer questions, although this is not always the case. Each application is either approved, not approved or – more commonly – approved subject to the applicant meeting certain conditions. In this latter case, further information may need to be provided or the research protocol amended in particular ways before final approval is given. Research which involves vulnerable groups – for example children, pregnant women, those who are unconscious and those in institutions such as care homes or prisons – must meet particularly strict ethical guidelines and may take more time to gain approval.[9]

BOX 3.4

Issues Considered by Ethics Committees when Looking at an Application

- Scientific design and conduct of the study: including the appropriateness of the design in relation to objectives, methodology, justification of predictable risks in relation to benefits, and provisions for monitoring and auditing the conduct of the study.

- Recruitment of research participants: including the characteristics of the population, the means of contacting and method of recruiting participants, and inclusion and exclusion criteria.

- Care and protection of research participants: including the safety of any intervention, the suitability of the investigators' qualifications and experience, the adequacy of health and social care support for participants, the appropriateness of any rewards or compensations given to participants, and any conflicts of interest that may affect the judgement of the researchers.

- Informed consent: including a full description of the process for obtaining consent, information sheet and consent forms, justification for including participants who cannot consent, and provisions made for responding to questions and complaints.

- Community considerations: including the relevance of the research to local and/or concerned communities and its likely impact on them, steps taken to consult them, the contribution to capacity building in the community, and the way in which the results of the study will be made available to participants and concerned communities.

Adapted from Department of Health (2001) *Governance Arrangements for NHS Research Ethics Committees* (London: Department of Health).

Once an application has been approved and a study has begun, researchers have a responsibility to report any adverse events that arise and to seek the REC's approval before changing any aspect of their protocol. RECs may also monitor the study as it progresses by requiring annual reports from the principal investigator and copies of any research publications.

Conclusions

Ethics is essential to good research. Indeed, research which does not meet high standards of ethics cannot be good research. Fundamental to ethical research are the values and attitudes, knowledge and skills of the researchers who carry it out and it is through education and experience, debate and reflection that these are formed. Ethical theories, principles and codes of practice or research conduct provide important 'tools' for researchers in considering what they should do and research ethics committees provide an alternative perspective and independent advice. Responsibility for ethical conduct, however, ultimately lies with researchers themselves and it is in their day-to-day actions and decisions that 'positively ethical' research is produced (Fallon and Long, 2007).

 # References

Alderson, P. and Morrow, V. (2004) *Ethics, Social Research and Consulting With Children and Young People* (Ilford, Essex: Barnardo's).

Bartlett, H. and Martin, W. (2001) 'Ethical issues in dementia research'. In Wilkinson, H. (ed.), *The Perspectives of People with Dementia: Research Methods and Motivations* (London: Jessica Kingsley).

Beauchamp, T. and Childress, J. (2001) *Principles of Biomedical Ethics*, 5th edn (Oxford: Oxford University Press).

Beecher, H. (1966) 'Ethics and clinical research', *New England Journal of Medicine*, **274**, 1354–60.

Berglund, C. (1998) *Ethics for Health Care* (Melbourne: Oxford University Press).

Boulton, M. and Parker, M. (2007) 'Introduction: Informed consent in a changing environment', *Social Science and Medicine*, **65**, 2187–98.

Boynton, P. (2005) *The Research Companion: A Practical Guide for the Social and Health Sciences* (Hove: Psychology Press).

Burgess, M. (2007) 'Proposing modesty for informed consent', *Social Science and Medicine*, **65**, 2284–95.

Department of Health (2001) *Governance Arrangements for NHS Research Ethics Committees* (London: Department of Health).

Edwards, R. and Mauthner, M. (2002) 'Ethics and feminist research: theory and practice'. In Mauthner, M., Birch, M., Jessop, J. and Miller, T. (eds), *Ethics in Qualitative Research* (London: Sage).

Fallon, D. and Long, T. (2007) 'Ethics approval, ethical research and delusions of efficacy'. In Long, T. and Johnson, M. (eds), *Research Ethics in the Real World: Issues and Solutions for Health and Social Care* (London: Churchill Livingstone Elsevier).

Gilligan, C. (1982) *In a Different Voice: Psychological Theory and Women's Development* (Cambridge: Harvard University Press).

Gillon, R. (1994) 'Medical ethics: Four principles plus attention to scope', *British Medical Journal*, **309**, 184–8.

Haigh, C. (2007) 'Getting ethics approval'. In Long, T. and Johnson, M. (eds), *Research Ethics in the Real World* (Edinburgh: Churchill Livingstone).

Humphreys, L. (1970) *Tearoom Trade: A Study of Homosexual Encounters in Public Places* (London: Duckworth).

Israel, M. and Hay, I. (2006) *Research Ethics for Social Scientists* (London: Sage).

Kampmeier, R. (1972) 'The Tuskegee study of untreated syphilis', *Southern Medical Journal*, **5**, 1247–51.

Kent, J., Williamson, E., Goodenough, T. and Ashcroft, R. (2002) 'Social science gets the ethics treatment: Research governance and ethical review', *Sociological Research Online*, **7** (4): www.socresonline.org.uk/7/4/williamson.html.

Murphy, E. and Dingwall, R. (2007) 'Informed consent, anticipatory regulation and ethnographic practice', *Social Science and Medicine*, **65**, 2223–34.

National Research Ethics Service (2007) *Information Sheets and Consent Forms: Guidance for Researchers and Reviewers*. Version 3.2 May 2007: http://www.nres.npsa.nhs.uk/rec-community/guidance/#InformedConsent.

Noddings, N. (2003) *Caring: A Feminine Approach to Ethics and Moral Education,* 2nd edn (Berkeley: University of California Press).

Oliver, P. (2003) *The Student's Guide to Research Ethics* (Maidenhead: Open University Press).

Pappworth, M. (1967) *Human Guinea Pigs* (Boston: Beacon Press).

Parker, B. (1994) 'Research ethics committees'. In Tschudin, V. (ed.), *Ethics Education and Research* (Harlow: Scutari).

Ramcharan, P. and Cutcliffe, J. (2001) 'Judging the ethics of qualitative research: Considering the "ethics as process" model', *Health and Social Care in the Community,* **9**, 358–66.

Renzetti, C. and Lee, R. (1993) *Researching Sensitive Topics* (London: Sage).

Ridley, A. (1998) *Beginning Bioethics: A Text With Integrated Readings* (New York: St Martin's Press).

Scullion, P. (1999) 'Critiquing the ethical aspects of research', *British Journal of Therapy and Rehabilitation,* **6**, 540–4.

Seale, J. and Barnard, S. (1999) 'Ethical considerations in therapy research', *British Journal of Occupational Therapy,* **62**, 371–5.

Tarling, M. (2002) 'Ethical issues'. In Tarling, M. and Crofts, L. (eds), *The Essential Researcher's Handbook for Nurses and Health Care Professionals,* 2nd edn (Edinburgh: Baillière Tindall).

Truman, C. (2003) 'Ethics and the ruling relations of research production', *Sociological Research Online,* **8** (1): www.socresonline.org.uk/8/1/truman.html.

Van der Arend, A.J.G. (2003) 'Research ethics committees and the nurse's role'. In Tadd, W. (ed.), *Ethics in Nursing Education, Research and Management: Perspectives from Europe* (Basingstoke: Palgrave Macmillan).

Williamson, T. (2007) 'The individual in research'. In Long, T. and Johnson, M. (eds), *Research Ethics in the Real World: Issues and Solutions for Health and Social Care* (London: Churchill Livingstone Elsevier).

Zimbardo, P. (1973) 'On the ethics of intervention in human psychological research: With special reference to the Stanford prison experiment', *Cognition,* **2**, 243–56.

Notes

1. *Nuremberg Code:* http://ohsr.od.nih.gov/guidelines/nuremberg.html.

2. *Declaration of Helsinki:* http://ohsr.od.nih.gov/guidelines/helsinki.html.

3. The *Belmont Report: Ethical Principles and Guidelines for the Protection of Human Subjects of Research:* http://ohsr.od.nih.gov/guidelines/belmont.html.

4. *International Ethical Guidelines for Biomedical Research Involving Human Subjects:* http://www.cioms.ch/frame_guidelines_nov_2002.htm.

5. For example, the Tuskegee study (Kampmeier, 1972), the Stanford 'prison' experiment (Zimbardo, 1973) and the *Tearoom Trade* (Humphreys, 1970).

6. Title 45 of the Code of Federal Regulations Part 46, Sub-part A: http://www.hhs.gov/ohrp/humansubjects/guidance/45cfr46.htm.

7. In other words, the individual must feel able to decide *not* to take part.

8. Van der Arend (2003) and Israel and Hay (2006) both review procedures in a wider range of countries.

9. Some types of study – for example, audits or service evaluations – may not require review by an ethics committee but clarification of whether this is the case, and what is considered an audit or service evaluation, is required before the study begins.

Part 2

Desk-based Research

Literature Reviews

4

MARTIN LEACH, JOANNE NEALE AND PETER A. KEMP

Introduction

A literature review brings together existing knowledge on a particular topic. In so doing, the general aim is to summarise, evaluate, synthesise and interpret previous research, arguments and ideas in order to make sense of current knowledge in the subject area being investigated. Unlike an annotated bibliography, which is simply a descriptive summary of the literature on a given topic, the literature review shows how individual publications link together and where any gaps in current knowledge lie.

In recent years, the terms 'traditional review', 'narrative review' and even 'journalistic review' have variously been used to lump together any method of reviewing that does not adhere to the very standardised procedures of a 'systematic review' (see Chapter 5). However, this grouping of 'other' types of review wrongly implies that literature reviews are unsystematic and therefore unscientific (Hammersley, 2001). Equally, it fails to capture the diverse nature of literature reviews, which vary considerably in their style and form depending on their purpose (for example, some literature reviews are intended to be stand-alone accounts of existing knowledge whilst others provide background information to set the scene for further research).

It is not necessary to be an expert on a topic in order to conduct a literature review. Indeed, undertaking a literature review can be a good way for students and researchers to familiarise themselves with existing knowledge and is often the first step towards developing expertise in a subject area. Nonetheless, high-quality reviews do tend to require the skills of an accomplished scholar who is familiar with a wide range of research designs and methodological traditions, as well as the practical, empirical and conceptual issues relating to the topic being reviewed (Hart, 1998: 44).

Historical Context

Although it is difficult to be precise about the origins of literature reviews, early intellectuals such as Bacon (*c*.1214–1294), Copernicus (1473–1543) and Galileo (1564–1642) all seem to have reviewed relevant theories that were in existence at the time they developed their ideas. Several centuries ago, students of Chinese medicine and science were also aware of, and built upon, theories that had been proposed by others before them (Sivin, 1988). The astronomers Halley (1656–1742) and Herschel (1738–1822) read and wrote scientific papers (Halley, 1683; Herschel, 1826), whilst 'journals' or diaries passed between small groups of scientists in mid-seventeenth century England and France (Dawes et al., 1999). It is debatable whether such individuals conducted 'literature reviews' as such. Yet, they clearly sought to inform themselves of the latest developments in their respective fields.

Until the late twentieth century, libraries – with their stacks of books, journals and records – were the obvious starting point for any individual wanting to familiarise themselves with current knowledge in a particular field. Many hours could be spent searching card catalogues by hand and poring over documents, but the amount of literature that could be reviewed was invariably constrained by the local availability of materials. Towards the end of the twentieth century, however, computers and electronic media rapidly revolutionised literature reviewing and increased its popularity. First, the number of academic journals and other electronic sources of information increased exponentially; second, it was suddenly possible to access and download much of this information, often in full-text format, without even leaving home.

Although the growth of electronic media has in many respects enabled literature reviewing to flourish, the academic credibility of the method has more recently been challenged by the emergence of systematic reviews and meta-analyses (see Chapter 5). Proponents of systematic reviews – which have largely focused on quantitative data obtained from randomised controlled trials (see Chapter 11) – have often claimed that other forms of literature reviewing are sloppy, biased and incomplete (Greenhalgh, 1997). In response to this, some academics have defensively argued that literature reviews should always be conducted in a very systematic and standardised manner, even if the detail required for a full systematic review is not present (Aveyard, 2007). Others have sought to devise systematic reviewing techniques that can accommodate the diverse forms of evidence, including qualitative data, used in more 'traditional' reviews[1] (Mays et al., 2005; Petticrew and Roberts, 2005).

Such developments have no doubt been useful in encouraging reviewers of all persuasions to reflect carefully on their methods and to be open and transparent about how their work has been undertaken. Nonetheless, those who have sought to make literature reviews highly standardised have often failed to appreciate that literature reviews and systematic reviews fulfil very different functions. For example, systematic reviews address very specific questions about the effects of a particular policy, practice or medical intervention and are consequently good for theory testing. In contrast, literature reviews address broader and more complex topics by providing a map of research in a particular field and are thus more suited to theory building and hypothesis generation (Baumeister and Leary, 1997; Hart, 1998; Hammersley,

2001). Literature reviews are not, in other words, a 'poor relation' to system-atic reviews. They are, and must be preserved as, an important and diverse method in their own right.

Current Use

Literature reviews commonly function as stand-alone reports, book chapters, journal articles or dissertations. Here, it is generally expected that the review will say something original. As Aveyard explains, the aim is to move from 'the known (the individual pieces of research and other information) towards the unknown (combining the results of the different information to reach new insights on a topic)' (Aveyard, 2007: 18). Reviews can also be undertaken to set the scene or provide the context for further evidence. For example, they are often the starting point for research grant applications (where it is usually necessary to demonstrate how the proposed study will relate to and develop existing understanding) or journal articles (where a topic must be introduced prior to presenting new empirical data). In addition, literature reviews might be used more loosely as the foundation for a commentary, opinion piece or policy document.[2]

A good literature review will identify and clarify the key concepts, ideas and theories relating to the topic being studied. It should also summarise and critique the evidence but then synthesise this to develop a fresh perspective. Ideally, the review produced will provide the reader with an overview of the topic; clarify and suggest explanations for any contradictory evidence; identify gaps in current knowledge and areas for further research; and offer conclusions that might inform future debate, theorising and practice. By revealing how others have defined and measured key concepts, undertaken related studies and struc-tured their findings, the literature review can also help those planning their own study to ascertain the significance of their topic or problem, focus their research question, and improve their methodology (Hart, 1998; Kumar, 2005).

Unsurprisingly, given their many forms and functions, literature reviews legitimately draw upon a wide range of materials. This can include published and unpublished scholarly writing, such as books; journal articles; confer-ence proceedings; abstracts; dissertations and theses; bibliographies; discus-sion papers; and government reports. It might also include documents that are not published in the conventional way, such as online information; consultation papers; strategy documents; bulletins; circulars; resource packs; expert opinion; letters; personal communication; newspaper articles; audio-visual items; and leaflets (Hek and Moule, 2006). This does not mean that all sources will be given equal weight or credibility in the review. Indeed, a good review will carefully evaluate the reliability of the sources included and prioritise those deemed most robust. However, being as inclusive as possible, at least at the outset, helps to capture the full range of perspectives and ideas currently in circulation.

BOX 4.1

Types of Question Addressed by Literature Reviews

- What is the current state of knowledge on topic X?

- What are the limitations of this knowledge base?

- What are the key concepts and theories underpinning topic X?

- How does the evidence on topic X vary between studies and sources and how might any contradictions be explained and resolved?

- What are the current gaps in knowledge on topic X?

- How might existing knowledge on topic X be used to inform policy, practice and theoretical debate?

- What should be the focus of future research on topic X?

- What might my research question add to the knowledge base on topic X?

- How important is my research problem in the context of what is already known about topic X?

- What can the existing literature teach me about how to conduct a new study on topic X?

Main Strengths of Literature Reviews

Literature reviews offer a much broader picture of a topic than a single study or piece of work. By summarising and synthesising a whole body of literature in a particular area, they provide a comprehensive overview of current knowledge or understanding and reduce the likelihood that false conclusions will be drawn. Furthermore, by critically evaluating the relative worth of each piece of information, it is often possible to clarify or explain discrepancies between authors. Equally, by locating each piece of information within the context of other pieces of information, new insights can be generated and theoretical issues that are beyond the scope of any individual output explored.

Literature reviews also have important practical strengths. Health and social care practitioners need to be up-to-date with the latest information in their field, but they are unlikely to have the time to read, assimilate and interpret every publication or to follow every debate. A good literature review will provide them with an accessible, balanced guide that allows them quickly to make sense of a particular topic (Aveyard, 2007). Undergraduate and postgraduate students can also find that conducting a literature review for their dissertation enables them to immerse themselves in a topic that interests them, but without having to succumb to the pragmatic challenges and unpredictability of securing research ethics and local governance approval (Aveyard, 2007; also see Chapters 2 and 3).

In addition to the above, literature reviews can address complex policy and practice issues that cannot be answered by systematic reviews. For example, they can trace the historical development of a scientific principle or clinical concept and increase understanding of institutions and processes (Baumeister and Leary, 1997; Hammersley, 2001). They are also able to deal with many different types of information collected from different disciplines and using different methodological approaches. As such, they are a very flexible technique that permits the researcher to exercise their interpretive and analytical skills. Moreover, their versatility means that they can be written and presented in different styles and formats to accommodate the needs of particular audiences (Hammersley, 2001).

Main Weaknesses of Literature Reviews

Literature reviews are not inevitably 'unsystematic' or 'unscientific' simply because they are not 'systematic reviews'. Nonetheless, they can – like any study – be done badly and it is easy for a reviewer to produce a piece of work that is difficult to verify because the methods of selecting, critiquing and analysing the material are not clearly documented (Greenhalgh, 1997; Aveyard, 2007). Furthermore, those who undertake a literature review without appropriate knowledge and training often produce reports that are incomplete or that simply document what each author said in turn without any attempt at analysis, synthesis or interpretation (Haywood and Wragg, 1982; cited in Bell, 1987).

It is also the case that literature reviews can be susceptible to the subjective judgements, preferences and biases of a particular reviewer's perspective. *In extremis*, a poor reviewer might deliberately omit evidence that is inconsistent with their preferred argument or theory (Aveyard, 2007). More subtly, the literature that is reviewed might be influenced by the reviewer's background and interests. Thus, a physiologist investigating the use of aromatherapy in health care is likely to draw upon literature and theories relating to the interaction of aromatic molecules with neurotransmitters, whereas a mental health nurse investigating the same topic might be more interested in literature and ideas relating to touch and interpersonal interaction.

Finally, there are some practical hurdles to overcome when undertaking a good literature review. For example, it is necessary to identify a topic or research question that is broad enough to generate interesting literature but not so broad that a search produces an unmanageable amount of data. This is particularly important for the student or novice researcher who may have limited time and resources and can easily be overwhelmed by the amount of available information. In recent years, the internet and computers have made searching faster and provided access to an enormous range of literature. This, however, means that reviewers must carefully plan their searching, budget for the costs of retrieving information not downloadable or held locally, and devise effective systems for storing sources and keeping notes. They must also build in time to update their searches so that the very latest materials can be included in their final report.

MAIN STRENGTHS AND WEAKNESSES
... OF LITERATURE REVIEWS

Strengths

- Literature reviews produce a much broader, comprehensive and accurate picture of a topic than a single study or piece of work. For example, they can clarify discrepancies between authors and explore theoretical issues that are beyond the scope of any individual document.

- Literature reviews can quickly provide health and social care practitioners with a balanced and accessible guide to the latest information on a particular topic.

- Literature reviews provide students with an ideal opportunity to immerse themselves in a topic, without having to succumb to the challenges of securing research ethics and local governance approval.

- Literature reviews are a flexible method which can address complex policy and practice issues, process diverse types of information, and be written in a style and format appropriate to the audience.

Weaknesses

- It is easy for a reviewer to produce a piece of work that is difficult to verify because the methods are not clearly documented.

- Those who undertake a literature review without appropriate knowledge and training often produce reports that are incomplete and lacking in analysis, synthesis and interpretation.

- Literature reviews can be susceptible to the subjective judgements, preferences and biases of a particular reviewer's perspective.

- Electronic searching means that it is easy to become overwhelmed by the amount of available information. Reviewers must therefore plan their work carefully.

Conducting a Literature Review

In this section, we describe how to conduct a stand-alone literature review, rather than one undertaken as a precursor to presenting new empirical data. As Cresswell (2003: 35) notes, there is no one way to conduct a literature review. Nonetheless, reviewers should seek to follow stages similar to those involved in conducting primary research.

Deciding on the research question

A literature review should begin with a clearly stated question, problem or puzzle. This should be focused, address a topic that interests and motivates the researcher, be achievable within the time frame, and answerable from the literature (Aveyard, 2007: 55). It does not need to be as tightly structured as it would in a systematic review (see Chapter 5), but researchers must be unambiguous about what they are aiming to achieve.

Preparing a search strategy

Once the research question, problem or puzzle has been formulated, a search strategy has to be devised. This involves specifying the parameters of the search; listing search terms (or keywords); and determining the databases and other resources that will be used. The parameters of the search might relate to the types of material to be included (for example only peer-reviewed journal articles, books and published reports); the language of publication (for example only materials written in English); the date of publication (for example only sources published after 2000); geography (for example only materials relating to North America); or even study design or methods (for example only qualitative research). These parameters – often referred to as the inclusion and exclusion criteria – ensure that the review focuses on the types of evidence that will best address the research question.

Search terms are chosen to reflect the most important ideas, concepts or variables for the review. In health and social care, these commonly relate to the population or group being studied, the intervention or treatment being received, and the kinds of measures or outcomes of interest.[3] However, to ensure that searching is inclusive, alternatives for each search term should also be listed. Thus, if the population of interest is teenagers, 'teens', 'youths', 'adolescents', 'young people', 'young adults' and so on should additionally be searched.[4] Researchers must likewise account for variant spellings and single versus plural nouns or nouns versus verbs. When searching electronically, this can, to an extent, be overcome by using symbols known as wildcards (such as ?, $ or *). Thus, 'orthop?dic' can be used to search for orthopedic or orthopaedic and 'inject*' to search for injector, injectors, injection or injecting).[5]

When conducting reviews that include publications from different countries, it is important to ensure that the literature search includes terms that may be country-specific. For example, programmes that enable older people and people with disabilities to purchase their own care have a variety of different names. They are known as 'direct payments' in the UK, 'long-term care allowances' in Austria, 'personal assistance budgets' in the Netherlands and 'consumer-directed personal assistance' in the USA. Some authors have also recently given them the generic name of 'cash for care' schemes (Ungerson and Yeandle, 2006). A literature search that included all of these terms, but not 'consumer-directed personal assistance', would probably fail to find many US publications.

In today's computerised world, the main resources for literature searching are likely to be electronic databases (such as ASSIA, MEDLINE, PsycINFO, CINAHL or Social Care Online). These databases provide direct access to journal articles and other key literature, but will not necessarily identify all relevant data. For example, many studies are not published and much information is not in the public domain or is very difficult to locate (such as research theses and information produced by commercial organisations). Additional strategies for searching are therefore required, including hand searching through journals and reference lists; speaking with experts in the field; and simply browsing library shelves.

Retrieving materials

In order to remember what has been done and to demonstrate a methodical approach, the reviewer should keep a record of when searches were undertaken, the keywords used, the databases searched or resources covered, and the quantity and type of potentially useful materials found. Retrieved items must also be carefully logged and filed. For example, each time a document is obtained, the reviewer should systematically record authors; date; title; place of publication; publisher; page numbers and so on. The databases or other sources from which the publication was retrieved should also be noted. These details might be recorded using a simple manual card filing system or a computer programme such as EndNote or Reference Manager (Hek and Moule, 2006).

Assessing relevance and rigour

The reviewer must next read[6] the retrieved literature to assess whether or not it is actually relevant to the research question or problem. If it is relevant, they should produce a short written summary of key information, such as the central aim or problem, research design, population or participants studied, and key findings. The reviewer should also make a judgement on the overall rigour and significance of each retrieved item in order to determine how much weight to accord it in the final review.[7] The process of critiquing a research paper, especially for the novice reviewer, is often best undertaken with the assistance of a critical appraisal tool.[8] Such tools, which can be generic or specific to a particular research design, help to ensure that the strengths and weaknesses of each study are assessed consistently (Oxman, 1994; MacAuley et al., 1998; Aveyard, 2007).

Analysing and interpreting the data

A good literature review should not simply be a descriptive summary of a series of publications. Rather, it involves analysing and interpreting ideas and arguments. This requires the reviewer to combine, classify and then organise all the information they have collected in order to make connections between individual documents, explain any differences or similarities between authors and find new meaning from the literature as a whole (Aveyard, 2007). To this end, the reviewer must not impose a priori categories on the data. Instead, they should scrutinise all the evidence creatively and flexibly, so allowing the main themes and theories to emerge.

One strategy that can assist with this process is to produce a literature map. This is a visual picture (usually in the form of a tree, flow chart or circles) which serves two main functions. First, it can provide an overview of all the relevant or the most important literature and ideas on a topic, illustrating what has been done, when, by whom and using what methods. Second, it can be annotated to show links between studies and ideas and to reveal how these relate to each other and where future research is needed (Hart, 1998; Cresswell, 2003).

Writing

If done well, the classification and organisation of the data should provide a framework for writing up the review. This will commonly involve the use of headings and sub-headings that relate to the key themes and sub-themes identified during the analyses. These headings and sub-headings should be arranged so that they link to each other and follow a logical order, collectively addressing the review's central research question or problem (Aveyard, 2007). Alternatively, it might be more appropriate to present the findings under broad headings relating to chronology; study purpose or objective; methodological approach; or authors' conclusions (The Writing Center, 2007). Again, though, there will likely be some ordering by sub-theme under these broader headings.

As it will seldom be either possible or necessary to discuss every single item that has been read, the reviewer should focus on those materials that are most directly relevant and methodologically robust or which have been the most widely cited on the topic. For some types of literature review, it can be helpful – whenever a new item is introduced – to provide brief contextual information about the type and quality of the evidence reported (Aveyard, 2007). In the discussion section of the review, it is common practice to highlight the strengths and weaknesses of the reviewing procedures adopted; discuss the meaning of the findings within the wider context of any relevant theory, policy and practice; identify questions that remain unanswered; and make suggestions for future research (Doherty and Smith, 1999).

An Example of a Literature Review

The literature review method can be illustrated by a study of carers' aspirations and decisions about work and retirement. This was part of a larger research project funded by the UK Department for Work and Pensions (DWP) and conducted by researchers based in the Social Policy Research Unit at the University of York, UK. The other elements of the study were qualitative, in-depth interviews with carers and focus groups with staff working for Jobcentre Plus,[9] local authority social services departments, and carers' organisations. The literature review was published as a chapter in the report written for the DWP (Arksey et al., 2005) and incorporated into a book chapter based on the project (Arksey and Kemp, 2006).

According to the 2001 Census, there were an estimated 5.6 million people in Britain looking after a relative or friend in need of support because of age or frailty, physical or learning disability or illness. Although many carers will be working when the need to care arises, combining work and care can be very difficult. Giving up work or working fewer hours can, however, cause carers severe financial, social and emotional hardships (Department of Health, 1999). The DWP commissioned the research in order to ascertain what can be done to assist carers to remain in work, or to return to work during or after an episode of caring. The remit of the literature review was broad; namely, to examine the existing evidence on carers in relation to employment and retirement.

For the purposes of the review, 'carers' were defined as adults below state pension age who provided unpaid care for sick, disabled or frail elderly people where the recipients of their care included chronically sick or disabled children, spouses, elderly parents, other relatives, friends or neighbours. Childcare and foster caring were excluded. Although the aim was to produce a narrative review of the existing evidence base, rather than a 'systematic review', the intention was to be transparent and systematic. To this end, the research team carried out an extensive search of academic, policy and professional databases, as well as internet sites belonging to carers' organisations and government departments. They also followed up references in cited publications and contacted leading researchers in the field. The software package EndNote was used to search for and manage references.

Geographical coverage was confined to the UK and, because of time and resource constraints, only articles published since 1985 were included. Both qualitative and quantitative research-based publications were included, but commentaries, opinion pieces, and consultation documents were excluded. Very short (1–2 pages) articles were also excluded on the grounds that they could not contain enough information to appraise the quality of the research. Over 150 full-text publications were retrieved and these were all evaluated using a quality appraisal tool, with only those which passed the quality appraisal being included in the final review.

Findings related to the incidence and nature of caring and the characteristics of carers; the nature of employment undertaken by people providing unpaid care; the impact of caring on paid employment; factors affecting decisions about combining work and unpaid care; workplace policies and practices that would help carers to combine care-giving and employment; and the income consequences of caring, including the impact on earning and pensions. Key points included:

- Most carers wish to remain in work and many are very reluctant to give up their jobs. However, many employed carers find it difficult to care at the same time as engaging in paid work and this seems to become more difficult once people provide more than about 20 hours of care per week.

- Co-resident, rather than extra-resident, carers face the biggest obstacles to combining work with their caring responsibilities.

- A range of factors influence carers' decisions about whether to remain in work or change their employment status, for example: being able to afford to give up work; job enjoyment; stress levels at work; being out of work; and access to support.

- Being able to retire early with a full occupational pension or favourable retirement deal can be a significant incentive to leave work in order to undertake caring duties, especially for men.

- Interrupted or short working careers, or moving from full-time to part-time work, have implications for earnings and subsequent pension entitlements, especially if the caring episode lasts for many years.

- Most employers give little consideration to carer-friendly work practices and where these do exist carers often feel unable to take advantage of them.

The research team used the findings emerging from the literature review to inform the design of the topic guides they used later in the in-depth interviews and focus groups. In addition, the review identified some important gaps in the existing evidence base and areas where more research is required. These were documented in the final report and included, *inter alia*, limited information on: the impact of caring on people from different ethnic groups; combining self-employment with caring duties; the role of services in helping carers to remain in, or take up, paid employment; and the role of voluntary work in carers' lives. The research team was also invited to present the findings of the literature review to the DWP in order to inform the development of its policy on carers.

Further Reading

Aveyard, H. (2007) *Doing a Literature Review in Health and Social Care: A Practical Guide* (Maidenhead: Open University Press).

Aveyard's book is primarily aimed at students writing a literature review for their undergraduate dissertation. However, it will also be useful to postgraduate students and health and social care practitioners new to the processes of reviewing. Aveyard advocates a highly standardised approach to reviewing and guides the reader logically through the key stages of developing a review question, searching, appraising, synthesising and presenting the findings in a dissertation. Chapters end with useful summaries and tips for writing a review and the book concludes with a short but helpful glossary of common research terms.

Baumeister, R.F. and Leary, M.R. (1997) 'Writing narrative literature reviews', *Review of General Psychology*, **1**, 311–20.

This article on narrative literature reviews is suitable for both novice and experienced researchers. It provides a very interesting account of the importance of literature reviews in knowledge development and clearly highlights some of the main advantages of narrative literature reviews over empirical reports (for example, narrative reviews are better able to tackle broad and abstract questions; engage in *post-hoc* theorising; and appreciate and use methodological diversity). The authors offer practical guidance on how to undertake a narrative literature review, including some common mistakes, and conclude that the method occupies a special and privileged place in the scientific enterprise.

Hammersley, M. (2001) 'On "Systematic" Reviews of Research Literatures: A "Narrative" Response to Evans and Benefield', *British Educational Research Journal*, **27**, 543–54.

This article is a gem for those seeking to defend the narrative literature review against the over-privileging of the systematic review. Although written primarily for those working in the field of education, its arguments apply equally to health and social care. Hammersley carefully identifies a series of flaws in the assumptions underpinning systematic reviews and contends that the priority given to this method is in danger of reducing research to collections of studies that can only answer single policy- or practice-relevant questions. Presenting the systematic reviewer as a mere 'technician' (in contrast to the 'thinking' narrative reviewer), Hammersely is simultaneously provocative, scholarly and entertaining.

Hart, C. (1998) *Doing a Literature Review: Releasing the Social Science Research Imagination* (London: Sage).

This is a standard text on literature reviewing which is primarily written for postgraduate research students at master's and doctoral level within the social sciences. However, it will be of interest to a much broader audience, including those within health and social care. The book markets itself as an 'introduction' rather than a 'manual' and its focus is on reviewing research literature as a basis for undertaking further primary research. The need for depth, breadth, rigour, consistency and effective analysis and synthesis are all emphasised and Hart responds to this by providing a comprehensive overview of the key aspects of reviewing, including classifying, organising, mapping, analysing and writing.

 # References

Arksey, H. and Kemp, P.A. (2006) 'Carers and employment in a work-focused welfare state'. In Glendinning, C. and Kemp, P.A. (eds), *Cash and Care: Policy Challenges in the Welfare State* (Bristol: Policy Press).

Arksey, H., Kemp, P.A., Glendinning, C., Kotchetkova, I. and Tozer, R. (2005) *Carers' Aspirations and Decisions Around Work and Retirement,* Department for Work and Pensions Research Report No. 290 (London: Department for Work and Pensions).

Aveyard, H. (2007) *Doing a Literature Review in Health and Social Care: A Practical Guide* (Maidenhead: Open University Press).

Baumeister, R.F. and Leary, M.R. (1997) 'Writing narrative literature reviews', *Review of General Psychology,* **1**, 311–20.

Bell, J. (1987) *Doing Your Research Project: A Guide for First-time Researchers in Education and Social Science* (Milton Keynes: Open University Press).

Cresswell, J.W. (2003) *Research Design: Qualitative, Quantitative and Mixed Methods Approaches,* 2nd edn (London: Sage).

Dawes, D., Davies, P., Gray, A., Mant, J., Seers, K. and Snowball, R. (1999) *Evidence-Based Practice: A Primer for Health Care Professionals* (London: Churchill Livingstone).

Department of Health (1999) *Caring about Carers: A National Strategy for Carers* (London: Department of Health).

Doherty, M. and Smith, R. (1999) 'The case for structuring the discussion of scientific papers', *British Medical Journal,* **318**, 1224–5.

Greenhalgh, T. (1997) 'How to read a paper: Papers that summarise other papers (systematic reviews and meta-analyses)', *British Medical Journal,* **315**, 672–5.

Halley, E. (1683) 'A theory of the variation of the magnetical compass', *Philosophical Transactions,* **13**, 208–21.

Hammersley, M. (2001) 'On "systematic" reviews of research literatures: A "narrative" response to Evans and Benefield', *British Educational Research Journal,* **27**, 543–54.

Hart, C. (1998) *Doing a Literature Review: Releasing the Social Science Research Imagination* (London: Sage).

Haywood, P. and Wragg, E.C. (1982) *Evaluating the Literature,* Rediguide 2 (Nottingham: University of Nottingham School of Education).

Hek, G. and Moule, P. (2006) *Making Sense of Research: An Introduction for Health and Social Care Practitioners,* 3rd edn (London: Sage).

Herschel, J.F.W. (1826) 'On the parallax of fixed stars', *Philosophical Transactions of the Royal Society of London,* **116**, 266 (published after his death in 1822).

Kumar, R. (2005) *Research Methodology: A Step-by-step Guide for Beginners,* 2nd edn (London: Sage).

MacAuley, D., McCrum, E. and Brown, C. (1998) 'Randomised controlled trial of the READER method of critical appraisal in general practice', *British Medical Journal,* **316**, 1134–7.

Mays, N., Pope, C. and Popay, J. (2005) 'Systematically reviewing qualitative and quantitative evidence to inform management and policy-making in the health field', *Journal of Health Services Research Policy,* **10**(S1): 6–20.

Oxman, A.D. (1994) 'Systematic reviews, checklists for review articles', *British Medical Journal,* **309**, 648–51.

Petticrew, M. and Roberts, H. (2005) *Systematic Reviews in the Social Sciences: A Practical Guide* (Oxford: Blackwell Publishing).

Sivin, N. (1988) 'Science and medicine in Imperial China – the state of the field', *The Journal of Asian Studies,* **47**, 41–90.

The Writing Center (2007) *Handouts and Links: Literature reviews* http://www.unc.edu/depts/wcweb/handouts/literature_review.html (accessed 30 November, 2007).

Ungerson, C. and Yeandle, S. (eds) (2006) *Cash for Care in Developed Welfare States* (Basingstoke: Palgrave Macmillan).

Notes

1 We use the term 'traditional reviews' here to distinguish them from 'systematic reviews'. However, we maintain that the term 'traditional reviews' does not adequately capture the diverse range of forms that literature reviews can take.

2 It is here that reviews are most likely to take an 'unsystematic' form, because the reviewer may select those items that best support their underlying proposition or argument.

3 These terms are often evident from the wording of the research question or problem.

4 Many bibliographic databases provide a thesaurus to help identify relevant synonyms.

5 For a comprehensive search, it is usually necessary to combine search terms using Boolean operators – 'AND', 'OR', 'NOT', 'NEAR'.

6 Preliminary scanning may indicate that an item can be discarded without a detailed read.

7 The reviewer should only include work that was undertaken in an ethical manner.

8 One very useful set of critical appraisal tools – free to download for personal use – is produced by the Critical Appraisal Skills Programme (CASP): http://www.phru.nhs.uk/Pages/PHD/CASP.htm.

9 Jobcentre Plus is the agency which provides social security benefits and employment advice to people of working age in the UK.

Systematic Reviews

LESLEY SMITH AND LORRAINE DIXON

Introduction

Health and social care professionals have to digest ever-increasing amounts of information in order to keep up with new research findings (see also Chapter 4). It can be difficult to assess and assimilate all the available information on a topic, particularly as individual studies often produce conflicting results. Yet today's emphasis on evidence-based practice requires practitioners to use the latest research to inform their decision-making. Systematic reviews have emerged as an important research method to meet this need. Systematic reviews use existing primary research for secondary data analysis, eliciting common themes and results, and providing a good evidence base to inform policy-making and practice. They have the advantage of bringing together what can be vast bodies of information, and they provide an easy-to-digest, considered synopsis of the latest evidence on a particular issue or intervention.

Oxman and Guyatt (1988) defined the systematic review as an approach that applies explicit scientific principles aimed at minimising both bias and random errors. A systematic review often includes a meta-analysis: a mathematical synthesis of the quantitative results of two or more studies that address a similar question in a similar way. The key features of a systematic review are: a clearly defined research question; transparent methods, defined a priori to include clear criteria for including and excluding studies; exhaustive searches for published and unpublished studies; explicit reporting of the methods used to appraise, abstract and synthesise information from individual studies, conducted in duplicate to minimise errors; and clear presentation of study findings (Khan et al., 2001).

Historical Context

Chalmers et al. (2002) have argued that 'efforts to reduce the likelihood of being misled by biases and chance in research synthesis have quite a long history' (p. 13). In the eighteenth century, for example, James Lind – a Scottish naval surgeon – sought to provide a 'critical and chronological' overview of the many published reports on the prevention and treatment of scurvy. In the early nineteenth century, the French statistician Legendre developed the method of least squares to combine data from different astronomical observations where the errors were known to be different. And by the end of the nineteenth century, Herbert Nichols had produced a detailed review of theories and experiments in psychology (all cited in Chalmers et al., 2002).

Although the need for methods to reduce the risk of bias and chance in research synthesis had been recognised for more than two centuries, it was not until the twentieth century that explicit methods were eventually developed. During the first half of the twentieth century, examples of research synthesis became available in medicine, education, physics and agriculture (ibid). Later, in 1976, Gene Glass introduced the concept of meta-analysis as a means to statistically combine results from different studies that investigated similar topics. Since that time, the practice and theory of literature synthesis has been dramatically transformed. Early meta-analyses, predominantly in the education and medical field, were vigorously criticised (Mulrow, 1987; Slavin, 1995), and this contributed to the development of the more systematic and robust approaches to evidence synthesis in practice today.

The rise of the systematic review is also closely linked to the rise of evidence-based medicine and, particularly, to the recognition of the importance of randomised controlled trials (RCTs) (see Chapters 1 and 11). In 1979, the British medical researcher and epidemiologist Archie Cochrane argued that medical professionals required critical summaries of all RCTs that could be updated periodically (Cochrane, 1979). Subsequently, professionals working in a range of medical fields began to produce registers of RCTs. As an example, by mid-1980, the National Perinatal Epidemiology Unit at the University of Oxford, UK, had coordinated the development of a large collection of systematic reviews on pregnancy and childbirth (Chalmers et al., 1989).

In 1992, the first Cochrane Centre was opened in Oxford, UK, in order to facilitate and coordinate systematic reviews of RCTs relating to healthcare. By 1993, the Cochrane Collaboration[1] had been established. The Cochrane Collaboration is an international, independent, not-for-profit organisation, which is dedicated to ensuring that up-to-date, accurate information about the effects of healthcare interventions are available worldwide. It comprises an international network of researchers, academics, practitioners and users, all of whom are committed to ensuring that healthcare knowledge is quality assured, accessible and cumulative. To this end, 'review groups' undertake systematic reviews of healthcare interventions across a diverse range of fields. These reviews are then published on the online Cochrane Library.[2]

Over the years, the value of systematic reviews has also been recognised within the broader social care field and social sciences more generally. In the UK, for example, the Evidence for Policy and Practice Information Co-ordinating Centre (EPPI-Centre)[3] was formed at the University of London in 1993. Since then, it has established a body of systematic review evidence for social science and public policy. Also, the National Health Service Centre for Reviews and Dissemination (CRD)[4] at the University of York was established in 1994 in order to produce high-quality systematic reviews for health and social care.

Further key developments have been the formation of two sibling organisations of the Cochrane Collaboration: The Campbell Collaboration[5] and the Human Genome Epidemiology Network (HuGENeT),[6] both in the USA. The Campbell Collaboration was set up by social scientists in 1999. It is a voluntary organisation, created to encourage positive social change and to improve the quality of global public and private services by preparing, maintaining and disseminating systematic reviews of social science evidence. The organisation focuses on reviews relating to education, social welfare, and crime and justice. HuGENet was established in 1998. It is a global collaboration committed to the evaluation of both the impact of human genome variation on population health and ways in which genetic information can be used to improve health and prevent disease. One aspect of HuGENet's work is the production of HuGE systematic reviews, which evaluate the association of a particular gene with a particular disease.

Current Use

For many years, synthesising other people's research was often seen by academics as an inferior and scientifically derivative activity (Chalmers et al., 2002). Today, it is increasingly accepted as a fundamental research method in its own right. Systematic reviews are now available in a wide range of disciplines, including agriculture; biology; chemistry; criminology; education; law; psychology; and public policy. Furthermore, the findings of systematic reviews are influencing policy and practice not only in healthcare, but also in the fields of education and criminal justice. Systematic reviews have now expanded the types of studies summarised to include research designs evaluating diagnostic accuracy, genetic epidemiology and qualitative outcomes.

Systematic reviews are especially beneficial in situations where there is a focused research question, a body of primary studies addressing this question, and uncertainty about the answer to the question. An individual study, on its own, rarely provides a definitive answer regarding the effectiveness of a particular drug or intervention. However, when the results of a number of similar studies are integrated in a systematic review, a clearer and more reliable result can be found. In this way, systematic reviews are a vital tool for providing the information needed to underpin evidence-based practice.

Over the past few decades, the quantity of primary research and published data has expanded rapidly. This explosion of information creates difficulties for practitioners and policy-makers who need to keep abreast of current research findings and who have to determine which findings are most reliable. By drawing together and summarising the results of multiple research studies, systematic reviews help make sense of the 'glut' of information frequently encountered (Parahoo, 2006). Indeed, as argued by Evans and Pearson (2001), systematic reviews have now become the gate-keepers of nursing knowledge – taking a pivotal role in healthcare and replacing primary research as a source of evidence on which decisions are made.

Systematic reviews play a key role in helping to guide the decisions of policy-makers and practitioners. They are also an important tool for researchers, who may use them to brief themselves both on a topic of interest and on gaps in current knowledge. They can be used – and some would say that they are essential – to support and substantiate new research proposals (Egger et al., 2001a; Chalmers et al., 2002). Systematic reviews are not, however, simply a means of synthesising existing evidence. A good systematic review, particularly one incorporating meta-analysis, can provide original insights and important new knowledge, which can improve the reliability and accuracy of research findings and recommendations.

BOX 5.1

Types of Question Addressed by Systematic Reviews

- How effective is a health or social intervention? For example: Do sexual abstinence-only programmes prevent HIV infection in high-income countries?

- How safe is a health or social intervention? For example: Is exposure to benzodiazepines during pregnancy associated with malformations in the new-born?

- How accurate is a diagnostic tool or questionnaire in measuring what it sets out to measure? For example: How accurate is the Alcohol Use Disorders Identification Test (AUDIT) when screening for alcohol dependence in a primary care population compared with a gold standard clinical interview?

- Does the presence of a particular factor increase or decrease the risk of subsequent ill-health? For example: Does poor academic attainment at school predict future social conduct disorder?

- Does a specific gene variant confer an increased risk of a particular disease? For example: Is DRD2 Taq1A allele associated with an increased chance of becoming alcohol dependent?

- What are people's perceptions about a particular service, intervention or package of care? For example: What are the help-seeking barriers for, and maternal treatment preferences of, women with postpartum depression?

Main Strengths of Systematic Reviews

A key strength of systematic reviews is that they provide a more objective appraisal of the available evidence compared with traditional narrative literature reviews (see Chapter 4). Narrative literature reviews are more prone to bias, and their conclusions may be influenced more by the subjective impressions of the reviewer (Mulrow, 1987; McAlister et al., 1999; Cipriani and Geddes, 2003). In contrast, systematic reviews use explicit methodology aimed at reducing the risk of bias. By systematically searching, appraising and summarising all relevant studies, a more objective assessment of the evidence is possible, and this improves both the reliability and the accuracy of conclusions.

A particular advantage of systematic reviews including a meta-analysis is their statistical power. Statistical power is the probability of detecting a significant difference between the groups being compared in a study. Individual studies are often too small to detect effects that may be clinically important. By pooling similar studies in a meta-analysis, the sample size (and thus the statistical power) is increased, allowing differences between interventions to be detected. This may lead to a more efficient introduction of effective treatments or to recognition of ineffective treatments. Even if there is more than one study conclusively demonstrating significant effects, by using a meta-analysis, the overall effect can be estimated more precisely.

A further strength of systematic reviews is that the consistency of results can be examined across studies – this is particularly facilitated when a meta-analysis is conducted. Where there are sufficient data, such exploratory analyses – which investigate whether treatment effects vary according to the particular characteristics of a given study or participant – can help to guide treatment decisions and future research questions. Systematic reviews allow a more thorough examination of all available data and enable reviewers to move beyond the conclusions of individual studies. They may also resolve disagreement between individual studies (Cipriani and Geddes, 2003).

Conducting a systematic review of the literature can be very time-consuming. However, it is usually more time- and cost-efficient than undertaking a new study. Systematic reviews are recommended before designing a new study because they can identify weaknesses in the methodology of existing studies and may prevent unnecessary replication. They may also usefully identify gaps in the evidence base and may be helpful in generating questions for future research.

Main Weaknesses of Systematic Reviews

Systematic reviews, like any review of the literature, are potentially subject to publication bias. Publication bias is when studies with statistically significant results are more likely to be published, or published more than once, in

English-language journals, and sooner than studies with non-significant results (Dickersin, 1997; Egger et al., 1997; Tramer et al., 1997; Ioannidis, 1998). This in turn leads to such studies being more frequently cited (Gotzsche, 1987; Ravnskov, 1992), and more frequently identified and included in reviews. Outcome reporting bias is a form of publication bias, where the most favourable outcomes from a study are reported and the less favourable outcomes are omitted (Chan et al., 2004a; Chan et al., 2004b; Chan and Altman, 2005). Systematic reviews with comprehensive literature searches can help to minimise the influence of publication bias.

Although systematic reviews are designed with methodological rigour in mind, there is still scope for introducing bias. Research protocol requirements determine study types, participants, interventions, outcomes and methods for their identification, appraisal and synthesis prospectively. Nonetheless, inevitably, many decisions are based on findings from the available data and this can introduce bias and produce erroneous results and conclusions. Additionally, systematic reviews are only as good as the primary studies used. If these are flawed, the findings of the systematic review may also be compromised. This is a common source of discordant findings from systematic reviews of the same topic.

Systematic reviews are often less expensive to undertake than primary studies. However, they may be more costly and time-consuming than traditional narrative reviews. For example, many of the stages of systematic reviews are conducted in duplicate to minimise bias, and acquiring primary publications and translating foreign language papers can prove expensive and can slow down the review process.

MAIN STRENGTHS AND WEAKNESSES
... OF SYSTEMATIC REVIEWS

Strengths

- Explicit and transparent methods limit bias and improve the reliability and accuracy of conclusions.

- Combining data in a meta-analysis increases the power to detect differences between interventions and produces more precise estimates.

- Systematic reviews and meta-analyses facilitate the examination of consistency of results between studies and may resolve uncertainty where individual studies disagree.

- Systematic reviews can help to identify gaps in the evidence base and weakness in the methodology of existing studies.

- Systematic reviews are usually cheaper and quicker than conducting new research.

Weaknesses

- Publication bias is a serious threat to the validity of a systematic review.

- Biased results and misleading conclusions can result where the reviewers' decision-making and methodology are influenced by the data reported in the studies under review.

- Systematic reviews are only as good as the primary studies used. If these are flawed, the findings of the systematic review may also be compromised.

- Systematic reviews can be more resource intensive than narrative reviews; it is easy to underestimate the amount of time and effort required.

Conducting a Systematic Review

The methods for undertaking systematic reviews of RCTs are supported by a body of empirical research and published guidelines (Egger et al., 2001b; Higgins and Green, 2005). However, methods for searching, appraising and synthesising other study designs are less established, and clear guidelines are lacking. In this section, we describe how to undertake a systematic review using RCTs. Readers undertaking systematic reviews of other quantitative and qualitative studies are likely to find Petticrew and Roberts (2006) a useful resource.

It is easy to underestimate the time and resources required to conduct a systematic review. Each stage requires much painstaking work, and a review is likely to take months, rather than weeks, to complete. The process is similar to primary research in that it requires methodical and thorough collection, measurement and synthesis of data. The steps involved in conducting a systematic review are outlined below.

Framing the question and writing a protocol

Having a clearly defined research question is fundamental to the success of a systematic review. Research questions may be quite broad, such as 'Do antibiotics improve wound healing?', or narrow, such as 'Do systemic antibiotics improve wound healing in women following a Caesarean section?'. In formulating the research question, it is useful to think about four key elements, commonly known as 'PICO'. These are:

1. **P**opulation or patients – for example women who have had a Caesarean section

2. **I**ntervention(s) or exposure(s) – for example systemic prophylactic antibiotics plus standard post-operative wound care

3. **C**omparator group(s) – for example standard post-operative wound care

4. **O**utcome(s) – for example complete wound healing, infection plus other relevant outcomes.

The aim is to be clear and comprehensive about each of these elements in order to formulate an unambiguous research question. This helps to determine the study designs that are most appropriate for inclusion. Once the question has been formulated, it is advisable to develop a protocol outlining the methods of the review, and the criteria that studies must meet in order to be included. A protocol facilitates transparency of the review methodology, ensuring rigour, and decreases the number of decisions driven by the data that are found. A peer-reviewed protocol is required for all Cochrane and Campbell Collaboration systematic reviews.[7]

Searching for studies

The steps involved in identifying potentially relevant studies include: selection of relevant databases, listing appropriate search terms[8] and retrieval of references. There are numerous searchable electronic databases available, such as: MEDLINE; EMBASE; CINAHL; CENTRAL; PsychInfo; AMED; and ASSIA. The website for each database provides information about the subject area and journals covered. The review question will determine the number and choice of databases to search. Although there is a degree of overlap between databases, searches across many databases decrease the likelihood of missing studies.

There are two main approaches to planning a search: 'high sensitivity, high yield' and 'high precision, low yield'. In practice, a balance somewhere between the two is recommended. In a 'high sensitivity, high yield' search, as many references as possible are identified, so as to minimise the possibility of missing potentially relevant studies. For example, a search for studies evaluating school-based drug education programmes for the prevention of illicit drug use in adolescents might include terms for the population of interest (such as, 'adolescent' OR 'child' OR 'youth' OR 'teenager') combined with terms for the intervention of interest (such as, 'primary prevention' OR 'drug education' OR 'counseling' OR 'peer group'). Although this approach increases the risk of identifying and retrieving studies that do not meet the inclusion criteria, it decreases the risk of missing studies that have been inadequately indexed on the databases.

In contrast, a 'high precision, low yield' search targets relevant studies more specifically. Thus, for the example above, a precise search might involve using one of the population terms AND one of the intervention terms AND an outcome term such as 'drug use' AND a particular study design, such as 'RCT'. The requirement that references should include at least one term in each concept will mean that fewer studies are identified, but that a greater proportion of them will be relevant. The more concepts that are added to the search, the more precise the search becomes. This approach risks missing some studies; which should be considered if there is a paucity of studies in the review area.

Inevitably, initial searches will miss potentially relevant studies and additional strategies must be employed. Studies identified by initial searches should be retrieved and reference lists scanned for articles that were not originally identified. A citation search should also be conducted to identify articles that have cited identified relevant studies and that may also be relevant. Writing to experts in the field, and to clinical trial registries, can also yield otherwise unavailable data. However, it is difficult to locate and obtain all studies, published and unpublished. Therefore, the reviewer must remain aware of the influence of potential publication bias on the findings and overall conclusions.

Assessing for eligibility

Once all potentially relevant articles are obtained, they are assessed to determine whether or not they meet the review eligibility criteria. Assessments are performed in duplicate by two independent assessors. Eligibility criteria are based on which studies definitely answer the question(s) posed by the review, and should be determined at the protocol stage.

Quality assessment

Assessing the studies for the likelihood of bias – sometimes referred to as quality assessment – plays an important role in the interpretation of the study findings. Each study is assessed using explicit and standardised procedures. Whilst the elements appraised will depend on the study design and the review topic, at least three potential sources of bias should be assessed (Jüni et al., 2001; Deeks et al., 2003). These are 'selection bias', which occurs when there are systematic differences between comparison groups in prognosis or responsiveness to treatment; 'ascertainment bias' or 'detection bias', which occurs when the investigators' knowledge of which group a participant was assigned to in a trial influences their assessment of the outcome; and 'attrition bias', which refers to differences in those who enter and remain in a study and those who are excluded or drop out.

Numerous checklists and assessment scales have been developed, many of which assign an overall score to each study in order to differentiate between studies of variable quality[9] (Moher et al., 1995). However, assigning a quality score is problematic, because the assessment is highly dependent on the scale used, with discordant results produced by different scales (Jüni et al., 1999). As with other stages of the review, it is important for the quality assessment to be conducted independently by at least two reviewers, with discrepancies resolved through discussion or consultation with another reviewer.

It is advisable to incorporate the outcome of the quality assessment within the systematic review. One approach is to exclude studies unless they meet a pre-determined quality threshold, for example only including studies where both the participant and the caregiver are unaware of group assignment (double blind).

Alternatively, a more inclusive approach may be preferable whereby studies are included regardless of blinding status, and the impact of the presence or absence of adequate blinding on the overall review findings is assessed through sensitivity analysis[10] (Smith et al., 2000). The latter approach avoids excluding potentially informative data. Jüni et al. (2001) provide a useful outline of the pros and cons of various ways of incorporating study quality into meta-analysis.

Data extraction

Data extraction involves recording relevant information from each study onto a proforma.[11] As with eligibility and quality assessment, decisions about the information to extract should ideally be decided at the protocol stage. Data extraction usually includes details such as: study design; population; intervention or exposure; comparison group(s); outcome measures; and results. Data extraction should be performed independently by at least two reviewers in order to improve reliability. Disagreements should be resolved by consensus or arbitration. Where agreement cannot be reached, the potential influence of any uncertainty should be investigated through sensitivity analysis.

Often a single study will generate a number of published articles, each reporting on different outcomes or different lengths of follow-up. However, these publications will sometimes include duplicate data – particularly if the results are positive (Tramer et al., 1997). Great care should be taken to exclude duplicate data as their inclusion would bias the results. In contrast, if key information has not been fully reported within a given article, it can be beneficial to contact the study authors so that the missing data can be incorporated.

Data synthesis

Data synthesis gathers and summarises results of included studies in order to provide an estimate of the average effectiveness, investigate if the effect varies between studies, and – if this does vary – to investigate possible sources of the differences. This may be achieved through a narrative synthesis, with or without the addition of meta-analysis. In some situations, meta-analysis may not be advisable, particularly if studies have disparate methodologies, populations, interventions or outcomes. Meta-analysis may also simply be impossible if insufficient data are reported. A meta-analysis is by no means essential in order to make a review 'systematic'. Although a quantitative synthesis has the advantage of producing an overall average effect of an intervention, a clear and comprehensive summary of the studies – including an overview of their characteristics in a table – will aid interpretation and facilitate making clear and constructive conclusions.

In a meta-analysis, data from similar studies are combined to estimate a weighted average effect, in which more weight is given to studies contributing more information (larger sample sizes and more precise estimates of treatment effects) than studies contributing less information. Studies are not, however, combined as if the data resulted from one large study, but combined in two stages. First, the effect size and 95% confidence interval[12] for each study are derived. Second, these are pooled to generate the overall effect. Decisions about which statistical method to use depend on the type of data to be analysed and the expected and observed variation in results between studies (Higgins and Green, 2005).

Interpretation of study findings

Findings of systematic reviews should be interpreted taking into account: clinical context, the strengths and weaknesses of the primary studies, and the potential for bias due to the review methodology. If a review finds no evidence of an effect, it is important to differentiate between the *absence of evidence* demonstrating an effect and the clear demonstration of an *absence of an effect*. To conclude that a potentially effective intervention is ineffective on the basis of insufficient data is wrong and potentially misleading. A more valid interpretation would be that current evidence is weak and more rigorous studies are required in order to answer the question with greater certainty.

An Example of a Systematic Review

A systematic review conducted for the Cochrane Pregnancy and Childbirth group evaluated the evidence for the effectiveness of continuous one-to-one support given during labour, compared with usual care (Hodnett et al., 2003). The reviewers also evaluated: whether effects of continuous support were affected by the birth institution's policies and routine practices; whether the caregiver was a family member or a member of staff; and whether the support was initiated at an early or late stage of labour.

The review was conducted according to guidelines recommended by the Cochrane Collaboration (Higgins and Green, 2005) according to a strict protocol, with pre-defined methods for searching, assessing and synthesising results. It was funded by academic institutions in South Africa, Canada and the UK, and by Childbirth Connection, USA, a consumer advocacy organisation that promotes continuous labour support.

The authors of the review carried out a comprehensive search for all RCTs published in any language, of continuous one-to-one support, compared with usual care, for women during labour, which evaluated the effects on mothers and their babies. Sources searched were MEDLINE, the Cochrane Central Register of Controlled Trials (CENTRAL) and 30 journals and major conference proceedings. The search was updated in April 2006.

Two authors independently extracted data from the relevant studies and checked for agreement. Additional information was sought from original trial authors if insufficient data were reported in the articles. Information was summarised on a range of outcomes including labour, birth or newborn events, immediate maternal psychological outcomes and long-term maternal outcomes.

The reviewers found 15 RCTs with 12,791 women that met the review inclusion criteria. The studies were conducted across a variety of care settings and cultures in Australia; Belgium; Botswana; Canada; Finland; France; Greece; Guatemala; Mexico; South Africa; and the USA.

In all studies, support was described as continuous or near-continuous presence during active labour. One-to-one support was provided by women who had either experienced childbirth themselves or who were nurses, midwives, doulas or birth educators. With the exception of one trial, all studies evaluated support by a woman who was not part of the childbearing woman's existing social network. Support was provided before active labour started in five studies, during active labour in six studies and during either early or active labour in four studies. The control group received 'usual care', as defined by the trial authors, and in no case did this involve continuous support.

Although the reviewers judged the susceptibility to bias of the studies included in the review to be low, blinding of participants and caregivers was not possible, so the potential for performance and detection bias could not be ruled out. However, some studies did attempt blind data collection, and only studies with <20% attrition were included in the meta-analysis.

The meta-analysis showed that women who were allocated to receive continuous support during labour were more likely to have a spontaneous vaginal birth and less likely to require pain medication during labour. They were also more satisfied with their childbirth experience than women who were allocated to usual care. Exploratory subgroup analyses suggested that benefits were greater when: support was provided by a family member rather than a member of staff; support was initiated early rather than in established labour; and support was given in units where epidural analgesia was not routinely available. There were no increased risks to the baby. The authors concluded that continuous support is a safe and effective intervention.

On the strength of the findings of the first publication of this review in 2003, clinical practice guidelines in Canada (SOGC, 1995), the UK (MIDIRS, 1999) and the USA (AWHONN, 2007) recommended that continuous support be available for all women during labour. The subsequent publication of a large RCT confirmed the main findings of the review and strengthened the original conclusions. Results of the subgroup analyses should be interpreted with caution and should be further explored in RCTs before firm recommendations are made.

Priorities for further research were identified. These included evaluations of the effects of continuous support on mothers' and babies' health and well-being in the postpartum period, in particular regarding outcomes associated with significant morbidity, such as urinary and faecal incontinence, painful intercourse and depression.

Further Reading

Egger, M., Davey Smith, G. and Altman D.G. (eds) (2001) *Systematic Reviews in Healthcare* **(London: BMJ Publishing Group).**

This book provides an introduction to the rationale and principles of systematic reviews. It also covers more advanced topics, such as reviews of diagnostic studies, prognostic studies and economic evaluation. Practical advice on meta-analysis using various statistical packages is given. The book concludes with a section on the Cochrane Collaboration and a chapter discussing unresolved issues and future challenges. Chapters 1, 18 and 19 are available free online at www.systematicreviews.com. As leaders in the field of healthcare evaluation, the authors have provided an invaluable resource for healthcare practitioners, researchers, consumers and policy-makers who want to understand the role of systematic reviews, critically appraise published reviews or perform reviews themselves.

Khan, S.K., Kunz, R., Kleijnen, J. and Antes, G. (2003) *Systematic Reviews to Support Evidence-based Medicine. How to Review and Apply Findings of Healthcare Research* **(London: The Royal Society of Medicine Press Limited).**

Whilst this is a good introductory text on how to conduct a review, it does not cover more advanced methods of analysis or how to deal with difficult issues. Written by veterans of numerous systematic reviews, the book is aimed at nurses, doctors, allied health professionals, public health personnel, new reviewers, and students of epidemiology and health technology assessment.

Higgins, J.P.T. and Green, S. (eds) (updated May 2005) *Cochrane Handbook for Systematic Reviews of Interventions 4.2.5* **http://www.cochrane.org/ resources/handbook/hbook.htm (accessed 27 October, 2007).**

This comprehensive manual, available online, provides step-by-step instructions on planning and conducting a systematic review. Special topics are also covered including: how to deal with cluster and crossover studies, unit of analysis issues, and indirect comparisons. Written by leaders in the science of conducting and reviewing biomedical research, the manual is an invaluable resource for anyone doing or thinking of doing a systematic review.

Petticrew, M. and Roberts, H. (2006) *Systematic Reviews in the Social Sciences: A Practical Guide* **(Oxford: Blackwell Publishing).**

In this book, Petticrew and Roberts have provided an overview of systematic literature review methods applied to the social sciences and other fields, including psychology, criminology, education, transport, social welfare, public health, and housing and urban policy. The book takes the reader through the process of conducting a review stage by stage and requires no previous knowledge. It includes detailed sections on assessing the quality of both quantitative and qualitative research; searching for evidence in the social sciences; meta-analytic and other methods of evidence synthesis; publication bias; heterogeneity; and approaches to dissemination.

References

AWHONN (Association of Women's Health, Obstetric and Neonatal Nurses) (2007) *Professional Nursing Support of Laboring Women.* http://www.awhonn.org (accessed 23 March, 2007).

Chalmers, I., Enkin, M. and Keirse, M.J.N.C. (eds) (1989) *Effective Care in Pregnancy and Childbirth* (Oxford: Oxford University Press).

Chalmers, I., Hedges, L.V. and Cooper, H. (2002) 'A brief history of research synthesis', *Evaluation and the Health Professions*, **25**, 12–32.

Chan, A.W. and Altman, D.G. (2005) 'Identifying outcome reporting bias in randomised trials on PubMed: Review of publications and survey of authors', *British Medical Journal*, **330**, 753.

Chan, A.W., Hrobjartsson, A., Haahr, M.T., Gotzsche, P.C. and Altman, D.G. (2004a) 'Empirical evidence for selective reporting of outcomes in randomized trials: Comparison of protocols to published articles', *Journal of the American Medical Association*, **291**, 2457–65.

Chan, A.W., Krleza-Jeric, K., Schmid, I. and Altman, D.G. (2004b) 'Outcome reporting bias in randomized trials funded by the Canadian Institutes of Health Research', *Canadian Medical Association Journal*, **171**, 735–40.

Cipriani, A. and Geddes, J. (2003) 'Comparison of systematic and narrative reviews: The example of the atypical antipsychotics', *Epidemiologia Psichiatria Sociale*, **12**, 146–53.

Cochrane, A.L. (1979) '1931–1971: A critical review, with particular reference to the medical profession'. In *Medicines for the Year 2000* (London: Office of Health Economics) pp. 1–11.

Deeks, J.J., Dinnes, J., D'Amico, R., Sowden, A.J., Sakarovitch, C., Song, F., Petticrew, M. and Altman, D.G. (2003) 'Evaluating non-randomised intervention studies', *Health Technology Assessment*, **7**, iii–x, 1–173.

Dickersin, K. (1997) 'How important is publication bias? A synthesis of available data', *AIDS Education and Prevention*, **9**, 15–21.

Egger, M., Smith, G.D. and O'Rourke, K. (2001a) 'Rationale, potentials and promise of systematic reviews'. In Altman, D.G. (ed.), *Systematic Reviews in Healthcare* (London: BMJ Publishing Group).

Egger, M., Davey Smith, G. and Altman D.G. (eds) (2001b) *Systematic Reviews in Healthcare* (London: BMJ Publishing Group).

Egger, M., Zellweger-Zahner, T., Schneider, M., Junker, C., Lengeler, C. and Antes, G. (1997) 'Language bias in randomised controlled trials published in English and German', *The Lancet*, **350**, 326–9.

Evans, D. and Pearson, A. (2001) 'Systematic reviews: Gatekeepers of nursing knowledge', *Journal of Clinical Nursing*, **10**, 593–9.

Glass, G.V. (1976) 'Primary, secondary, and meta-analysis of research', *Educational Researcher*, **5**, 3–8.

Gotzsche, P.C. (1987) 'Reference bias in reports of drug trials', *British Medical Journal (Clinical Research Education)*, **295**, 654–6.

Higgins, J.P.T. and Green, S. (eds) (updated 2005) *Cochrane Handbook for Systematic Reviews of Interventions 4.2.5.* Cochrane Library. http://www.cochrane.org/resources/handbook/hbook. htm (accessed 27 October, 2007).

Hodnett, E.D., Gates, S., Hofmeyr, G.J. and Sakala, C. (2003) 'Continuous support for women during childbirth', *Cochrane Database of Systematic Reviews*, Issue 3. Art. No.: CD003766.

Ioannidis, J.P. (1998) 'Effect of the statistical significance of results on the time to completion and publication of randomized efficacy trials', *Journal of the American Medical Association*, **279**, 281–6.

Jadad, A.R , Moore, R.A., Carroll, D., Jenkinson, C., Reynolds, D.J.M., Gavaghan, D.J. and McQuay, H.J. (1996) 'Assessing the quality of reports of randomized clinical trials: Is blinding necessary?', *Controlled Clinical Trials*, **17**, 1–12.

Jüni, P., Altman, D.G. and Egger, M. (2001) 'Systematic reviews in health care: Assessing the quality of controlled clinical trials', *British Medical Journal*, **323**, 42–6.

Jüni, P., Witschi, A., Bloch, R. and Egger, M. (1999) 'The hazards of scoring the quality of clinical trials for meta-analysis', *Journal of the American Medical Association*, **282**, 1054–60.

Khan, K.S., Ter Riet, G., Glanville, J., Sowden, A.J. and Kleijnen J. (eds) (2001) *Undertaking Systematic Reviews of Research on Effectiveness*, 2nd edn, CRD report no. 4 (York: NHS Centre for Reviews and Dissemination).

McAlister, F.A., Clark, H.D., van Walraven, C., Straus, S.E., Lawson, F.M., Moher, D. and Mulrow, C.D. (1999) 'The medical review article revisited: Has the science improved?', *Annals of Internal Medicine*, **131**, 947–51.

MIDIRS (Midwives Information and Resource Service) (1999) *Support in Labour: Informed Choice for Professionals* leaflet (York: MIDIRS and the NHS Centre for Reviews and Dissemination).

Moher, D., Jadad, A.R., Nichol, G., Penman, M., Tugwell, P. and Walsh, S. (1995) 'Assessing the quality of randomized controlled trials: An annotated bibliography of scales and checklists', *Controlled Clinical Trials*, **16**, 62–73.

Mulrow, C.D. (1987) 'The medical review article: State of the science', *Annals of Internal Medicine*, **106**, 485–8.

Oxman, A.D. and Guyatt, G.H. (1988) 'Guidelines for reading literature reviews', *Canadian Medical Association Journal*, **138**, 697–703.

Parahoo, K. (2006) *Nursing Research: Principles, Process and Issues*, 2nd edn (Basingstoke: Palgrave – now Palgrave Macmillan).

Petticrew, M. and Roberts, H. (2006) *Systematic Reviews in the Social Sciences: A Practical Guide* (Oxford: Blackwell Publishing).

Ravnskov, U. (1992) 'Cholesterol lowering trials in coronary heart disease: Frequency of citation and outcome', *British Medical Journal*, **305,** 15–19.

Slavin, R.E. (1995) 'Best evidence synthesis: An intelligent alternative to meta-analysis', *Journal of Clinical Epidemiology*, **48,** 9–18.

Smith, L.A., Oldman, A.D., McQuay, H.J. and Moore, R.A. (2000) 'Teasing apart quality and validity in systematic reviews: An example from acupuncture trials in chronic neck and back pain', *Pain*, **86,** 119–32.

SOGC (Society of Obstetricians and Gynaecologists of Canada) (1995) 'SOGC policy statement: Fetal health surveillance in labour', *SOGC News*, 41–5.

Tramer, M.R., Reynolds, D.J., Moore, R.A. and McQuay, H.J. (1997) 'Impact of covert duplicate publication on meta-analysis: A case study', *British Medical Journal*, **315,** 635–40.

Notes

1 http://www.cochrane.org/index.htm

2 http://www3.interscience.wiley.com/cgi-bin/mrwhome/106568753/HOME

3 http://eppi.ioe.ac.uk/cms/

4 http://www.york.ac.uk/inst/crd/

5 http://www.campbellcollaboration.org/index.asp

6 http://www.hugenet.org.uk/

7 Some examples of protocols can be found at: http://www.mrw.interscience.wiley.com/ cochrane/clsysrev/articles/CD005557/frame.html and http://www.campbellcollaboration. org/doc-pdf/Ass_children_w_phys_impairments.pdf.

8 Search terms are identified using free text (terminology generated by the author of the reference) and MeSH (database specific thesaurus terminology).

9 One such scale commonly used is the Jadad scale (Jadad et al., 1996).

10 This is an analysis to assess how robust the results are to uncertain decisions or assumptions about the data and the methods that were used.

11 Examples of data extraction forms can be found at: http://www.york.ac.uk/inst/crd/report4. htm and http://epoc.cochrane.org/en/handsearchers.html

12 The 95% confidence interval refers to the range of values within which it is possible to be 95% certain that the true effect size lies.

6 Content Analysis

MICHELLE JACKSON

Introduction

There are almost as many definitions of 'content analysis' as there are texts written on the topic. However, for a representative definition we might turn to Berelson, who states that, 'Content analysis is a research technique for the objective, systematic, and quantitative description of the manifest content of communication' (Berelson, 1952: 18). Put another way, we can summarise the aim of content analysis as being to turn words into numbers (c.f. Franzosi, 2004). In fact, content analysis can be carried out on any form of communication, whether it contains written or spoken words, or even film or pictures. In this chapter, the focus is mainly on the content analysis of written material.

Content analysis is often considered to be a quantitative method, as the purpose is to turn complex material into a set of numbers within a relatively small set of categories. However, in some senses content analysis lies between the quantitative and qualitative divide – it embodies the qualitative features of interpretation and close reading of texts, and then turns these features into quantitative data.

Historical Context

Research using what we would today consider to be a form of content analysis was carried out long before the term 'content analysis' was invented. Indeed, one of the first reported uses of content analysis dates back to the 1740s.[1] Dovring (1954) describes a religious controversy in Sweden surrounding the publication of a collection of hymns, titled *Songs of Zion*. The collection was not part of the official Hymnal of the State Church, but the State Censor decided that it could be published (p. 389). However, when a second edition was put forward for publication some years later, the State Church objected, as they felt that the first edition had had a pernicious influence on the people's religious devotion. Although the *Songs* were republished, an argument raged regarding how far they contained sinful material. This event became important to the history of content analysis when, to try to settle the argument, various individuals carried out a systematic and quantitative analysis of the content of the *Songs*, to examine how far their content was in fact sinful and whether the content differed significantly from that in the established Hymnal. As Dovring writes, 'In fact, if not in name, participants in this debate were concerned with many of the problems which concern today's content analyst: the identification of key symbols, the division of content into favourable, unfavourable and neutral categories, the coding of values, and other related problems' (1954: 389).

A number of other small-scale content analysis studies can be identified in the history of the method (for a description of other small-scale studies see Krippendorff, 1980: Ch. 1). But while these smaller scale projects are undoubtedly important to the history of content analysis, the method did not become a recognised part of the researcher's toolkit until more recently.[2] The 1940s saw the term 'content analysis' first appearing in journal articles, and around the same time the work of Harold Lasswell and his associates was arguably the final step in establishing the method as we know it today (Franzosi, 2004: 33). Lasswell's interest was in the systematic study of political language to uncover, 'Who says what in which channel to whom with what effect?' (Lasswell, 1948: 50). He headed a research group working on the influence of propaganda and political communication (Experimental Division for the Study of Wartime Communications). The work of the group is reported in the seminal book, *Language of Politics*, which contains both methodological guidance and examples of content analysis in practice (Lasswell et al., 1949). One such example shows how content analysis was used to detect pro-Nazi propaganda in books and periodicals published in America in the 1940s. The evidence was then used to prosecute the culprits in federal court cases (see Lasswell et al., 1949, Ch. 9 for a detailed discussion of the use of content analysis in the detection of propaganda).[3] By the end of the Second World War content analysis had therefore been firmly established, and spread to a whole range of academic disciplines.

The recent history of content analysis is defined by the increasing use of computers, which have allowed researchers to carry out content analysis research more quickly and easily than they might have done previously. The first computer program dedicated to the analysis of text was developed in Harvard in the 1960s with the General Enquirer project, and today there are any number of computer programs available to content analysis researchers. While not all content analysis researchers will use computers to analyse text, the possibility only increases the flexibility and attractiveness of the method.

Current Use

Content analysis is used across the social sciences, for many and varied purposes. As content analysis can be used to examine any form of communication – verbal, written, audio, visual – the range of material analysed is understandably large. In health and social care research, content analysis has often been used to analyse media content and written material.[4]

The media are of evident interest to health and social care researchers, as for many people the media are the primary source of information on health and illness. Researchers have examined media content, such as representations of health issues on television (for example Johnson and Johnson, 1993), to investigate how far the media present a realistic picture of health issues. Studies of magazine advertisements for pharmaceuticals have also employed content analysis, asking whether, for example, advertisements are biased, whether they rely on stereotypical images, and whether the content of advertisements might have an impact on people who see the advertisements. In one such study, Cline and Young argue that:

> In summary, beyond promoting social stereotypes lies the potential for [advertising's] visual cues to reinforce already existing disparities in access to health information and, to the extent that ads promote visits to physicians, disparities in access to health care. (2004: 154; see also Cline and Young, 2005).

Expanding on this, Young and Cline (2005) argue that direct-to-consumer advertisements (DTCA) contain 'textual cues' that, 'associate medical and identity rewards with products and their use, and associate punishments with failure to use' (p. 363). These textual cues might include claims about rewards which would be expected when using the product, such as 'relieves fears' or 'clears up skin', and implied punishments if the product is not used, which might include 'outcome X happens if left untreated' (p. 355).

Purely textual material is also relevant to content analysis researchers interested in health matters. Newspaper articles can be analysed for bias (for example Philo, 1996); governmental and pressure group materials can be analysed for commonalities and differences in approach and opinion (for example Pandiani et al., 1996); and emails between doctors and patients can even be analysed to document and understand communication regarding healthcare (Anand et al., 2005).

Content analysis has also been extremely influential in political science, where Lasswell's tradition of analysing political communication continues to this day. Notably, the Manifesto Research Group (later known as the Comparative Manifestos Project) has used content analysis to uncover the ideological positions of political parties from their election manifestos (Budge et al., 2001). An election manifesto can be seen as setting out a political party's position on a whole range of issues, including those relating to health and social care. Data from the analysis of manifestos can therefore be used to measure what a political party stands for, to compare the positions of parties within and across countries, and to examine how these positions change over time. Furthermore, the data can then be used to address questions about the relationship between party positions and, say, public opinion (see also Budge et al., 1987; Gabel and Huber, 2000; Laver, 2001). In addition to the content analysis of party manifestos, other political scientists have used content analysis to derive information about party positions from parliamentary speeches (for example Hobolt and Klemmemsen, 2005) or to examine the content of political advertising (Prior, 2001).

Within other disciplines, such as sociology, content analysis is used to answer a range of research questions. Cultural sociologists have analysed personal ads (for instance, newspaper advertisements placed by people looking for partners) to document the characteristics that individuals highlight as being desirable in a mate, as well as which of their own characteristics they choose to promote (Buchmann and Eisner, 1997; Johnson, 2003). One study, for example, shows a sharp decrease in the percentage of advertisements in which the author described themselves as 'domestic' alongside a sharp increase in those in which the author described themselves as 'sensitive' over the course of the twentieth century (Buchmann and Eisner, 1997: 166–7). Sociologists interested in employment have similarly analysed job advertisements to uncover the types of characteristics that employers require when recruiting for new employees (Jackson et al., 2005; Sacchi et al., 2005; Jackson, 2007).

BOX 6.1

Types of Question Addressed by Content Analysis

- Lasswell's definition of the aims of content analysis serves as a useful summary of the questions which can be addressed using the method: 'Who says what in which channel to whom with what effect?' (1948: 50). Any researcher interested in the analysis of communication should consider content analysis as a research tool.

- One form of communication of particular interest to content analysis researchers is the mass media. Content analysis is used to document the contents of the media, to simplify media messages and to identify main themes. Knowledge of the content of the media can then be used to understand how public perceptions of health issues are influenced by the media.

- Content analysis is particularly valuable when a researcher has a question which must be addressed using quantitative data (for instance, a 'how much?' question). It can be used to transform qualitative data, such as that gained through interviews or observation, into quantitative data.

Main Strengths of Content Analysis

An obvious strength of content analysis is its capacity to turn words into numbers. Any question asking 'how much?', 'how often?', or 'to what extent?' will usually require access to quantitative data. Using content analysis, a researcher is able to extract information from qualitative sources (such as newspaper articles, television broadcasts and political party manifestos) to provide quantitative measures. To take a simple example, we might call to mind recurring debates about reducing the time limit for abortions from 24 weeks and ask whether the content of British newspaper articles focusing on this issue differs depending on the publication in which they appear. From casual observation, we could argue that some newspapers print articles which seem to support a reduction in the limit, while others appear to be more strongly in favour of the status quo. One way to examine whether the content of articles differs depending on the newspaper in which they are printed would be to read the articles closely, and then provide an impressionistic report of the contents of each newspaper, illustrating their position by using representative quotations from the articles or writing a very detailed description. However, an impressionistic account of this type is always open to criticism from other researchers: how should we judge whether one researcher's impression of the content is correct? On the other hand, if we carried out a content analysis of the newspaper articles, counting how many times particular words appeared, we could show the differences between the newspapers more transparently. We could, for example, compare how many times different newspapers mention the words 'life', or 'baby', or 'right to choose', or 'reproductive rights'. These comparisons would allow a researcher to make strong and persuasive claims about whether articles in different newspapers do indeed offer different perspectives on abortion.

A further strength of content analysis is that researchers can analyse data that they have already gathered using other research methods, so that maximum information can be obtained from those data. A researcher using interviews might address one aspect of their research question using representative quotes from the interviews, but then content analyse the interview data to identify the major themes. This allows the researcher to combine the strengths of different research methods, as well as providing a certain amount of flexibility in the types of research questions that the data can be used to address.

A final strength of the method which should be mentioned is its use in generating hypotheses and theories, which can then be tested. Content analysis can provide an extremely detailed description of a form of communication, and identify relationships which may need to be investigated further. Through the process of designing a coding frame (for instance, a set of coding categories), and conducting the analysis, the researcher gains an in-depth knowledge of the communications of interest, and this can stimulate new ideas and help with the interpretation of findings.

Main Weaknesses of Content Analysis

Lasswell's classic definition of the purpose of content analysis as being to find out, 'Who says what in which channel to whom with what effect?' (Lasswell, 1948: 50) highlights the types of question which a content analysis can address. But to identify the weaknesses of the method, it is worth thinking about what Lasswell's definition leaves out. Importantly, content analysis is not helpful in understanding *why* someone would say what they did. The motivations behind the production of the material are impossible to pin down using content analysis alone. A researcher interested in these motivations therefore needs either to use other research methods to uncover them, or to use pre-existing theory and evidence to hypothesise about them.

Another limitation of content analysis is that, rather obviously, a researcher is only able to analyse *existing* content. Anything not included in the material cannot, by definition, be analysed. This could potentially be a problem when dealing with material which is biased in some way. For example, propaganda material might leave out certain pieces of information or present biased accounts of the information included. If a researcher does not consider possible biases in their material, a content analysis might lead to them drawing false or incomplete conclusions.

While the weaknesses highlighted so far can be problematic to the researcher, they are only weaknesses if the method is applied to inappropriate research questions, without due care and attention. A final weakness identified here, however, is likely to apply every time content analysis is employed; that is, that content analysis is both time-consuming and hard work. The process of designing a coding frame, and subsequently coding a sample of material to it, requires a great amount of effort. This effort is likely to be rewarded, however, with a unique data set well-suited to answering the research questions.

MAIN STRENGTHS AND WEAKNESSES
... OF CONTENT ANALYSIS

Strengths

- Material originally in qualitative form (such as words) can be transformed into numbers to allow researchers to answer quantitative questions.

- Researchers can analyse data collected using other research methods so that maximum information can be obtained from those data. This allows the researcher to combine the strengths of different research methods and increases the scope of questions that can be answered.

- In the process of carrying out a content analysis, the researcher gains an in-depth knowledge of the material. This can help in both generating new hypotheses and interpreting findings.

Weaknesses

- Content analysis can only provide information about what is in a communication, not why it got there.

- Content analysis can only provide information about what is contained within the material of interest. This can be a problem if there is bias in the material analysed. For example, a common propaganda tool is to remain silent about information that is unfavourable while emphasising information that is desirable. Content analysis will pick up only the emphasis, not the silence.

- Content analysis can be extremely time-consuming.

Conducting a Content Analysis

If a content analysis is the appropriate method for answering a research question, the researcher will usually proceed as follows.

Consider the empirical and theoretical background to the research question

The first, extremely important, step in carrying out a content analysis is to familiarise oneself with the theoretical and empirical background to the research question. It is impossible to design a coding frame without understanding the conceptually relevant distinctions that need to be maintained in order to make sense of the source data; it is *meanings of words* not *words in themselves* that content analysts aim to code. For example, if we look at the words 'blue', 'yellow', 'white' and 'brown', we might categorise all four words as colours. But in another context, such as an analysis of descriptions of drug addiction, 'blue' and 'yellow' might refer to different strength diazepam pills, while 'white' and 'brown' might be categorised as types of heroin. Without background information and a clear research question, a content analysis is unlikely to yield useful results.

Decide on the appropriate sample of material to be coded from the entire universe of material available

The researcher must also consider the sample of material that will be coded.[5] In many content analysis projects the sampling population might be very difficult to define as the universe of symbolic communications is very large (including, for example, newspapers, books, government records, recorded audio or video material, internet sites or even research material initially collected using a different methodology). Therefore, most content analysis projects will have two sampling stages. In the first, the researcher employs all the knowledge that they have about the question so that they can distinguish between relevant and irrelevant material. In the second, a sample of the available material is selected for analysis. This second stage is familiar to many types of research, and a range of different established sampling designs can be used, including random sampling, stratified random sampling and systematic sampling (See Krippendorff, 1980: Ch. 6 for more information on sampling).

To take an obvious example, if we were interested in how information about cancer was presented in the British mass media, we would first rule out any communications published outside Great Britain as well as communications which could not be considered as part of the mass media. If, after considering the relevancy of the available material, the field was still too large, we would use a second stage of sampling in which a selection of the available material was chosen for analysis. In the case of information about cancer, we might gather a randomly chosen sample of 10% of all television programmes on the subject, 5% of all radio programmes and 20% of all newspaper articles.

Develop a coding frame and carry out the content analysis, paying attention to questions of reliability and validity

Having clarified the research question and chosen a sample for analysis, the next step of the project is to design a coding frame and code material to it. During this process, the content analysis researcher is aiming to take a huge amount of complex material and simplify it. Most content analysis projects will proceed by working through the following stages:

● *Develop broad categories grouping together similar words and phrases*

Before designing coding categories, it is important for the researcher to establish what types of words and meanings appear in the material. An effective coding frame can only be designed by someone who understands the whole range of content. Therefore, a sensible strategy is to begin by simply going through a large amount of the relevant material, noting down each word or phrase that appears.

After creating this list of words and phrases, the researcher will begin to group together words and phrases which have similar meanings in the context of interest. At this point, the aim is to produce very broad categories of a general nature. While this is only the first stage in designing the coding frame, the researcher must keep the research question in mind so that the broad categories do not overlap. For example, in our study of how information about cancer is presented, we might group together all of the words referring to cancer itself in one broad group, all of the words referring to particular individuals in another group, all of the words referring to organisations in another group and so on. We continue to develop these broad categories until all of the words and phrases can be placed somewhere. In common with many other pieces of social science research, we maintain an 'Other' category, for words and phrases that do not seem to fit anywhere else.

● *Within those broad categories, distinguish more specific (sub-)categories*

Having developed broad categories which group together the words and phrases of interest, the researcher will next move on to create much smaller categories. These categories must distinguish between themes of theoretical interest, be exhaustive so that every word and phrase has a place somewhere and, finally, be mutually exclusive so that no word or phrase can be included in more than one category. To develop these smaller categories, the researcher repeats the previous stage, this time looking to create categories within the broad ones created earlier. In our cancer study, we might break down the 'Cancer' category into different types of cancer, the 'Individuals' category into 'Men', 'Women', 'Young', 'Old' and so on, and the 'Organisations' category into 'Health Organisations', 'Governmental Organisations',

'Charitable Organisations' and so on. (See Holsti, 1969 for a description of the types of categories that might be employed in a content analysis).

● *Finalise the coding frame and carry out the content analysis*

Once the coding categories have been finalised, we have the coding frame which will be used in the analysis. But before using the coding frame in the research, it is essential to test it by coding to it material similar to that to be used in the final research. Often, it is only when testing a coding frame that problems with it become clear. If the coding frame is difficult to use – for example, it is not clear where certain words or phrases should fit or some categories seem to include too many different words – the coding categories should be rethought.

Throughout the content analysis process, the researcher must pay attention to issues of reliability and validity. Thinking first about reliability (a prerequisite for validity), the researcher must ensure that the findings are both stable and reproducible. For the findings to be *stable*, the researcher must be able to code the same material into the same coding frame more than once and obtain the same results. For the findings to be *reproducible*, the researcher must code material using their coding frame, and a second coder must be able to code that same material using the same coding frame and obtain the same results (for this reason, reproducibility is also known as inter-coder reliability). As Weber writes:

> High reproducibility is a minimum standard for content analysis. This is because stability measures the consistency of the individual coder's private understandings, whereas reproducibility measures the consistency of shared understanding (or meaning) held by two or more coders. (Weber, 1990: 17; see also Kaplan and Goldsen, 1949; Krippendorff, 1980, for more information on inter-coder reliability)

Turning to validity, a content analysis can be seen as valid to the extent that it measures what it is intended to measure. The validity of a content analysis is usually studied by comparing the results or measures obtained from it with those obtained by another method, the validity of which has already been established for measuring the same characteristic (Janis, 1949). For more information on validity in content analysis, see Krippendorff (1980).

Analyse the data using an appropriate technique and relate the results to the research question

The final step of a content analysis project is to analyse the data and relate the findings to the research question. The specific techniques that are used to analyse the data will depend entirely on the form of the data and the types of question that are of interest, but content analysis researchers might use anything from basic descriptive statistics to advanced multivariate statistics (Neuendorf, 2002: Ch. 8 contains useful information about the techniques available for the analysis of content analysis data).

An Example of a Content Analysis Study

The media constitute the primary source of information about health matters for the majority of people, and with this role comes the power to define the public agenda on these matters (Karpf, 1988). Even without taking a position on whether the media act to manipulate public opinion, or simply reflect it, the content of the media is evidently of great interest. I now describe a study carried out by the Glasgow Media Group, in which content analysis is used systematically to record and understand the portrayal of mental illness in the British media. The study is reported in the book *Media and Mental Distress* edited by Greg Philo (Philo, 1996).[6]

In *Media and Mental Distress* (1996), the Glasgow Media Group (GMG) analyse images of mental illness portrayed in the media in the early 1990s. In the introduction, they describe their aim as follows:

> The research examines the content of media images and shows how conditions such as schizophrenia are portrayed and routinely stigmatised. The research also illustrates the impact of such images on public belief and on the attitudes and responses of carers, as well as on those of users of mental health services (Philo, 1996: xi)

The book uses a range of methods to examine different aspects of these research topics; results of a content analysis are reported in Chapter 4 'Media Content' (Philo et al., 1996: 45–81).

To examine the content of media images of mental illness, the GMG defined a sample which included television news reports (for example BBC and ITV main evening news broadcasts), fictional television programmes (for example soap operas, *Casualty*), newspapers (for example *The Sun, Daily Mirror*), popular magazines (for example *Cosmopolitan, GQ*) and children's literature (for example *Jackie* comic) (1996: 45–6). Both national and local media were sampled, for the period of one month (April 1993).

The sample of media output contained large numbers of words and phrases which were used in relation to mental illness, and content analysis was used to, 'show the dominant messages which are being given about mental illness across a variety of media' (1996: 46). Words such as 'barmy', 'neurotic', 'deranged' or 'schizophrenic' are present in a whole range of media output, and the purpose of the analysis was to identify the major themes, grouping references to similar words together into the same categories. The categories chosen for categorisation of the words were:

> (1) 'comic images'; (2) violence/harm to others; (3) violence to self; (4) prescriptions for treatment/advice/recovery; (5) criticisms of accepted definitions of mental illness (1996: 47)

Figure 6.1 illustrates the frequency of words in each of the categories for the total sample (adapted from Philo, 1996: 47, Figure 4.1a).

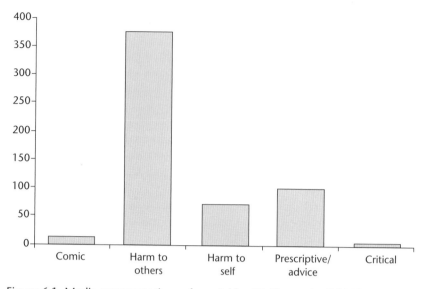

Figure 6.1 Media representations of mental health/illness, April 1993

As the figure shows, the content of media presentations of mental illness is clearly heavily skewed towards words and phrases which are associated with violence/harm to others, with far fewer words and phrases mentioned indicating harm to oneself. As the authors note, 'This is a media world populated by "psychopaths", "maniacs" and "frenzied knife men" … Such media images contrast sharply with the actualities of mental illness' (1996: 50). In sum, negative images of mental illness are far more likely to be presented than positive images.

Having identified that words representing violence are often associated with mental illness in the content analysis, the GMG then conducted focus groups in which people were asked to talk about their perceptions of mentally ill characters depicted in the media (for example characters in soap operas who had suffered mental illness). This additional qualitative component complemented the quantitative analysis of media content by providing detailed information on presentations of mental illness.

In sum, the study shows that it is important to record media content in a systematic way. As the authors argued, 'Such representations … can alter perceptions of the "dangerous" nature of mental illness as well as affecting beliefs about the risks of random attacks by the "maniacs" who are presented as populating the world' (Philo, 1996: 80).

Further Reading

Holsti, O.R. (1969) *Content Analysis for the Social Sciences and Humanities* (Reading, MA: Addison-Wesley).

As the author states in the preface, this book should be used by researchers considering using content analysis and wanting to learn more about it rather than by those who hope for a 'step-by-step formula for every research question'. Research designs, the uses of content analysis and inferences that can be made on the basis of such data, as well as the mechanics of the method are covered.

Krippendorff, K. (1980) *Content Analysis: An Introduction to its Methodology* **(Beverly Hills: Sage).**

This book is, quite simply, the bible for content analysis researchers. Exceedingly clear, well-written, and comprehensive, the book introduces the method, deals with the conceptual and methodological essentials (including sampling, reliability and validity) and provides a practical guide to carrying out an analysis. While the book is indispensable for the beginner content analyst, it also has plenty to offer to more advanced researchers. A second edition published in 2004 includes sections on computing and content analysis software.

Lasswell, H.D., Leites, N. and Associates (eds) (1949) *Language of Politics. Studies in Quantitative Semantics* **(New York: George W. Stewart).**

Lasswell et al.'s volume is an important step in the history of content analysis, but offers more than historical interest. The book is helpfully divided into three sections: introduction, technique and applications. In the introduction, Lasswell outlines the method, describing the circumstances under which content analysis might be used and the value of the method for empirical research. The technique is covered in much greater detail in the chapters comprising the second section, in which Lasswell and his co-authors discuss reliability, validity and sampling amongst other topics. Finally, the applications section shows how content analysis was used to detect propaganda in communication. The book is far from a basic introduction, so would be best read in conjunction with the other recommended texts.

Neuendorf, K.A. (2002) *The Content Analysis Guidebook* **(Thousand Oaks, CA: Sage).**

This is a good introductory textbook for those wishing to learn about the key concepts in content analysis. In addition to the methodological discussions, the book contains a helpful chapter on appropriate statistical techniques for the analysis of data derived from a content analysis. The use of computers in content analysis is also well-covered, with a description of the packages available. A website accompanies the book (http://academic.csuohio.edu/kneuendorf/content/).

Weber, R.P. (1990) *Basic Content Analysis*, **2nd edn (Newbury Park, CA: Sage).**

This book is part of the *Quantitative Applications in the Social Sciences* series by Sage, and discusses the method in the clear and concise manner typical of books in that series. Although the book deals with the basics of content analysis, the amount of detail provided on each topic is understandably curtailed, so a beginner might find it useful to read a more basic introduction first.

Acknowledgements

I would like to thank Sara Hobolt and Jo Neale for their very helpful advice.

 References

Anand, S.G., Feldman, M.J., Geller, D.S., Bisbee, A. and Bauchner, H. (2005) 'A content analysis of e-mail communication between primary care providers and parents', *Pediatrics*, **115**, 1283–8.

Berelson, B. (1952) *Content Analysis in Communication Research* (Glencoe, IL: Free Press).

Buchmann, M. and Eisner, M. (1997) 'The transition from the utilitarian to the expressive self: 1900–1992', *Poetics*, **25**, 157–75.

Budge, I., Robertson, D. and Hearl, D. (eds) (1987) *Ideology, Strategy and Party Change: Spatial Analyses of Post-War Election Programmes in 19 Democracies* (Cambridge: Cambridge University Press).

Budge, I., Klingemann, H.-D., Volkens, A. and Bara, J. (eds) (2001) *Mapping Policy Preferences: Estimates for Parties, Electors and Governments, 1954–1998* (Oxford: Oxford University Press).

Cline, R.J.W. and Young, H.N. (2004) 'Marketing drugs, marketing health care relationships: A content analysis of visual cues in direct-to-consumer prescription drug advertising', *Health Communication*, **16**, 131–57.

Cline, R.J.W. and Young, H.N. (2005) 'Direct-to-consumer print ads for drugs: Do they undermine the physician–patient relationship?' *Journal of Family Practice*, **54**, 1049–57.

Dovring, K. (1954) 'Quantitative semantics in 18th century Sweden', *Public Opinion Quarterly*, **18**, 389–94.

Eldridge, J. (ed) (1995) *Glasgow Media Group Reader, Volume 1: News Content, Language and Visuals* (London: Routledge).

Franzosi, R. (2004) *From Words to Numbers: Narrative, Data, and Social Science* (Cambridge: Cambridge University Press).

Gabel, M.J. and Huber, J.D. (2000) 'Putting parties in their place: Inferring party Left–Right ideological positions from party manifestos data', *American Journal of Political Science*, **44**, 94–103.

Hobolt, S.B. and Klemmemsen, R. (2005) 'Responsive government? Public opinion and government policy preferences in Britain and Denmark', *Political Studies*, **53**, 379–402.

Holsti, O.R. (1969) *Content Analysis for the Social Sciences and Humanities* (Reading, MA: Addison-Wesley).

Jackson, M. (2007) 'How far merit selection? Social stratification and the labour market', *British Journal of Sociology*, **58**, 367–90.

Jackson, M., Goldthorpe, J.H. and Mills, C. (2005) 'Education, employers and class mobility', *Research in Social Stratification and Mobility*, **23**, 3–34.

Janis, I.L. (1949) 'The problem of validating content analysis'. In Lasswell, H.D., Leites N. and Associates (eds) *Language of Politics: Studies in Quantitative Semantics* (New York: George W. Stewart).

Johnson, C.A. and Johnson, B.E. (1993) 'Medicine on British television: A content analysis', *Journal of Community Health*, **18**, 25–35.

Johnson, M. (2003) *Partner Search: Preferences and Presentation* M.Sc. Thesis (Oxford: University of Oxford).

Kaplan, A. and Goldsen, J.M. (1949) 'The reliability of content analysis categories'. In Lasswell, H.D., Leites, N. and Associates (eds) *Language of Politics: Studies in Quantitative Semantics* (New York: George W. Stewart).

Karpf, A. (1988) *Doctoring the Media: The Reporting of Health and Medicine* (London: Routledge).

Krippendorff, K. (1980) *Content Analysis: An Introduction to its Methodology* (Beverly Hills: Sage).

Lasswell, H.D. (1948) 'The structure and function of communication in society'. In Bryson, L. (ed.) *The Communication of Ideas* (New York: Institute for Religious and Social Studies).

Lasswell, H.D., Leites, N. and Associates (eds) (1949) *Language of Politics: Studies in Quantitative Semantics* (New York: George W. Stewart).

Laver, M. (ed.) (2001) *Estimating the Policy Position of Political Actors* (London: Routledge).

Neuendorf, K.A. (2002) *The Content Analysis Guidebook* (Thousand Oaks, CA: Sage).

Pandiani, J.A., Murtaugh, M. and Pierce, J. (1996) 'The mental health care reform debate: A content analysis of position papers', *Journal of Mental Health Administration*, **23**, 217–25.

Philo, G. (ed.) (1995) *Glasgow Media Group Reader, Volume 2: Industry, Economy, War and Politics* (London: Routledge).

Philo, G. (ed) (1996) *Media and Mental Distress* (London and New York: Longman).

Philo, G., McLaughlin, G. and Henderson, L. (1996) 'Media content'. In Philo, G. (ed.) *Media and Mental Distress* (Harlow: Addison Wesley Longman).

Pope, C., Ziebland, S. and Mays, N. (2000) 'Qualitative research in health care', *British Medical Journal*, **320**, 114–6.

Prior, M. (2001) 'Weighted content analysis of political advertisements', *Political Communication*, **18**, 335–45.

Sacchi, S., Salvisberg, A. and Buchmann, M. (2005) 'Long-term dynamics of skill demand in Switzerland from 1950–2000'. In Kriesi, H., Farago, P., Kohli, M. and Zarin-Nejadan, M. (eds) *Contemporary Switzerland: Revisiting the Special Case* (Basingstoke: Palgrave Macmillan).

Weber, R.P. (1990) *Basic Content Analysis*, 2nd edn (Newbury Park, CA: Sage).

Young, H.N. and Cline, R.J.W. (2005) 'Textual cues in direct-to-consumer prescription drug advertising: Motivators to communicate with physicians', *Journal of Applied Communication Research*, **33**, 348–69.

Notes

1   In fact, the roots of content analysis can be traced back much further than this. Rhetorical analysis, in which communication is analysed to understand how persuasive arguments are constructed, can be traced back to ancient Greek times (Neuendorf, 2002).

2   Krippendorff argues that one reason why the influence of the earlier studies was not greater was because they were only discovered many years later (1980: 13).

3   Another group that should be mentioned in this context is the American Federal Communications Commission (FCC), headed by Hans Speier between 1942 and 1948. In their work, the FCC analysed German radio broadcasts in an attempt to uncover 'preparatory propaganda' and therefore aid the war effort.

4   Many researchers who carry out interviews will also explore their data by developing broad categories which identify the main themes of the data. Pope et al. (2000) summarise what they see as the distinctiveness of this approach compared to traditional content analysis, arguing that, 'The key point about this process is that it is inclusive; categories are added to reflect as many of the nuances in the data as possible, rather than reducing the data to a few numerical codes' (p. 114). A content analysis researcher would, however, argue that traditional content analysis coding categories can and should reflect nuances in the data.

5   In reality, decisions about sampling are likely to be made throughout the research process, and even after the coding frame has been designed, but I describe all of the sampling decisions that need to be made within a project at this point.

6   The Glasgow Media Group has analysed media content for many years. They are particularly well-known for their analyses of the content of British news broadcasts, focusing on news content, language and the role of visual images in news reporting. Classic articles published by the Group can be found in two volumes of collected works (Eldridge, 1995; Philo, 1995).

7

Discourse Analysis

DEBORA OSBORNE AND JOANNE NEALE

Introduction

Discourses are ways of thinking, talking, acting and reacting within particular contexts that are accepted and understandable by others within the same culture. In other words, discourses allow what we say and do to be comprehensible to others. Within health and social care, these might include biomedical discourses; nursing discourses; caring discourses; psychological discourses; managerial discourses; lay discourses; disease discourses; and illness discourses. For example, biomedical discourses assume that illnesses are biologically rather than socially determined, that doctors have knowledge and authority, and that patients are relatively powerless. In contrast, illness discourses focus on patient experiences, including the meaning of illness, the complexity of living with illness, and the responses of the sick person's wider social network.

'Discourse analysis is concerned with how an individual's experience is socially and historically constructed by language' (Crowe, 2005: 56). That is, how social relations, identities, knowledge and power are created through what is said and written (Crowe, 2005: 55). To this end, the focus for the discourse analyst is the texts in which language is located. Within health and social care, these might include medical and nursing books; written medical notes; government health and social care policies and strategy documents; service protocols; patient and service leaflets/information sheets; patients' diaries; newspaper and magazine articles; art and literature; advertisements for health products; and the transcripts of interviews or conversations undertaken with professionals, patients, carers or service users. The discourse analyst does not assume that these texts are in any way representative of an essential truth. Rather, they are understood as cultural representations of the discourses that frame normal practices.

Historical Context

Discourse analysis originated in the field of linguistics where it was applied to the way sentences and utterances merged to form discourses. During the 1960s and 1970s, it developed within and across the humanities and social sciences, combining with new sub-disciplines such as semiotics, socio-linguistics, psycholinguistics, text linguistics and pragmatics. By the end of the twentieth century, discourse analysis had been employed within a wide range of disciplines, including psychology, social psychology, sociology, social policy, geography, anthropology, international relations, communication studies, and nursing, as well as health and social care more generally. A key factor in this progression to a much broader range of subject areas was the demise of the Age of Enlightenment and the emergence of postmodernism and post-structuralism.

During the Age of Enlightenment, scientists and philosophers alike attempted to make sense of the world in humanist, rational terms – primarily underpinned by a belief that a central 'truth' was out there to be discovered and questions posed by the human condition could be answered empirically and objectively. Existence could be traced back to an origin and history moved purposefully forwards on a continuous natural trajectory. In the 1960s, however, a new school of intellectual and critical thought, broadly termed 'post-structuralism', emerged in France. This was part of a larger postmodernist movement, the major proponents of which were Roland Barthes, Gilles Deleuze, Jacques Derrida, Friedrich Nietzsche, Julia Kristeva and Michel Foucault.

Postmodernists were critical of the dominant Western culture and philosophy that prevailed at the time. They argued that there could be no objective revelation of some pre-existing truth because truth and reality shifted and meant different things at different times to different people. Thus, there were no grand theories, no authoritative voice, and no unified self that advanced on a continuous, necessary trajectory. Instead, existence was random and often accidental. Indeed, history was divergent and incorporated marginalities and disunities. It was this marginality and the possibilities of transcendence that enabled the post-structuralists to question and analyse dominant ways of thinking, talking and acting (Ramazanoglu and Holland, 2002).

By the 1980s and 1990s, the flexibility and versatility inherent in discourse analysis had made it attractive to a range of postmodern approaches. For example, Derridean theory sought to deconstruct prevailing oppositional binaries (such as healthy/sick, masculine/feminine, young/old) that bestow dominance in Western cultures and permit some knowledges (healthy, masculine, young) to become privileged over others (sick, feminine, old). A genealogical or Foucauldian paradigm examined relations of power and the ways in which specific knowledges (such as medical knowledge or the knowledge of the state penal system) acted on and through the body to produce certain identities (such as patient or prisoner). Meanwhile, Fairclough's critical discourse analysis revealed oppressive practices and different ways of seeing what is often opaque to those within a culture – for example the need for a socio-cultural, as well as biomedical, understanding in the diagnosis of ill-health.

Each of these approaches attested to multiple realities 'knowable only through representations of culture or deconstructions of language and discourse, with no single truth or accessible reality' (Ramazanoglu and Holland, 2002: 152). Furthermore, they recognised that discourses were culturally and historically contingent so that their influences and how they themselves were influenced changed across time and context. The way Western society has referred and responded to people with learning disabilities offers a good example. Historically, terms such as 'idiots', 'imbeciles', and 'mental defectives' were all in common usage and hospitalisation was considered the best practical response. Today, under the discourse of community care, such terms are considered derogatory and it is widely accepted that people with learning disabilities are quite capable of living in the community, provided they are offered appropriate support.

Current Use

Whilst many research methods attempt to isolate the data from the context within which they are collected, discourse analysis emphasises both the data and its context (Crowe, 2005). In other words, discourse analysis illustrates how meaning is conveyed through language and words, but also through the cultural and social conventions that are constructed as 'normal' in any culture. Since cultural and social conventions are ever-changing, no particular experiences, practices or inequalities are necessary, natural or inevitable. Accordingly, discourse analysis reveals how it is possible to challenge dominant discourses and, in turn, argue for and promote social change. Such analytical exposure is attractive to those who wish to open up for scrutiny those taken-for-granted policies, actions and institutions that set up binaries that can privilege or oppress individuals, groups or practices. For these reasons, discourse theory has become particularly attractive to those seeking to expose oppressive and hence limiting discourses. Over the years, this has included feminists, queer theorists and others who have identified oppressive regimes or practices within their fields of existence, be that at work or in their social lives.

Discourse analysis is not a research method in any traditional unified way, but is rather a process. It is a way of critically thinking about circumstances of possibility or a way of understanding reflections of aspects of realities particular to time and culture. This enables the researcher to open up for scrutiny the common assumptions that are deeply culturally embedded and therefore rendered invisible and so taken for granted as true or prediscursive. Being multidimensional and multifunctional in its approach, discourse analysis facilitates historical interpretation and enables the researcher to investigate social change. It also permits the exploration of cultural hegemonies and their role in 'constituting social ... relations' (Fairclough, 1992: 12). The latter was neatly captured by Rudge and Morse (2001) who showed how individuals living with diagnoses of schizophrenia embraced biomedical discourses relating to their illness, but then used metaphor to undermine medical science's ownership of their situation.

Within discourse analysis, conventional data collection techniques are used to generate texts that are 'analysed discursively from a particular understanding of discourse analysis and driven by a certain theoretical frame' (Cheek, 2004: 1145–6). This might be deconstruction, genealogy, critical discourse analysis, feminism, postmodernism, linguistic anthropology, ethnomethodology and so on. In fact, the theoretical base can sit within a number of epistemological paradigms. For example, post-structuralist feminists might argue that there is a dominant male discourse that subordinates and marginalises the experiences of women, but also recognise the immense hetereogeneity of female experiences which means that some women (such as women from black and minority ethnic groups, older women or women who are unwell) are more marginalised than others.

Within discourse analysis, the aim of a study, the type of analytic techniques to be employed and the knowledge produced cannot be divorced from the epistemological position adopted by the researcher (Crowe, 2005). Indeed, the researcher's epistemological stance is just as much a part of the context of 'reading' the data, as are the data themselves. So, discourse analysis undertaken from a post-structuralist epistemology will likely identify different key discourses from discourse analysis undertaken by a queer theorist or Foucauldian analyst or ethnomethodologist. Despite this, all types of discourse analysis are united by a mission to explore how some discourses are deemed or understood to be culturally more legitimate than others. For example, why the doctor's account of illness is credited with more weight than the patient's or why the care home manager's view of how the day should be structured is considered more important than the residents' opinions.

BOX 7.1

Types of Question Addressed by Discourse Analysis

- Discourse analysis enables the researcher to scrutinise common assumptions that are deeply culturally embedded and thus taken for granted. It also facilitates the investigation of social change and the exploration of cultural hegemonies. Examples of discourse analysis questions might include:

  - What do the policy and procedure manuals reveal about the dominant discourses in a hospital?

  - How do media reports construct families seeking asylum in Britain?

  - How is heterosexuality privileged in popular texts in modern Western culture?

  - What discourses are employed by family members to describe their problems in family therapy?

Main Strengths of Discourse Analysis

Perhaps the most provocative strength of discourse analysis is that it can lead to fundamental changes in the practices of an institution, a profession, or society as a whole. This has become increasingly appealing as societies (and particularly Western societies) have evolved into more complex mixes of race and cultures in recent years, and as marginalised groups have begun to challenge the dominant discourses that work to discriminate against them by privileging other groups and practices. Such change has been evidenced in the health and social care field where discourse analysis is gaining momentum as a research philosophy that opens up to scrutiny the dominant ways of thinking and talking and the taken-for-granted practices both within professions and in relation to caring for a diverse client base (Crowe, 2005).

A second strength of discourse analysis is that it provides a holistic method for understanding complex socio-cultural phenomena. This provides a welcome alternative to more traditional positivist paradigms that have often examined society overly simply through the eye of the culturally privileged Western white middle-class male and failed adequately to account for the diverse experiences of those many groups marginalised within society. For example, discourse analysis has successfully exposed and critically analysed the cultural beliefs and practices that have impinged negatively on groups as diverse as women, those who are mentally ill, poor people, substance abusers, people who are HIV positive, and gay, lesbian and transgendered populations.

Thirdly, discourse analysis has a strong theoretical base that gives it weight and authority and enables it to expose and traverse diverse intellectual terrains. Nevertheless, the theoretical base that underpins research utilising discourse analysis is always clearly and transparently articulated to the research consumer. This includes an open justification of why particular texts and discourses are included and what epistemological assumptions are driving the analyses. Such candidness means that complex theoretical ideas are conveyed unambiguously and provide readers of discourse analysis with understandable, accessible and highly readable examinations.

Main Weaknesses of Discourse Analysis

One of the major criticisms of discourse analysis research is that it can suffer from under-analysis or indeed no analysis (Antaki et al., 2003). From the discussion thus far, it should be evident that anyone employing the technique has to subscribe to a highly theoretical epistemological base, and this requires extensive reading and engagement with a range of prevailing discourses. As such, discourse analysis can be both time-consuming and challenging for the novice researcher. Yet, without a sound theoretical base to underpin the research, discourse analysis can be seriously flawed. This danger is heightened by the fact that discourse analysis is a relatively new technique which can embrace a number of paradigmatic approaches and be used in very disparate areas of enquiry. As such, there is a propensity for self-teaching (Burman, 2004) and this can lead to inconsistency, inappropriate or inadequate argumentation, and misunderstandings (Antaki et al., 2003).

A second weakness of discourse analysis is that it does not adhere to any 'scientific', rationalist rules and thus tends to be unreplicable and non-generalisable. It is instead a purely subjective technique and this can give it an overall appearance of being a method that is partial and perhaps one where it seems 'anything goes' (Antaki et al., 2003). This criticism has come particularly from quantitative quarters, but also from some corners of qualitative research, exacerbated by the fact that it is a relatively novel approach with few teachers and little support from the wider community. As such, it has often been ghettoised and deemed weak or groundless research.

Perhaps the most pervasive criticism levelled against discourse analysis is that it offers no solutions. Unlike many other methods, it does not profess to seek truth or untruth; it merely aims to reveal and disrupt that which is taken for granted and accepted as normal and inevitable, so that cultural change is possible. Thus, it can expose hegemonic practices and how these work to oppress and privilege within a culture. Yet, it does not offer anything in their place. When and how change occurs are simply not addressed by the discourse analyst.

MAIN STRENGTHS AND WEAKNESSES
... OF DISCOURSE ANALYSIS

Strengths

- Discourse analysis challenges dominant ways of thinking, talking and acting that discriminate or marginalise and it can thus lead to socio-cultural change.

- Discourse analysis provides a holistic method for understanding complex socio-cultural phenomena.

- Discourse analysis has a strong theoretical base which it translates into understandable and accessible examinations of phenomena for the reader.

Weaknesses

- Discourse analysis can suffer from under-analysis or no analysis, particularly at the hands of the novice researcher.

- Discourse analysis is a highly subjective technique that does not adhere to any 'scientific' rationalist rules and, as such, tends to be unreplicable and non-generalisable.

- Discourse analysis does not search for truth claims and offers no solutions to the injustices of dominant discourses which oppress and privilege.

Conducting a Discourse Analysis

As a theoretical approach, discourse analysis can be utilised within any discipline and can employ a broad range of methodological devices, such as speech act theory, critical discourse analysis, conversational analysis, political analysis and so on (for more examples, see Wetherell et al., 2001, and Wodak and Meyer, 2001). The aim is not to discover a pre-existing truth (indeed, the existence of pre-existing truths is denied), but rather to understand how discourses construct and maintain realities, as they are themselves being constituted. Thus, by employing discourse analysis, the researcher seeks different – not better – ways of 'seeing' the world in which we exist. In order to achieve this, a number of common stages are generally followed (see also Crowe, 2005).

Identifying a research question

A discourse analysis study usually begins with the researcher questioning a particular form of social practice and its relationship to social structure (Fairclough, 1995) – for example dominant hospital discourses; the state's relationship with asylum seekers; or the privileging of heterosexuality in modern Western culture. The objectives are then to ascertain how discourses construct and are constructed by social and political inequality, power relations or hegemonic practices. Unlike most other methodological approaches, the researcher does not need a clear research question or statement of enquiry at the outset – this can be formalised later. A general topic or problem will permit the researcher to explore key discourses and the context in which they emerge.

Selecting or creating texts

The next task of the discourse analyst is to decide which types of text will be analysed. The primary starting point for the selection or creation of texts will usually be the researcher's area of interest or the domain of practice to be deconstructed. For the asylum seekers' study, this would likely be policy and legislative documents, but might also include newspaper articles or interviews with asylum seekers and government officials. This choice of texts may be a purely practical matter that is dependent on the researcher knowing what is 'out there' and how to access it. However, the process tends to be executed best if the researcher has insider or intimate knowledge of the domain of practice to be researched and can access persons within the discipline who can offer key information.

The choice of texts to be included in a discourse analysis is vitally important since it is these texts that actually enable the researcher to make 'connections and inferences, in accordance with relevant interpretive principles, necessary to generate coherent readings' (Fairclough, 1992: 84). In practice, any type of text or textual feature is a potentially valuable source (Fairclough, 1992: 74) and a diverse range of texts can be used (for example books, novels, film, government documents, medical notes) or created (for example interview transcripts, diaries and so on). In fact, the greater the number and type of data sources included, the better as this facilitates the possibility for multiple understandings that do not necessarily privilege dominant discourses (Crowe, 1998).

Reviewing the texts to identify discourses and noting connections to other discourses

Once the texts have been identified and collated, they should be reviewed to identify key discourses and any connections with other relevant discourses. These interconnections are known as 'intertextuality' (Fairclough, 1992). For example, systematic and repeated readings of six patient information leaflets on osteoarthritis by Grime and Ong (2007) identified three main areas of discourse:

- Osteoarthritis as a disease and as an illness

- Causality, lifestyle and ageing in osteoarthritis

- Osteoarthritis management.

Within their analyses, Grime and Ong reflected on the dominance of the disease discourse and the limited discourse on illness. This was evidenced by the fact that five of the six leaflets focused on bodies rather than people, with advice centred on the biological rather than the social effects of osteoarthritis. In addition, the authors noted a contradiction between the discourse of the bioscientist which showed ageing to be a risk factor in osteoarthritis and the discourse of the NHS therapist which sought to encourage patient responsibility for averting osteoarthritis by establishing it as a preventable condition.

Identifying the values and assumptions that underpin social practices

Any text may be 'read' or 'interpreted' differently by each person who interacts with it. Thus, the researcher must clearly articulate their epistemological stance in the identification of texts as well as in their analysis. In so doing, the context and the 'reading' of the researcher can legitimately become part of the process of generating meaning. In addition, the researcher must be alert to the context in which the texts used in the analysis were created. To this end, they should acknowledge why and by whom texts were produced and who, if anyone, was the intended audience. The inclusion of verbatim text to illustrate key issues when writing up the findings is also a way of helping to ensure transparency and legitimacy.

Establishing rigour

In terms of establishing the methodological robustness of a discourse analysis study, the largely qualitative nature of the technique limits strict approaches to reliability or validity testing. Nonetheless, these are not unimportant questions and Crowe (2005) makes various suggestions in relation to both methodological and interpretative rigour. The researcher can, for example, ask themselves a number of key questions, such as: Is the research question appropriate for a discourse analysis?; Has a sufficient range of resources been reviewed (for example historical, political, clinical, lay)?; Have the interpretative paradigm, data gathering and analytical processes been clearly described?; and Are the linkages between discourse, findings and interpretation suitably explained and plausible?

Suggesting change

Finally, and as stated previously, a key strength of discourse analysis is its ability to challenge existing social practices and hierarchies and to promote social change. Thus, the researcher should reflect carefully on what their findings mean in real-world terms and, where possible, identify how discourses (or texts and talk in social practices) might be changed. For example, in their study of osteoarthritis, Grime and Ong (2007) concluded that the focus of written information needs to shift from joint biology to helping patients live with osteoarthritis in order to promote self-care. This means moving away from a disease discourse in patient leaflets to incorporate an illness discourse that values patients' experience of osteoarthritis.

An Example of a Discourse Analysis Study

The process of undertaking discourse analysis is perhaps best illustrated by examining in more detail a recent research study that used the method. For this purpose, the research paper: Crowe, M. (2002), 'Reflexivity and detachment: A discursive approach to women's depression', *Nursing Inquiry,* **9**(2): 126–32 has been selected.

Marie Crowe was the primary researcher and her study was conducted as part of her Ph.D. thesis which was awarded by Griffith University School of Film, Media and Cultural Studies in 1998. The study was a discourse analysis of women's experiences of mental distress and involved interviews with 12 female inpatients receiving treatment for mental disorders at a private psychiatric hospital. The texts analysed were transcripts from all the women's interviews, supplemented by biographical and fictional accounts. Detachment and reflexivity, and how these worked as contradictions in the lives of women, were central themes. The research was unfunded.

Crowe bases her analytic approach on Fairclough's (1992) critical discourse analysis and, in so doing, emphasises 'the cultural and linguistic construction of [the women's] experiences' (p. 126). She argues that Western culture privileges discourses of reflexivity and detachment over relationality, cooperation and connection with others. Yet, the subject positions traditionally available to women in modern Western culture have involved nurturing and caring for others. This generates a tension for women who are given a double message – that is, to focus on the needs of others whilst living in a culture that privileges self-objectivity and individuality. This places women in a more vulnerable position than men for experiencing alienation, which – within the dominant discourses of psychiatric medicine and the wider culture – is 'read' as depressive illness.

Crowe cites the *Diagnostic and Statistical Manual of Mental Disorders-IV* (*DSM-IV*) (American Psychiatric Association, 1994) as the authoritative text over what is deemed mental health/ill health in Western culture. Over time, this text has become widely accessible and is utilised by medical, nursing and lay people to diagnose and manage mental illness. Its allegiance with an alleged biomedical rationality allows the *DSM-IV* to be consumed as a true indicator of symptoms of mental disorders. Behaviours that then fall outside such discourses are either rendered invisible because they cannot be 'read' or they are given no authority. Crowe argues that the lives of women are categorised by such discourses and rarely, if ever, does this categorisation consider the socio-cultural context of individual women's lives.

In her analysis, Crowe explores the explicit use of the *DSM-IV* text and its process for claiming authority. However, she also considers connections with other texts/discourses. These include academic books and articles published in peer-reviewed journals of mental health, as well as nursing literature. This is complemented by psychoanalytical critical theory: specifically Lacan's theory of language and its role in constituting subjectivity (Lacan, 1979), but also Foucault (1977, 1988), Butler (1990), Kristeva (1989) and Fee (2000), who are all postmodern in their epistemologies. Crowe additionally connects these discourses to more popular culture, for example Frame (1980), Sechehaye (1951), and Schiller and Bennet (1994), who write of 'madness', typically their own.

Thus, Crowe uses other texts/discourses to argue that there is a wider context in which women's mental health should be considered. In exploring the 'intertextuality' of discourses, she challenges the authority of the *DSM-IV* and builds up an analysis of the major concepts of cultural expectation and the construction of particular roles for women in order to reveal how their mixed messages can lead to an alienation that, if not understood in context, can be 'read' as depression. Additionally, she unpicks the ways in which discourses of mental health and illness allow a categorisation and naming of some behaviours as normal and others as abnormal. This process dominates her interviewees' construction and understanding of their lives as being different from cultural expectations and, so, abnormal. Thus, the women find themselves in the subject position of depressed woman, with all of the cultural connotations that this position and concomitant label bestows.

The dominant cultural discourses analysed by Crowe illuminate the ways in which the interviewees understand what is psychiatrically normal and not normal. Her analyses also reveal how the women utilise appropriate language from within the discourses of depression to make sense of their alienation and to understand how others also 'read' their behaviours within the same discursive conventions. So, the interviewees assume that they are depressed and people treat them as depressed, but this is only because of a particular contextual 'reading'. Crowe's study cleverly reveals how discourses work to make us believe that this is natural and inevitable.

Finally, Crowe's multidimensional analysis leads her to a discussion about the possible implications for mental health nurses' practice. She argues that mental health nurses could assist individuals to recognise 'the symbolic meaning embedded in their language and behaviour and the role that language plays in constructing their experiences'. She also suggests that mental health nurses could accept difference and promote 'multiplicity in individuals' responses to their social world', whilst simultaneously promoting 'social responsibility, communality and connection with others as a form of resistance to detachment and reflexivity' (p. 131). In this way, mental health nurses would be able to provide a more appropriate form of holistic care than is currently often the case.

Ultimately, Crowe argues that if mental health nurses understand the cultural context in which some women feel at variance and unable to be understood as 'normal', then they will be more able to deliver care that is meaningful to those women. In so doing, she has performed what Fairclough suggests is an approach that 'enables relationships between discursive and social change to be assessed, and detailed properties of texts to be related systematically to social properties of discursive events of social practice' (Fairclough, 1995, p. 8). As a result, we – as the consumers of such analyses – can view a practice in its completeness rather than merely viewing its surface.

Further Reading

Discourse & Society (Sage Publications).

This is a bi-monthly international journal that explores the relevance of discourse analysis to the social sciences. Its aim is to stimulate 'a problem-oriented and critical approach', with a particular focus on 'the political implications of discourse and communication'. Whilst the journal will enable the newcomer to discourse analysis to understand more about what discourse analysis is and is not, it is also suitable for the more advanced researcher. Recent papers have explored topics such as: 'Life stories used as evidence for the diagnosis of addiction in group therapy'; 'Size matters: Constructing accountable bodies in NSPCC helpline interaction'; and 'Narrative reflexivity as a repair device for discounting "cognitive distortions" in sex offender treatment'.

Jaworski, A. and Coupland, N. (eds) (1999) *The Discourse Reader* **(London: Routledge).**

This collection of over 30 writings includes contributions by many key names in the field. Various modern approaches to discourse analysis – including conversation analysis, narrative analysis, and critical discourse analysis – are covered. The text is divided into discrete sections that explore, *inter alia*, the meaning and context of discourse analysis; methods and resources for analysing discourse; identity and subjectivity; and power, ideology and control. Each section has an editors' introduction and discussion points so that readers can engage with important issues in practical ways. The book is very suitable for students from undergraduate level upwards.

Ramazanoglu, C. with Holland, J. (2002) *Feminist Methodology: Challenges and Choices* (London: Sage).

Although this text is not purely about discourse analysis, it explores feminist methods and epistemologies in terms that make the analysis of discourse clear and appropriate for health and social care professionals who often function within oppressive institutions of language and practice. The book contextualises discourse analysis nicely and begins to unravel the complexity of feminist epistemologies. Its highly accessible style and clear explanations of difficult concepts mean that it can be enjoyed by students and novice researchers.

Wetherell, M., Taylor, S. and Yates, S. (eds) (2001) *Discourse as Data: A Guide for Analysis* (London: Sage Publications).

This edited book is relevant for anyone who knows a little and wants to learn more about discourse analysis. The Introduction and Conclusion provide a broad overview of discourse analysis, including common methodological issues as well as some evaluation and application of the technique. The six intervening chapters are each written by an expert in a particular discourse analysis approach (such as conversation analysis, socio-linguistics and corpus analysis, and genealogical analysis). The book introduces key concepts and leads the reader through appropriate methods for analysing different types of text. It also offers practical opportunities to try out analytic concepts on real data.

Wodak, R. and Meyer, M. (2001) *Methods of Critical Discourse Analysis* (London, Sage Publications).

Methods of Critical Discourse Analysis introduces the various theories and methods associated with discourse analysis, including semiotics; socio-linguistics; critical discourse analysis; and historical approaches. The authors assume that the reader has minimal knowledge and this makes the text particularly useful for newcomers to the field. In addition to introducing the leading discourse analysts, the book provides ample descriptions of individual methods as well as an understanding of the theories that underpin them. There is also some comparative treatment of each of the methods so that the reader is assisted in deciding which may be the most appropriate to select for their particular research topic.

References

American Psychiatric Association (1994) *Diagnostic and Statistical Manual of Mental Disorders-IV* (Washington, DC: American Psychiatric Association).

Antaki, C., Billig, M., Edwards, D. and Potter, J. (2003) 'Discourse analysis means doing analysis: A critique of six analytic shortcomings', *DAOL (Discourse Analysis On-Line), **1**, 1.

Burman, E. (2004) 'Discourse analysis means analysing discourse: Some comments on Antaki, Billig, Edwards & Potter: Discourse analysis means doing analysis: A critique of six analytic shortcomings', *DAOL*, **1**, 1.

Butler, J. (1990) *Gender Trouble: Feminism and the Subversion of Identity* (London: Routledge).

Cheek, J. (2004) 'At the margins? Discourse analysis and qualitative research', *Qualitative Health Research*, **4**, 1140–50.

Crowe, M. (1998) *Doing What No Normal Woman Would Do* Ph.D. thesis (Griffith University, Brisbane: School of Film, Media and Cultural Studies).

Crowe, M. (2002) 'Reflexivity and detachment: A discursive approach to women's depression', *Nursing Inquiry*, **9**(2): 126–32.

Crowe, M. (2005) 'Discourse analysis: Towards an understanding of its use in nursing', *Journal of Advanced Nursing*, **51**, 55–63.

Fairclough, N. (1992) *Discourse and Social Change* (Cambridge: Polity Press).

Fairclough, N. (1995) *Critical Discourse Analysis: The Critical Study of Language* (Harlow: Pearson Education).

Fee, D. (ed) (2000) *Pathology and the Postmodern* (London: Sage).

Foucault, M. (1977) *Discipline and Punish: The Birth of the Prison* (London: Tavistock).

Foucault, M. (1988) *The History of Sexuality: Vol. 1, An Introduction* (Harmondsworth: Penguin).

Frame, J. (1980) *Faces in the Water* (London: Women's Press).

Grime, J.C. and Ong, B.N. (2007) 'Constructing osteoarthritis through discourse – a qualitative analysis of six patient information leaflets on osteoarthritis', *BMC Musculoskeletal Disorders*, **8**, 34.

Kristeva, J. (1989) *Black Sun: Depression and Melancholia* (New York: Columbia University Press).

Lacan, J. (1979) *The Four Fundamental Concepts of Psycho-analysis* (Harmondsworth: Penguin).

Ramazanoglu, C. with Holland, J. (2002) *Feminist Methodology: Challenges and Choices* (London: Sage).

Rudge, T. and Morse, K. (2001) 'Re-awakenings?: A discourse analysis of the recovery from schizophrenia after medication change', *Australian and New Zealand Journal of Mental Health Nursing*, **10**, 66–76.

Schiller, L. and Bennett, A. (1994) *The Quiet Room* (New York: Time Warner).

Sechehaye, M. (1951) *Autobiography of a Schizophrenic Girl* (New York: Grune and Stratton).

Wetherell, M., Taylor, S. and Yates, S. (eds) (2001) *Discourse as Data: A Guide for Analysis* (London: Sage Publications).

Wodak, R. and Meyer, M. (2001) *Methods of Critical Discourse Analysis*, (London: Sage Publications).

Service Audit

JOHN HALL AND ANNETTE K. DEARMUN

8

Introduction

Audit compares what a service actually does with what it should be doing and then seeks to identify and implement changes in order to improve practice. Although audit is not technically research, it is included in this volume because of its many similarities with research and because of its increasing use in health and social care. For example, audit employs many of the same techniques of planning, sampling, data collection, analysis and dissemination as research. Like research, audit answers specific questions relating to the quality of care. Additionally, a well-conducted audit will often raise important issues that can then be pursued through research. Because of such similarities, research and audit are often confused. However, whereas research is primarily undertaken to create new knowledge (for example about what professionals should be doing), audit seeks to ensure that agreed best practice is being followed.

A number of definitions of audit exist, but one that is widely used in the UK is:

> A quality improvement process that seeks to improve patient care and outcomes through systematic review of care against explicit criteria and the implementation of change. Aspects of the structure, processes and outcomes of care are selected and systematically evaluated against explicit criteria. Where indicated, changes are implemented at an individual, team, or service level and further monitoring is used to confirm improvement in healthcare delivery. (The National Institute for Health and Clinical Excellence and Commission for Health Improvement, 2002: 1)

The above definition is applicable to both health and social care settings and emphasises that audit is a process – hence the term 'the audit cycle'. After any changes have been implemented, practice should subsequently be re-audited in order to ensure that improvement has resulted. A defining feature of audit is that it assesses current practice against a previously agreed set of criteria or standards (Hill and Small, 2006). Hence, audit implies that there is already an evidence base against which to compare services and service delivery. This evidence may be epidemiological, experimental, or developed through the consensus of experts and published in a professional best practice guideline.

Historical Context

The term 'audit' can be traced back to medieval times and originally referred to the settling of accounts. For example, an audit house was an appendage to a cathedral where business was transacted. Over time, audit came to mean an official examination of accounts, particularly by an independent body, that would ensure financial probity and reassure shareholders that an enterprise was being run honestly. In the United Kingdom, the earliest known reference to the existence of a public official auditing government expenditure is the Auditor of the Exchequer in 1314 (National Audit Office, 2007). It was not, however, until the 1866 Exchequer and Audit Departments Act that government departments were required to produce annual financial accounts and report back formally to parliament (ibid.). Today, government audit in the UK is exercised by the National Audit Office, an independent body established in 1983.

An important early example of the application of audit principles to healthcare was provided by Florence Nightingale (1820–1910) at Scutari Hospital in the Crimea during the Crimean War of 1853–1855. Nightingale kept meticulous records of mortality rates among the wounded soldiers and sailors. By comparing observed practice with best available evidence and making sure that changes occurred, Nightingale was able to reduce mortality in a military hospital from 40% to 2% (Ougrin and Banarsee, 2006). Another early and complementary example of audit is provided by the American surgeon Ernest Codman (1869–1940). He tracked the outcomes of the treatment of patients by individual surgeons at Massachusetts General Hospital in order to identify 'clinical misadventures'. Codman called his approach the 'end results system', and he is the founder of what is now known as patient outcome management (Spiegelhalter, 1999).

It was not until many years later that medical and clinical audit[1] became part of routine health care management in Britain. Initially, medical audit was based only on the voluntary peer-review of work undertaken by doctors and the findings produced were confidential rather than open to public scrutiny. This changed in 1990 after the UK Government White paper *Working for Patients* (Department of Health, 1989) increased funding to introduce audit for all professions throughout the British National Heath Service (NHS).

In 1992, the Department of Health established a Clinical Outcomes Group for England, the purpose of which was to give strategic direction to the development of clinical rather than merely medical audit. This Group adopted a multidisciplinary approach in order to identify and achieve improved healthcare outcomes in the widest sense possible. From this point, successive British governments issued guidance on assessing health outcomes, with the most recent guidance included within a wider Quality and Outcomes Framework (QOF) (Department of Health, 2004). Since 1999, each nation within the UK has issued its own guidance on clinical outcome monitoring, as illustrated by a report from Scotland with major sections on lung cancer and hospital emergency re-admissions (Clinical Outcomes Working Group, 2002).

The application of audit to social care has been slower than to clinical care, one reason being that it is much harder to establish clear links between interventions and outcomes for social care. Despite this, the importance of measuring and comparing the provision of social care against set criteria in order to improve service organisation and delivery is widely recognised and has increasingly been carried out in a coordinated multiprofessional context. For example, the Commission for Social Care Inspection (CSCI) was established in 2004 as the single inspectorate for social care in England, combining the previously separate work of the Social Services Inspectorate (SSI), the SSI/Audit Commission Joint Review team, and the social care work of the National Care Standards Commission.

Current Use

The need for audit in health and social care arises from a concern that services may not be providing the level and quality of care that they are supposed to be providing. The presence of skilled staff, good intentions and adequate equipment do not by themselves ensure high quality and sustainable services. Problems may arise because of inadequate levels of staffing, changed clinical priorities, unforeseen crises, the lack of well-organised appointment systems, insufficient aftercare services and so on. There may also be considerable variations in practice between individual professionals or services.

Three important aims of audit are *monitoring, comparing* and *promoting quality.* Through the process of *monitoring*, audit seeks to clarify what exactly is happening in a service – such as, how many patients or clients are being seen or how long they have to wait for treatment. By *comparing,* audit investigates similarities and differences between services, and between services and previously agreed standards, in order to identify how and why one service might be performing to a higher or lower standard than expected, a process also known as benchmarking. In order to *promote quality,* audit seeks to ascertain whether a service is leading to good outcomes and how better outcomes might be achieved.

Audits may be both self-initiated and mandated. Self-initiated audits can occur if any health or social care practitioner or service manager becomes concerned about their personal effectiveness or the effectiveness of the team or service in which they work. For example, they may be concerned that too many clients are dropping out of their treatment programmes prematurely or they might feel that a similar service nearby is attracting more referrals. This may prompt them to carry out a relatively small-scale internal audit focusing on specific questions, such as how many treatment sessions are actually being carried out by each therapist or whether the service they are providing is unattractive to particular age or diagnostic groups.

Other forms of audit are, conversely, mandatory. For those working in statutory health and social care services (and for many working in the independent sector or in private practice), some categories of information need to be provided as a condition of a service contract or by law. This might include data required by an Act of Parliament or as a result of government policies and their associated management and practice guidance. Examples would include mandatory data collection under the Mental Health Act 1983, such as the provision of annual statistics by each Mental Health Trust on the number of people who have been sectioned (that is, compulsorily detained), or under the Children Act 2004, such as the requirement of a regular performance rating of local authorities with respect to the services they provide for young people.

Within the UK, a practical handbook prepared by the Department of Health (Copeland, 2005) now effectively constitutes an official guide to NHS audit practice. This handbook has been endorsed by a number of government bodies and is designed to give advice and guidance to those organisations where local clinical audit is proving difficult to embed. Some events are deemed so important that national reporting systems, known as National Confidential Enquiries, have been established. This has, for example, been the case in respect of neonatal deaths (CEMACH, 2004) and suicides (Royal College of Psychiatrists, 1995). Furthermore, when very serious negative incidents – such as deaths or serious injuries – occur, services will often have their own standard reporting procedures.

Decisions about which aspects of service should be audited will reflect the needs, priorities and concerns of a range of stakeholders, including the Government, those paying for services, professionals providing services and patients and clients using services. Nonetheless, the priorities of these groups may differ, and historically it is service users who have had the weakest voice in determining what is audited and when. This has, though, begun to change. During the 1990s, many public services took important new steps to increase user involvement and user choice in service delivery and this has now fed into auditing processes, ensuring that the wishes of the service users and patients are always taken into account, unless there is a very good reason for them being overridden (see Farrington-Douglas and Allen, 2005).

Audit is, of course, not a process specific to the UK. Rather it occurs at a national, local and service level in countless countries across the globe. In Australia, for example, an audit toolkit for maternal health in women from ethnic minorities has been prepared by the Healthy Life Healthy Community programme of the Australian government (Department of Health and Ageing, 2007). In North India, meanwhile, clinical audit has been used to improve the quality of obstetric care (Mercer et al., 2006). Equally, international audits are commonly undertaken by agencies such as the World Health Organization (WHO). An example of the latter is a review of long-term care for older people in Europe, which was undertaken in the light of the projected 77% increase in the number of people aged 65 and over between 2004 and 2050 (Sorenson, 2007).

Clearly, it can be helpful to make practice comparisons between countries, and this is assisted by using the same standards and measures. Nonetheless, interpreting data at an international level can be difficult because there is usually wide variability in the type and quality of data collected, the diagnostic criteria used, and the ways services are resourced and organised. Furthermore, broader socio-economic factors – such as poverty, levels of unemployment and educational provision – can have dramatic impacts on health and social care outcomes independent of how services are provided.

BOX 8.1

Types of Question Addressed by Audit

- What is going on? For example: How long does it take for clients to be seen? How many staff have qualifications that enable them to undertake specified responsibilities?

- What is the quality of the service? For example: Are service users satisfied with the services they receive? In residential settings, are the domestic arrangements – including catering – meeting the expectations of residents?

- What are the outcomes of the service? For example: How many looked-after children are entering further or higher education? Do people leaving hospital with long-standing mental health problems access employment services?

- How does the service compare with similar services elsewhere? For example: Are the rates of referral to specialist children's services similar in different areas? Are there any significant variations in patterns of funding and staffing at substance misuse services in different cities?

Main Strengths of Audit

An important advantage of audit is that it often uses data that are already being collected as part of routine service delivery and monitoring. As a result, information can be obtained quickly and at relatively low cost. Moreover, answers to potentially important issues can be provided and positive service changes implemented much sooner than would be the case if a full research project had to be designed and conducted. The relative speed of undertaking audit compared with research is particularly useful when trying to address current or emergent policy and practice issues, especially those that may be of media interest.

Audit methods of collecting information about a service can also have high face validity. That is, they tend to be meaningful to those who are participating. This is because audits involve a wide range of stakeholders (managers, professionals, service users) from the very outset – in deciding what is to be audited, establishing best practice standards, collecting data, assessing performance, and identifying and implementing change. Such involvement helps to make the processes of audit transparent to all concerned. Additionally, the routine participation of staff in audit provides them with an opportunity to learn about service evaluation, and can encourage them to think critically about their practice and how it might be improved.

A further important strength of audit is its simplicity. Audit does not seek to provide definitive evidence of what works or what is best practice. It rather offers an account of what is happening in a service. Thus, it does not demand large samples or complex statistical analyses. As a result, the data generated by audit can be presented in the form of accessible tables and charts that are easily digested by busy policy-makers and managers. The simplicity of audits also means that they can easily be repeated, so providing numerical measures to indicate progress from one audit to another.

Main Weaknesses of Audit

Perhaps most obviously, the tendency for audits to be focused on local procedures and practices means that findings should not be generalised beyond the services involved. Additionally, the lack of formal experimental methods and strict comparison groups limits the power of the technique to uncover complex relationships between different procedures or measures. Furthermore, the apparent simplicity of the data collection tools commonly used – such as activity data, questionnaires and surveys – can mean that they are developed by individuals or groups who have little formal research training. This can lead to poor instrument design, with ambiguous questions or unclear response categories that only come to light once the audit has commenced.

The relative speed and ease of undertaking audits can also have drawbacks. For example, because audits do not generally need to proceed through a formal ethics committee (see Chapters 2 and 3), it is possible to undertake them without giving due consideration to potentially salient ethical issues. The selection of participants in audit procedures can additionally be opportunistic, depending on who happens to be present and willing at the time, or even who can be persuaded to participate by managers. Furthermore, the lack of peer review (see Chapter 1), both in the planning and writing up of audits, can increase the likelihood of methodological flaws, misunderstandings and errors. Together these can result in audit being seen as a 'short-cut' or 'quick and dirty' way of accessing data.

Finally, in selecting aspects of services to be evaluated in an audit, it is usual to adopt those which demand fairly objective and quantifiable measures (such as waiting times or number of clients or patients seen). This can fail to capture the more subjective and qualitative aspects of care (such as how people feel about the way they were treated, and whether or not they feel that their needs have been addressed). Consequently, the simplicity of audit data collection procedures and analyses can produce relatively superficial findings that do not generate theory and that, by themselves, are unlikely to lead to innovation in practice (although they may support it).

MAIN STRENGTHS AND WEAKNESSES

… OF AUDIT

Strengths

- Routinely collected data can be used, so offering a way of obtaining information quickly and at relatively low cost to address potentially important and very topical practice-focused issues.

- Audit methods tend to have high face validity.

- The routine involvement of staff in audit provides them with an opportunity to learn about service evaluation, and can encourage them to think critically about their practice and how it might be improved.

- Audits are relatively simple to undertake. This means that they can easily be repeated to monitor change over time. Moreover, findings can be presented in the form of accessible tables and charts which are easily digested by busy policy-makers and managers.

Weaknesses

- The tendency for audits to be focused on local procedures and practices means that findings cannot be generalised beyond the services involved.

- The lack of formal experimental methods and strict comparison groups limits the power of audit to uncover complex relationships between different procedures or measures.

- The relative speed and ease of undertaking audits can result in the method being seen as a 'short cut' or 'quick and dirty' way of accessing data.

- In selecting aspects of services to be evaluated, it is usual to adopt those which demand objective and quantifiable measurement, thus neglecting more subjective and qualitative aspects of care.

- The simplicity of audit data collection procedures and analyses can produce relatively superficial findings that do not generate theory and that, by themselves, are unlikely to lead to innovation in practice.

Conducting an Audit

This section describes how to conduct an audit. These stages collectively comprise the audit cycle.

Deciding on a topic or aspect of a service or practice that needs to be scrutinised

Decisions about which issues should be audited will depend on a range of factors. These include the relevance of a topic, usually from a national or local perspective, taking account of whether there is a perceived problem; whether new guidelines, evidence-based criteria or standards have recently become available; and whether the issue represents a high-risk, high-volume, high-profile and/or costly aspect of care. Aspects of care known to be weak or not meeting accepted standards can also constitute important audit topics. Meanwhile, decisions will often be shaped by unanticipated local events, such as serious adverse incidents, complaints or high complication rates in a specific unit (Copeland, 2005).

Crucially, an audit topic should be one which is amenable to improvement. There is little point in auditing an area where there is little chance of change – perhaps because resources are not available, managers are not interested in the problem, clinicians are unlikely to change their practice, or the problem only affects a very small number of patients. Once an audit topic (for example condition X) has been selected, the main aim of the audit then needs to be stated (for example to improve practice in relation to condition X or to ensure that best practice is being followed in relation to X). Following this, more specific objectives should be defined. These will relate to the quality of care around condition X (such as whether it is appropriate; accessible; effective; and provided in a timely fashion).

Defining the criteria and standards against which the service or practice should be judged

The next stage of an audit is to identify or create criteria or standards against which the service or practice can be judged. These can come from several sources. For example, they may already be available locally or nationally within a relevant policy or professional document, with audit items clearly specified, or they may be implicit within existing recommendations. If these do not exist, a literature review can be undertaken to identify any underpinning research evidence that will help to clarify and establish best practice. If no clear evidence base is identified, focus groups or interviews with professionals and, if possible, service users can be undertaken to agree appropriate standards.

Standards can relate to three main aspects of the topic or aspect of service or practice being scrutinised. These include *the structures* in place within an organisation to support a particular outcome (such as the number of staff appropriately trained); the *process of care* (such as the amount of time taken to undertake an initial assessment); and the *outcome* of a specific intervention (such as, client satisfaction with the service). On balance, audits tend to be most effective when they focus on processes since these tend to be more amenable to change than structures or outcomes (UBHT Clinical Audit Central Office, 2005).

Ideally, standards and criteria should be conveyed via definitive unambiguous statements that identify the exact level and quality of care expected. Examples would include, 'All staff will have attended a recent training day'; 'All initial assessments are conducted within one hour'; and 'All clients score 6 or more in a satisfaction survey'. However, even apparently simple standards can prove ambiguous. Thus, the assertion 'All patients will have their urgent blood results recorded in their notes within thirty minutes' raises the question of what is meant by 'urgent'. Equally, there may be a tension between what is perceived to be 'ideal' and what is deemed to be 'the minimal acceptable standard'. For example, there may be evidence that thirty minutes is the optimal time, but one hour is acceptable and realistic given current resources.

Collecting data to establish what is happening in the service or practice

The next step involves collecting data on performance in order to ascertain what is actually happening in the service or practice. Audit generally involves the collection of relatively routine quantitative data that are recorded on an audit form or proforma. That said, the data collection process may still involve a number of different approaches. These commonly include reviewing existing records or documentation, the direct observation of current practice, and conducting a survey.

Existing records or documentation are a particularly valuable source of audit data as they are often compiled as part of routine day-to-day practice. Consequently, they can be gathered quickly and cheaply. However, they are not without their drawbacks. Whilst records and documentation often comprise anonymous data, they might also contain personal, sensitive and highly confidential information about individual patients or clients. In many countries, data protection legislation and research governance guidelines will restrict or prevent access to such data unless formal research ethics procedures are followed (see Chapters 2 and 3). Furthermore, the auditor may need to evaluate the quality of the documentation in terms of its legibility, content and any omitted items.

Some audits will, meanwhile, be amenable to *direct observation*. For example, if the intention is to discover whether professionals actually carry out a particular practice or activity, observation will normally yield more valid information than relying on them to describe their own practice. An example of this is a recent audit of hand-washing techniques in clinical or food preparation areas undertaken by the English Department of Health, where observing practice was deemed preferable to self-reports of staff compliance with hand-washing guidelines (Department of Health, 2007).

If a broad overview of a service or number of services is required, it can also be useful to conduct a *survey* (see Chapter 9). Problematically, preparing and conducting a survey can be time-consuming, so slowing down the auditing process. Additionally, surveys – particularly those using self-report questionnaires – can be prone to poor response rates. However, this can be improved by keeping questions simple and by preparing translated versions for non-native language speakers and large font versions for those with impaired vision. It is also sensible to arrange an effortless process for returning the information to the auditor, such as a clearly marked questionnaire return box within the service and the provision of stamped addressed envelopes for those wishing to take them away to complete.

Although audits do not tend to require formal ethical approval, it is important to decide in advance whether or not the data to be collected will be of a sensitive or confidential nature and then address this accordingly (including seeking formal ethical approval if this seems necessary). It is also crucial to consider who will be best placed to collect and analyse the data. This will largely depend on who has the necessary capacity and skills and will not necessarily be the same staff who designed the audit. For example, an observational audit of cleanliness could be undertaken by a ward housekeeper and analysis of the data by an administrative assistant. To ensure that these processes proceed smoothly, clear instructions should be provided to all involved and data collection procedures should be piloted.

Assessing the performance of the service or practice against the identified criteria and standards

Irrespective of the actual data collection method, the performance of the service or practice needs to be assessed using the data collected. If a standard audit form is not being used, it will usually be necessary to enter the data into a spreadsheet (such as Excel) or a standard quantitative data analysis package (such as SPSS). The data can then be described and analysed, and findings can be printed off and compared with the criteria or standards previously specified. For example, the data collected in Service A may show that 90% of staff had attended a recent training day, whereas this is only 50% in Service B and 30% in Service C.

Inevitably, assessing performance against objective and numeric criteria is easier than measuring how well an agency or service is complying with more vague directives (such as, 'There should be evidence that senior management are committed to the importance of safeguarding and promoting children's welfare' or 'The service development is informed, where appropriate, by the views of children and families').[2] Where criteria are vague, those undertaking the audit should have enough experience and knowledge of the topic being explored to be able to make judgements about the extent to which standards have been met. However, they may also consult other key stakeholders (practitioners, managers, clients/patients and so on) to reaffirm their views.

Identifying any changes that are required

Comparing the standards achieved by a service against the standards expected of it will help to identify the extent to which a service is actually doing what it is supposed to be doing. The auditors will be able to use the analysed data to reveal both the nature and extent of shortfalls. Meanwhile, the shortfalls should suggest areas where change is needed. Again, however, suggestions for change are best made in joint consultation with other key stakeholders to ensure that local contextual information is taken into account. Such contextual information might include factors both internal and external to the agency being audited (such as a temporary unforeseen reduction in funding or the unexpected departure of a key member of staff). This background information may help to explain underperformance but also affect decisions about how performance can and should be improved.

Effective change requires clear decisions about the nature of the required changes. Following consultation, the decisions must be authorised by a team leader or manager with the authority to allocate resources, to change working procedures as required, and to require the continuation of audit data collection. The outcomes of the audit and the recommended changes must be put in writing and communicated to those who have been audited and to any others whose working practices may need to be modified.

Implementing changes to effect positive change

If the audit process reveals that a change in policy or practice seems necessary, the next stage is to produce – again in consultation with the relevant stakeholders – a clear action plan highlighting what measures should be taken by whom, by when and to what end. Once this has been operationalised, the audit process should be repeated to ensure that positive change has indeed occurred and to identify further possibilities for improvement.

An Example of an Audit

Probably the majority of audit studies are carried out locally, and are intended only for local purposes. This makes it difficult to find examples published in peer-reviewed journals. However, an interesting paper by Sparkes (2005) reports on an audit of adherence to standards of care for patients with low back pain conducted in 1996. The paper is doubly helpful in that, unusually, it also provided data on a follow-up audit carried out five years after the first. The work was undertaken by a physiotherapist from Cardiff University, using data from the outpatient physiotherapy department at Addenbrooke's NHS Trust Hospital in Cambridge, UK. It was funded by the Clinical Audit Department and the Physiotherapy Department of the same Trust and was, thus, an 'in-house' audit.

Back pain is one of the most common causes of disability in developed countries, leading to high levels of both medical consultation and absence from work. Ensuring that services for people with low back pain conform to evidence-based standards clearly has the potential to relieve pain and reduce the financial costs associated with absence from work. The standards used in the first audit were developed from clinical standards on back pain published by the Royal College of General Practitioners (1994), taking into account other research on the principles of management of back pain and local guidelines on waiting times. They included seven specific audit standards relating to: waiting times; advice given to the patient; evidence of diagnostic triage following assessment; referral for rehabilitation; and consideration of the need for manipulation. A 'red flag' alerting system was also available to indicate the possible presence of serious underlying medical pathology.

In the first audit, the notes of a sample of 100 patients on the waiting list, referred for acute or chronic low back pain, were scrutinised. Data were obtained for 84 patients. If no information was given in the notes, then the standard was considered unmet. The extent to which each of the specific audit standards were attained ranged from 59% to 100% for six items; one item – consideration of the need for manipulation – was met in none of the notes. No patient was identified with possible serious pathology, so no red flags were used.

After the first audit, an improved appointment system was put in place and the clinical guidelines were actively disseminated through staff education programmes. By the time of the second audit in 2001, the original clinical guidelines had been modified, with the addition of a 'yellow flag' alert for relevant psychosocial factors. In addition, a further standard had been added to the orginal audit schedule and two of the original items had been slightly modified. In the second audit, the notes of only 30 patients were identified (because of lack of funding), and 24 sets of notes were scrutinised. This time, the extent to which the specific audit standards were attained ranged from 52% to 100% for seven items; with consideration of the need for manipulation again not met in any of the notes. No red flags were used, but 30% of patients were considered for yellow flags.

The discussion of the two audits highlighted both areas of good practice, and areas of practice in need of development. It was noted that some of the audit items related to very low frequency events – such as the presentation of severe pathology – and were therefore not sensitive enough to identify change in practice. Furthermore, patients in the audits suffered from both acute and chronic back pain, although the clinical guidelines from which the standards were derived were designed for acute low back pain only. This highlighted how the published guidelines did not match the case mix found in routine practice. The author concluded that the benefit of the audit was its ability to monitor service quality, identify problems and act as an impetus for service change. Equally, it encouraged the implementation of research-based practice guidelines and a commitment to evidence-based practice.

Further Reading

Baker, R., Hearnshaw, H. and Robertson, N. (1999) *Implementing Change in Clinical Audit* **(Chichester: John Wiley and Sons).**

Chapters within this edited volume relate, *inter alia*, to the role of clinical audit in changing performance; evidence and audit; managing change; implementing change; overcoming obstacles to changes; audit and learning; and audit and teamwork. The text is written for audit staff, healthcare managers, policy-makers and clinicians. With the help of case studies, it provides practical suggestions regarding how audit can be used to implement change in clinical practice.

Chambers, R. and Wakley, G. (2005) *Clinical Audit in Primary Care: Demonstrating Quality and Outcomes* (Oxford: Radcliffe Publishing).

Using a practical 'how-to-do-it' approach, this manual is targeted at those undertaking audit within the primary care setting. It utilises examples from around 20 different clinical fields and offers tips and advice that would enable audit data to be collected and analysed easily and meaningfully. Whilst it is likely to be of most interest to nurses, clinical staff, doctors and managers, the content is relevant to others working as part of multi-disciplinary health teams.

Copeland, G. (2005) *A Practical Handbook for Clinical Audit* (London: Clinical Governance Support Team, Department of Health).

This relatively short handbook is available online and free of charge at: http://www.cgsupport.nhs.uk/downloads/Practical_Clinical_Audit_Handbook_v1_1.pdf. Although it has been developed for individuals working within the NHS in the UK, it should appeal to a wider audience. It outlines various models for clinical audit and provides examples of good practice. A key objective of the handbook is to give advice and guidance to organisations where local clinical audit is proving difficult to embed and to improve the integration of audit into clinical governance. The website describes the handbook as an evolutionary document, indicating that updates – in particular examples of good practice with contact details – will be regularly added.

Malby, B. (1995) *Clinical Audit for Nurses and Therapists* (London: Scutari Press).

This is a widely used introductory text, specifically written for nurses, therapists, service commissioners and those undertaking audits. It seeks to present audit theories in an accessible manner.

Sale, D. (2003) *Understanding Clinical Governance and Quality Assurance* (Basingstoke: Palgrave Macmillan).

This book covers broader governance issues (such as evidence-based practice, integrated care pathways, and clinical risk management), as well as offering an excellent guide to audit. The text is written for healthcare professionals and utilises examples from practice to support the theory presented.

References

CEMACH (Confidential Enquiry into Maternal and Child Health) (2004) *Stillbirth, Neonatal and Post Neonatal Mortality 2000–2002, England, Wales and Northern Ireland* (London: CEMACH).

Clinical Outcomes Working Group (2002) *Clinical Outcome Indicators Report* (Edinburgh: the Scottish Government).

Copeland, G. (2005) *A Practical Handbook for Clinical Audit* (London: Clinical Governance Support Team, Department of Health).

Department of Health (1989) *Working for Patients* (London: Department of Health).

Department of Health (2004) *Quality and Outcomes Guidance – Updated 2004* (London: Department of Health).

Department of Health (2007) *Saving Lives: Reducing Infection, Delivering Safe and Clean Care* (London: Department of Health).

Department of Health and Ageing (2007) *Healthy for Life* Service Toolkit – Section 8: Maternal and Child Health Clinical Audit Tools and Systems Assessment Tool. Healthy Life Healthy Community programme of the Australian Government (Canberra: Department of Health and Ageing).

Farrington-Douglas, J. and Allen, J. (2005) *Equitable Choices for Health* (London: Institute for Public Policy Research).

Hill, S.L. and Small, N. (2006) 'Differentiating between research, audit and quality improvement: Governance implications', *Clinical Governance: An International Journal*, **11**, 98–107.

Mercer, S.W., Sevar, K. and Sadutshan, T.D. (2006) 'Using clinical audit to improve the quality of obstetric care at the Tibetan Delek Hospital in North India: A longitudinal study', *Reproductive Health*, **3**, 4.

National Audit Office (2007) *About Us: The History of the National Audit Office* http://www.nao.org.uk/about/history.htm (accessed 2 August, 2007).

Ougrin, D. and Banarsee, R. (2006) 'Clinical audit', *British Medical Journal Careers*, **333**, 68–9.

Royal College of General Practitioners (1994) *Clinical Standards Advisory Guidelines – Back Pain* (London: HMSO).

Royal College of Psychiatrists (1995) *Report of the Confidential Inquiry into Homicides and Suicides by Mentally Ill People* (London: RCP).

Sorenson, C. (2007) 'Quality measurement and assurance of long-term care for older people', *Euro Observer*, **9**, 1–4.

Sparkes, V. (2005) 'Treatment of low back pain: Monitoring clinical practice through audit', *Physiotherapy*, **91**, 171–7.

Spiegelhalter, D.J. (1999) 'Surgical audit: Statistical lessons from Nightingale and Codman', *Journal of the Royal Statistical Society: Series A (Statistics in Society)*, **162**, 45–58.

The National Institute for Health and Clinical Excellence and the Commission for Health Improvement (CHI) (2002) *Principles for Best Practice in Clinical Audit* (Oxford: Radcliffe Medical Press Ltd).

UBHT (United Bristol Healthcare NHS Trust) Clinical Audit Central Office (2005) *How to Choose and Prioritise Audit Topics*. http://www.ubht.nhs.uk/clinicalaudit/docs/HowTo/Topics.pdf (accessed 7 August, 2007).

Notes

1 'Medical audit' describes assessments of medical care, whilst 'clinical audit' describes the assessment of total care – including the resources available and used, the procedures for diagnosis and treatment, and the results of clinical interventions.

2 These two examples are taken from Section 11 of the UK Children Act 2004.

Part 3

Quantitative Research

Surveys

MARION WATSON AND LINDSEY COOMBES

Introduction

A survey is a method of collecting relevant descriptive data from a number of individuals, groups or representatives of groups in order to answer a research problem or question. This chapter concentrates on quantitative surveys, but surveys can be qualitative or mixed method depending on the research question and the questioning strategy used (Trochim, 1999). Quantitative surveys aim to describe a population by collecting large amounts of factual or categorical information on sufficient numbers of that population to provide representative data which can then be statistically analysed.

In a quantitative survey, respondents are always asked the same questions in the same order and are given the same set of fixed options for their answers. There is now a wide variety of quantitative survey techniques, but two of the most common in health and social care research are the self-administered paper questionnaire and oral surveys. Oral surveys can be conducted face-to-face or by telephone (Barriball et al., 1996) and are also known as structured or standardised interviews. In recent years, developments in information technology have added electronic surveys via email or the internet (Piamjariyakul et al., 2006) and automated telephone surveys via a digital (touch-tone) phone (Baer et al., 1995).

Historical Context

The earliest documented survey was probably carried out in 500–499BC by the Persian military to determine land grants and taxation (Kuhrt, 1995). Strictly speaking, this was a census as the entire population, rather than a sample, was surveyed. The census as a survey tool is prevalent throughout history, notably across the Roman Empire. In England, one well-known early example was the Domesday Book. This was conducted for William I of England in 1086 in order to determine who owned land so that they could be appropriately taxed (http://www.domesdaybook.co.uk/). Today, national censuses are conducted in many countries, often every ten years, to help governments monitor society and plan for future needs.

Surveys have long been part of health and social care research as a tool for epidemiology; the study of the health and illness of groups and populations. The most famous early epidemiological survey is that of Dr John Snow who, in 1854, identified cholera as a waterborne disease rather than an airborne disease as previously thought. By surveying where people collected their water, Snow successfully linked an outbreak of cholera across London's Soho district to the use of a single water pump. The pump handle was removed and an immediate reduction in cholera cases followed (Paneth, 2004).

Surveys first became influential in market research through the American company ACNielsen. Founded in 1923, this company surveyed consumer activity and advertising in order to provide its business clients with reliable, objective information on the impact of their marketing and sales programmes and their competitive performance. In 1939, the company became international and, since then, has had a major influence on national survey and data analysis techniques including trend analyses, modelling to predict population behaviours, and measures of confidence in survey outcomes (http://www2.acnielsen. com/site/index.shtml).

The earliest scientifically designed large-scale surveys were, however, the political opinion polls of the American statistician George Gallup (1901–1984). Gallup sought to survey representative samples of the voting population, taking into account sampling error and potential biases, such as selection bias (minimised by large samples and random sampling) and analytical bias (minimised by strict interviewing protocols and staff training). In 1936, Gallup correctly predicted Roosevelt's landslide US presidential victory and, in 1945, Clement Atlee's surprise labour party victory in the UK. The Gallup organisation (founded in 1958) now carries out polls worldwide focusing on people's views of political issues, the economy, health and education (http://www.gallup.com/).

While early surveys were largely restricted to counting individuals' responses to fixed questions and predicting their future behaviour or outcomes of their behaviour, the development of more complex statistical techniques has in recent years resulted in more meaningful ways of analysing survey data and correspondingly increased the rigour and scientific validity of the method. In particular, the development and application of probability theory means that researchers no longer need to survey a whole population (that is, a census) – they can now be confident that their results will be accurate so long as they collect data from an appropriately selected sample of the target population (this is discussed in more detail later).

Current Use

Quantitative surveys are appropriate when researchers can clearly define questions that it is possible to answer using a limited range of responses. Survey questions often seek factual information relating to respondents' characteristics and behaviour and, in health and social care, might also aim to clarify individuals' use or knowledge of services; treatment preferences; and satisfaction with services. Questions relating to the reasons 'why' individuals think or behave as they do are usually limited to those where the main types of response have already been established by previous research or are fairly easy to determine. Survey data are then analysed to describe the characteristics or opinions of the population, differences between subgroups of the population, and correlations between pertinent variables (for example whether men or women are more likely to experience a particular health condition or whether treatment satisfaction is associated with age, gender or healthcare provider).

As indicated above, surveys can take a variety of written and oral forms. Written surveys might be administered by post, email or internet; while oral surveys can be delivered face-to-face or via the telephone. The method of delivering a survey will depend on the purpose of the research project and the population being researched. For example, postal, email, internet and telephone surveys are particularly suited to collecting data from individuals who are geographically dispersed. Nonetheless, there are limitations. Common sense dictates that a postal survey is not appropriate for individuals who have no fixed address; an email or internet survey is unsuitable for population groups who are likely to have limited access to a computer; and a telephone survey is inappropriate for individuals with hearing problems.

In contrast, face-to-face surveys are particularly useful for those with literacy problems or those who are too ill, frail or young to complete questionnaires (Smeeth et al., 2001). They can also be effective when there is a need to ask complex questions or when there are long or confusing lists of response choices. This is because face-to-face interviewers can present participants with flash cards or other visual aids to facilitate the responding process. Furthermore, a skilled interviewer can adopt a conversational style that puts participants at their ease, yet guides them smoothly along the prescribed path of questions and response alternatives (Hyman, 1955).

Surveys can also be 'cross-sectional' or 'longitudinal' in design. Cross-sectional surveys collect information once from each respondent and are sometimes described as 'snapshot' surveys. Effectively, they describe the population of interest at the time of the survey. Longitudinal surveys collect information about the same issue or same respondents at several time points to identify change (for example to follow the rehabilitation needs of patients with long-term or progressive conditions such as arthritis) (see also Chapter 10). Performance tables (such as hospital care ratings and school league tables), which are now common across the public sector, have elements of both cross-sectional and longitudinal data. So, hospital care ratings provide cross-sectional information that allows healthcare providers to be compared nationally and longitudinal data to demonstrate any changes in provision over time.

Types of Question Addressed by Surveys

- Survey questions often seek factual answers relating to respondents' characteristics and behaviour. For example a survey of adolescent drinking habits might ask:

  - Are you male/female?

  - How old were you at your last birthday?

  - How many units of alcohol do you drink per week?

  - How often do you drink more than 14 units per week?

  - Do you drink mostly wine/beer/spirits/other (please specify)?

- Surveys might also provide information on patients' use or knowledge of services, treatment preferences and satisfaction with services. For example:

  - Is there a support group for parents of children with epilepsy in your area? Yes/No/Don't Know

  - Would you say that the help you get from your social worker is: Very helpful/ Quite helpful/Neither helpful nor unhelpful/Unhelpful/Very unhelpful?

- 'Why' questions are usually limited to those where information on the main types of response has already been established by previous research or is fairly easy to determine. For example:

  - What was your main reason for travelling to the hospital by public transport today? It is too difficult to park a car/I don't have my own transport/It is quicker by public transport/It is cheaper by public transport/Public transport is more environmentally friendly/Other (please specify)

Main Strengths of Surveys

An important strength of the survey is its familiarity and simplicity. We have all experienced surveys and seen the types of information they produce (for example the national census, consumer satisfaction surveys, opinion polls and league tables). Such familiarity and simplicity are advantageous for researchers, but also for those accessing or acting on survey findings. This is because it is easy for everyone to understand what the results represent and how they have been derived. Related to this, surveys are relatively easy to conduct. Considerable amounts of data can be obtained quite rapidly from large numbers of respondents with a diverse range of characteristics, even when they are widely dispersed geographically. Furthermore, the cost of conducting a survey can be relatively low – other than researcher time, the costs may just be printing and postage.

From a research ethics perspective (see Chapters 2 and 3), surveys tend to be less intrusive for the participants than other research methods such as interviews (Trochim, 1999). Participants who do not want to complete a paper or electronic questionnaire can simply ignore it and any reminders. In addition, responses to surveys are often collected in anonymised form or can be readily anonymised after data collection (by removing the respondent's name and any other identifying details and replacing these with a code).[1] Moreover, many health and social care surveys are distributed by a third party and returned by post, so there is no direct contact between the researcher and the respondent. Such procedures meet international data protection requirements[2] and prevent individuals from being linked to their answers or identified in publications.

A further strength of quantitative surveys relates to the fact that data collection and analysis are robust to various types of bias. For example, anonymity of participants can help to promote honest responses – particularly for sensitive topics or those relating to illegal behaviours (Scott and Sechrest, 1993). In addition, researcher bias is generally low. In paper surveys, this is largely limited to poorly worded 'leading' questions,[3] which should easily be avoided by a trained researcher. Meanwhile, interviewer bias in oral surveys can generally be minimised by training and clear instructions on how questions or responses can be explained. Once collected, survey data can be analysed quickly and easily with a high level of statistical precision using a modern computer programme, such as SPSS (http://www.spss.com/spss/) or SAS (http://www.sas.com/).

Main Weaknesses of Surveys

An important problem with surveys is that, once developed and distributed, the questions and format are fixed. It is not possible to change questions midway through a survey because all the respondents need to be asked the same questions in the same way. Furthermore, there is often no contact between the researcher and respondents so problems might not emerge until the questionnaires start to be returned. These problems might be trivial typographical or numbering errors, but they might affect the results or scientific integrity of the study. Anyone who has carried out a survey will have seen that people can easily interpret the same question very differently. For example, participants' responses to 'Do you take aspirin regularly?' will be highly dependent on their interpretation of 'regularly' (for example 'every four hours', 'daily', 'weekly', 'monthly' or 'every time they are in pain').

Beyond this, responses to survey questions – and thus to surveys more broadly – lack depth and detail. Participants are presented with only limited response categories and there is generally no opportunity for them to expand, clarify or justify their answers (Wall et al., 2002). Qualitative questions or boxes for respondents to add their own comments may be included, but will usually not be completed by all participants. Equally, in a large survey, there might only be the time and resources to analyse a sample of these. Inclusion of the response options: 'don't know', 'not applicable' and 'other'[4] are often necessary for completeness, but can reduce the number of individuals providing analysable data, especially in a small survey. Overall lack of depth means that surveys often need to be supplemented by qualitative methods – such as in-depth interviews (see Chapter 14) or focus groups (see Chapter 15) – to provide richer information.

Finally, response rates to surveys are often low, despite reminders and follow-up letters (Edwards et al., 2002). In today's world, we are often bombarded by people wanting us to ask us questions while we are shopping or 'pop-up' electronic surveys while we are using the internet. This can lead to respondent fatigue, whereby people ignore surveys entirely or only half complete them. Because of this, researchers need to find ways of motivating people to complete their particular survey (including offering rewards, such as a book token or the chance to win a gift). Such procedures can, however, bias responses by attracting particular groups of participants more than others (Perneger et al., 2005). Low response levels remind us that while a survey may be distributed to a representative sample of the population, there is no control over who will complete it and so no guarantee that the returns will be representative.

MAIN STRENGTHS AND WEAKNESSES
... OF SURVEYS

Strengths

- Surveys tend to be relatively easy to conduct and to understand.

- Considerable amounts of data can be obtained quite rapidly from large numbers of geographically dispersed respondents.

- The costs of conducting a survey can be quite low.

- Surveys are relatively non-intrusive for participants (they can be easy to ignore and anonymity is usually ensured).

- Data collection and analysis are robust to various types of bias.

Weaknesses

- Once the survey has been distributed, errors cannot be corrected and questions open to misinterpretation cannot be changed or clarified.

- Quantitative surveys lack depth and may need to be supplemented by other methods, such as in-depth interviews or focus groups, to provide richer data.

- Response rates to surveys are often low. Even if a survey is distributed to a representative sample of the population, the returns may not be representative.

Conducting a Survey

The main stages in conducting a survey are described briefly below.

Clarifying the research question/study aims and target population

A survey must begin with a clear research question and/or aims and objectives (see Chapter 2), from which the researcher can determine exactly who needs to be surveyed (the target population). 'A survey of asthma incidence in children' is vague, whereas 'Comparison of rural and urban asthma incidence among 11–16-year-olds in North West England' is precise. The purpose of the survey must be communicated clearly to potential participants in order to meet ethical requirements (see Chapters 2 and 3) and, hopefully, to motivate people to take part. For example, the asthma survey may be important for the planning of services and respondents should be told this.

In clarifying the purpose of the study, the researcher should also determine what data need to be collected. In the 'Comparison of rural and urban asthma incidence among 11–16-year-olds in North West England' study, information will be required on both the incidence of asthma and factors that might logically be associated with, explain, or predict the incidence of asthma. Here, the incidence of asthma is the main variable of interest or the 'dependent' variable and factors that might be associated with, explain or predict the incidence of asthma – such as whether a young person lives in a rural or urban area, their exact age, their gender, the type of accommodation they live in, whether they smoke and whether their parents smoke and so on – are the 'independent' variables.

Ethics and governance

As with any study, ethical and governance issues must be addressed early in the development stage (also see Chapters 2 and 3). For surveys, it is important to remember that having access to names and addresses or medical notes for the provision of care does not entitle access for research purposes and so permission from the care organisation will be required. In addition, telephone surveys must comply with telephone preference regulations.[5] Although the completion of a paper or electronic survey can be taken as consent in itself, those completing an interview survey will need to provide written or recorded verbal consent.

Preparing the questionnaire

Questions for a quantitative survey can be drawn from the existing literature (including other surveys), focus groups (see Chapter 15), expert knowledge or any combination thereof. Because a quantitative survey needs to be highly structured, all questions should be numbered to ensure that they are asked in the right order and all responses should be coded to facilitate data entry and analysis. A unique identifier should also be given to each participant's questionnaire so that information is not lost or duplicated and so that any apparent inaccuracies discovered during data entry can be checked back to their source (see below on data entry and cleaning).

To facilitate statistical analyses, the data collected by the questionnaire should be continuous (numbers including decimals), categorical (non-overlapping categories, such as men or women) or ordinal (categories which have an order but no numerical value, such as tall, medium, short). These forms of data can be provided by a variety of question types, including:

● *Multiple-choice questions* – the most appropriate response is ticked or circled; for example, 'Have you ever been given access to your own medical health records?' Yes/No/Can't remember.

● *Multi-response questions* – all responses that are appropriate are ticked or circled; for example, 'Who have you consulted for healthcare in the past 12 months?' GP/Practice Nurse/Hospital Doctor/Pharmacist/Complementary Therapist/Other (please specify).

● *Likert-type scales* – these typically require the respondent to choose from one of five options on a progressive scale; for example 'strongly agree', 'agree', 'neither agree nor disagree', 'disagree', 'strongly disagree'.

● *Guttman scales* – the respondent chooses from a series of questions which form a hierarchy. These are used in social science to identify depth of understanding of a topic or extent of agreement with an issue; for example 'I believe that smoking:' May shorten my life/May make me seriously ill/May harm my health/May affect my social life /Does not have much effect on me.

● *Visual analogue scales* – the respondent identifies their position on a line or scale; for example patients might be asked to indicate the level of pain they are experiencing following treatment, where 1 is no pain at all and 10 is the worst pain imaginable. Here the numbers are indicators rather than actual measurements so they can only be used to rank responses and cannot be used for statistical calculations.

● *Rating scales* – these are similar to visual analogue scales but discrete numbers, letters or images are used rather than a continuous scale. A series of 'smilies and frownies' may work well with children. ☺ ☺ ☹ (Read et al., 2002).

In addition, some questions can be included to indicate the internal consistency of responses (that is, how consistently individuals respond to questions about the same topic). This can be achieved by asking related questions at different points and then checking the responses to ensure they are similar and the results are thus robust. For example, the question 'Are you satisfied with current training provision?' might be asked in the middle of a questionnaire and the question 'How much of a concern for you is improving training?' might be asked towards the end (see Chapter 13 for a more detailed discussion of internal consistency).

Although the number of questions asked needs to be as few as possible to minimise time and effort, there must be sufficient questions to meet the research aims. Using a variety of question types to reduce question fatigue is important because participants may answer early questions carefully but then pass over later questions or abandon the questionnaire if they become tired or bored. Sometimes, however, the researcher will actually want participants to skip questions that do not apply to them. In such situations, 'routing questions' can be used to direct the respondent to the next applicable question. For example, 'Do you take vitamin supplements? If Yes, go to question 28; if No, go to question 32'.

Simple language and a logical ordering of topics are essential to maintain participants' interest, avoid confusion, and instil confidence that the survey is well-designed and worth completing. For example, in an evaluation survey, questions on past care should ideally lead into present experiences followed by expectations for future care. Complex, difficult or sensitive questions should be placed at a point where the participant's interest is likely to have been established but before respondent fatigue has set in. Requests for demographic information (and particularly income) can make people feel uncomfortable so are often best placed at the end when the respondent is likely to feel more relaxed and less threatened (Trochim, 1999). Leading questions (see above) and questions that involve two concepts (such as 'How kind and helpful did you find the therapist?'[6]) should always be avoided since they are confusing and can jeopardise the analysis.

Any instructions to participants must also be clearly stated both at the start of the questionnaire and, as necessary, in relation to individual questions. One of the first pieces of information that needs to be conveyed is who should complete the survey. If the target population is parents of teenagers, this needs to be stated at the outset so that others do not waste their time by continuing. Once the questionnaire has been drafted, the researcher must test it out or 'pilot' it. This involves asking a small number of people from the relevant target population to fill it in and comment on its ease of understanding, content and presentation. If numerous changes are needed, the pilot stage should be repeated (as many times as necessary) with the amended survey before distribution to the final population.[7]

Sampling

Except in a census, when the entire population is questioned, most surveys investigate a sample of a population. Practical considerations, such as access to participants or their availability, may skew or compromise the quality of the sample. However, a good sample is one that is, in so far as is possible, representative of the population of interest and selected without bias. Probability sampling offers a useful approach since it utilises random selection to ensure that every member of a population has an equal probability or chance of being chosen (Altman, 1991). Probability samples include:

● *Simple random samples* – for example tossing a coin, random number generation, computer-generated random lists

● *Cluster random samples* – for example everyone attending a clinic on a particular day

● *Systematic samples* – for example every nth patient seen by a clinician

● *Stratified random samples* – the population (for example patients of a family practice) is divided into sub-categories of interest (for example gender, then age groups) and participants are randomly sampled from each group or 'stratum' separately.

Non-probability samples may also be used but are weaker methodologically since they are not likely to be representative of the population of interest. Non-probability samples include:

● *Convenience samples* – for example passers-by or visitors in a hospital canteen who just happen to be present on the day of the survey

● *Purposive samples* – selected according to predetermined criteria, for example one person from each professional role in a health centre

● *Quota samples* – a set number of participants in each of several categories are selected, for example 20 students from each year of a 3-year course

● *Snowball sampling* – where a participant is asked to pass information to others who might be interested. This is not used very often in surveys but is useful for some groups, such as patients with rare diseases, who may know others with the same condition.

If the sampling strategy employed is likely to result in a biased sample, this should be carefully justified and reporting must clearly state that the findings may not be truly representative of the study population.

Sample size

The number of participants will inevitably be tempered by pragmatism, including the availability of the target population, time and resources. Nonetheless, the sample must be big enough to have a reasonable chance of generating statistically reliable results. Sample size for individual questions can be estimated using power calculations (estimates of the likelihood of detecting differences) (Altman, 1991). A detailed discussion of power calculations is beyond the scope of this chapter but they are discussed in more detail in Chapter 11 and a useful description and illustration of sample size formulas, including the formula for adjusting sample sizes for smaller populations, is provided by Bartlett et al. (2001).

Where it is not possible to calculate statistical power, sample size is based on a careful reading of the literature to determine what has, and what has not, been sufficient for previous similar research. As indicated above, response rates to surveys are often disappointing despite reminders; usually less than 50% (Edwards et al., 2007). This must be allowed for in selecting sample size. Thus, if 200 responses are needed, a sample size of at least 500 would be advised. If, however, the sample is unnecessarily large, participant time, resources and researcher time will be wasted, which is inefficient as well as unethical.

Data entry and cleaning

For small surveys, data entry is likely to be manual (that is, typed into a spreadsheet such as Microsoft Excel or SPSS) or, for very small surveys, written by hand into a table. For larger studies, response sheets that can be scanned into a computer are ideal. Electronic surveys can, meanwhile, be programmed so that responses to all the questions are automatically fed into a spreadsheet or database ready for the researcher. Once entered, the data then have to be cleaned to remove any obvious inaccuracies.[8] To ensure that this is undertaken systematically, each question should be separately reviewed. Computer spreadsheets facilitate this by allowing the data for any selected question to be ordered (or 'sorted') and thus more easily scanned. This will quickly reveal any obvious gaps in the data or impossible answers (such as someone with an age of 208 or a height of 20 metres). Equally, frequencies (see below) for each answer can be generated to similar effect. Any corrections made must then be recorded and stored with the original data.

Data analysis

Data analysis should always be considered from the outset of a survey to guarantee that the individual questions asked will collectively generate the right information to answer the study's main question or aim and objectives. For large surveys, it is also important to seek advice from experienced survey researchers and statisticians and to identify an appropriate statistical software programme. In undertaking the analysis, a researcher can use relatively simple 'descriptive statistics' to produce basic summary information about the data and the sample and more complex 'inferential statistics' to try to draw broader conclusions about the population from the sample (for example to test whether two sample means come from the same population or to estimate or predict the properties of the broader population from the properties of the sample).

Some common descriptive statistics used in quantitative surveys include:

- *Frequencies* – counts of each reply, such as number of males or females.

- *Standard deviation (SD)* – a measure of how much the data vary from the mean, for example, the heights of all children in a school will have a higher SD than the heights of children in a single year group.

- *Standard error (SE)* – a measure of variation of sample means. The SE is effectively a type of standard deviation which measures the precision of the sample mean.

- *Confidence interval (CI)* – these are calculated from the sample mean and standard error to provide a range of values within which it is expected the true value for the entire population lies, for example if the mean age of starting to walk amongst a sample of 200 toddlers in the UK is 12 months with a 95% CI of +/– 2 months, then there is a 95% probability that the mean for all toddlers in the UK is somewhere between 10 months and 14 months.

Some common inferential statistics used in quantitative surveys include:

- *T-test (t)* – assesses whether the mean scores of two groups are statistically different from each other. There are two different *t*-tests: the independent samples *t*-test, used when the scores are provided by two separate groups; and the paired-samples *t*-test, used when the scores originate from the same group measured on two separate occasions.

- *One-way analysis of variance (ANOVA) (F)* – an extension of the independent samples *t*-test, this typically tests whether the mean scores of three or more independent groups are statistically different from each other.[9]

- *Chi-square test (χ^2)* – tests whether two or more samples, each consisting of frequency (categorical) data, differ from each other. To this end, observed frequencies are compared with what we would expect to obtain according to a specific hypothesis. For example, a chi-square test could be used to test whether the number of asthmatic young people living in an urban area is greater than would be expected if those living in urban and rural areas were equally likely to be asthmatic.

- *Correlation coefficient (r)* – describes the strength and direction of the relationship between pairs of values from two different variables and indicates how much of a change in one variable is explained by a change in the other. A correlation of +1 means that there is a perfect positive relationship, a correlation of –1 means that there is a perfect negative relationship and a correlation of 0 means that there is no relationship.

An Example of a Survey

An interesting survey on the use of herbal therapies by older, community-dwelling women in Turkey was conducted by S. Gözüm and A. Ünsal from the

Ataturk University School of Nursing in Erzurum, Turkey. The study was funded by the Ataturk University and was published in the *Journal of Advanced Nursing* (Gözüm and Ünsal, 2004).

The aims of the study were to determine the prevalence of herbal therapy use among women over 65 years of age who were living independently in the community, and to compare the socio-demographic characteristics and health status of older women who were using herbal therapies and those who were not. For the purpose of the study, herbal therapy was defined as the use of plants for medicinal purposes rather than for food consumption.

A cross-sectional design was adopted, using a random sample from primary healthcare centres in one region of Turkey. In total, 383 older participants were interviewed at five primary healthcare centres. The inclusion criteria were: being female; non-institutionalised; at least 65 years old; able to communicate verbally; and agreeing verbally to participate in the study.

The interview schedule was reviewed by three research experts for face validity (to ensure that it seemed likely to measure what it set out to measure). It was then piloted with seven older women in order to estimate the time needed for administration and to test for clarity and logical flow. The schedule included questions on perceived health status and whether conventional care was being used in conjunction with herbal therapy. Socio-economic measures included participants' age; education level; current marital status; the place where they had spent the majority of their life; whether they had any health insurance; and economic status. Questions regarding perceived health status used a visual analogue scale that ranged from one (poor) to five (excellent). Other health-related questions were designed to be similar to those in earlier prevalence studies on the use of alternative therapies.

Statistical analysis was undertaken using SPSS. Frequencies were tabulated for categorical data and mean values and standard deviations were calculated for continuous data. Participants were categorised into two groups: women who used herbal therapies and women who did not. Differences between the two groups were investigated using student *t*-tests[10] and chi-square tests.

Findings showed that 160 different types of herbal products had been used by a total of 186 respondents. Nettle and nettle seeds, lemon and lemon peel, parsley, linden and mint were the most frequently consumed herbal preparations. Herbal therapies had been used by 48.3% of the sample in the previous 12 months, but no differences in the demographic characteristics of the users and non-users were identified. Herbal therapy use was, however, substantially higher among older women who:

- reported any disability in activities of daily living

- had poor self-reported health

- had frequent physician visits

- had chronic conditions such as cardiac problems, diabetes, stroke, cancer, asthma, pneumonia or urinary problems.

The study was the first to determine the prevalence of the use of herbal therapies by older women in Turkey. Knowing that nearly 50% of older women use herbal therapy is important because healthcare providers are often unaware of this and because herbal therapy can be problematic (for example as a result of interactions with prescription drugs, delays in seeking needed care and inadequate product control). Since community health nurses are often the first healthcare providers to have contact with people seeking medical assistance, they need to understand the herbal therapies that people use. Although the study was conducted in only one area of Turkey, it could have implications for nurses working with older Turkish women who have migrated to other countries. In addition, the findings could be relevant to younger patients, as older women may recommend treatments to other family members.

Further Reading

Altman, D.G. (1991) *Practical Statistics for Medical Research* (London: Chapman and Hall).

Altman's highly regarded book is well-organised and includes descriptions of types of data, the nomenclature of describing data, and chapters on analysis. It makes good use of real data and worked examples and there is also a useful chapter on research design. The book covers much more than the kinds of statistics that survey researchers are likely to use and is quite heavy on theory – so perhaps more suited to the experienced survey researcher.

Buckingham, A. and Saunders, P. (2004) *The Survey Methods Workbook* (Cambridge: Polity Press).

This book is aimed at beginners and covers quantitative survey design, data collection and data analysis, as well as offering a useful glossary of terms. The data analysis section is particularly helpful in providing a clear overview on presenting data, applying statistical tests, using SPSS and interpreting results. The book is supported by a dedicated website http://www.surveymethods.co.uk which gives additional examples, advanced information on statistical tests and a guide to further reading.

Oppenheim, A.N. (1992) *Questionnaire Design, Interviewing and Attitude Measurement*, 2nd edn (London: Pinter).

Often recommended to students, this book provides an excellent discussion of key issues in survey design with an especially useful chapter on standardised interviews. The thorough description of survey processes is particularly useful at postgraduate level and beyond.

Schuman, H. and Presser, S. (1981) *Questions and Answers in Attitude Surveys: Experiments on Question Form, Wording and Context* (New York: Academic Press).

This is a classic book, which draws upon more than 30 national surveys to provide interesting and valuable information on both survey design and analysis. Chapters explore issues such as the effects of question order and response order; open versus closed question formats; assessing no-opinion ('don't know') responses; measuring middle opinions; acquiescence in responses; strength of opinion; and wording strategies. It is suitable for both novice and experienced survey researchers alike.

References

Altman, D.G. (1991) *Practical Statistics for Medical Research* (London: Chapman and Hall).

Baer, L., Jacobs, D.G., Cukor, P., O'Laughlen, J., Coyle, J.T. and Magruder, K.M. (1995) 'Automated telephone screening survey for depression', *The Journal of the American Medical Association*, **273**, 1943–4.

Barriball, K., Christian, S., While, A. and Bergen, A. (1996) 'The telephone survey method: A discussion paper', *Journal of Advanced Nursing*, **24**, 115–21.

Bartlett, J.E., Kotrlik, J.W. and Higgins, C.C. (2001) 'Organizational research: Determining appropriate sample size for survey research', *Information Technology, Learning and Performance Journal*, **19**, 43–50.

Edwards, P., Roberts, I., Clarke, M., DiGuiseppi, C., Pratap, S., Wentz, R. and Kwann, I. (2002) 'Increasing response rates to postal questionnaires: Systematic review', *British Medical Journal*, **324**, 1183.

Edwards, P., Roberts, I., Clarke, M., DiGuiseppi, C., Pratap, S., Wentz, R., Kwan, I. and Cooper, R. (2007) 'Methods to increase response rates to postal questionnaires', *Cochrane Database of Systematic Reviews*, 2007, (2): MR000008.

Gözüm, S. and Ünsal, A. (2004) 'Use of herbal therapies by older, community-dwelling women', *Journal of Advanced Nursing*, **46**, 171–8.

Hyman, H.H. (1955) *Interviewing in Social Research* (Chicago: University of Chicago Press).

Kuhrt, A. (1995) *The Ancient Near East c.3000–330BC* Vol 2 (London: Routledge).

Paneth, N. (2004) 'Assessing the contributions of John Snow to epidemiology: 150 years after removal of the broad street pump handle', *Epidemiology*, **15**, 514–6.

Perneger, T.V., Chamot, E. and Bovier, P.A. (2005) 'Nonresponse bias in a survey of patient perceptions of hospital care', *Medical Care*, **43**, 374–80.

Piamjariyakul, U., Bott, M.J. and Taunton, R.L. (2006) 'Issues in nursing: Strategies for an internet-based, computer-assisted telephone survey', *Western Journal of Nursing Research*, **28**, 602–9.

Read, J.C, MacFarlane, S.J. and Casey, C. (2002) *Endurability, Engagement and Expectations: Measuring Children's Fun*, paper presented at the International Design and Children Workshop, Eindhoven, The Netherlands.

Scott, A. and Sechrest, L. (1993) 'Survey research and response bias', *Proceedings of the Survey Research Methods Section* American Statistical Association, p. 238–43. http://www.amstat.org/sections/srms/proceedings/papers/1993_036.pdf (accessed 14 December, 2007).

Smeeth, L., Fletcher A.E., Stirling, S., Numes, M., Breeze, E., Ng, E., Bulpitt, C.J. and Jones, D. (2001) 'Randomised comparison of three methods of administering a screening questionnaire to elderly people: Findings from the MRC trial of the assessment and management of older people in the community', *British Medical Journal*, **323**, 1403–7.

Trochim, W.M.K. (1999) *Research Methods Knowledge Base* (Ohio: Atomic Dog Publishing). Available at: http://www.socialresearchmethods.net/kb/contents.php

Wall, C.R., DeHaven, M.J. and Oeffinger, K.C. (2002) 'Survey methodology for the uninitiated', *Journal of Family Practice*, **51**, 573–85.

Notes

1 Only an independent person who has no access to participants' responses will know how to match the code to an individual's identity.

2 The Council of Europe signed a convention on anonymity for personal data in 1981. This was followed by enactment of laws in all European countries. Similar protection of personal data is required in developed countries worldwide for the use and storage of personal data.

3 These are questions that 'lead' the respondent to a particular response. For example, 'Did you find the dosage instructions complicated?' clearly invokes the response 'Yes'.

4 The response option 'other' should normally be followed by a request that the participant 'please specify' what the 'other' was.

5 Under UK Government legislation, the Privacy and Electronic Communications (EC Directive) Regulations 2003, it is unlawful to make unsolicited direct marketing calls to individuals who have indicated that they do not want to receive such calls. http://www.tpsonline.org.uk/tps/. In the USA, similar regulations are enforced by the Federal Communications Commission http://www.fcc.gov/.

6 This double question needs to be split into two: 'How kind did you find the therapist?' and 'How helpful did you find the therapist?' This will be more meaningful to those who found the therapist kind but not helpful or helpful but not kind.

7 If the pilot study is large enough, the data analysis can also be piloted to check the validity of the questionnaire: that is, does it measure what it is supposed to measure? (see Chapter 13 for further details on validity testing).

8 This might relate to the mixing of units (such as months and years or feet and metres), typographical errors or data entry in the wrong column of a spreadsheet.

9 There are various types of ANOVA and it is important to be familiar with these in order to ensure that the right test is selected.

10 Student's t-test is used when sample sizes are small.

Cohort Studies

HAMED A. ADETUNJI, JOANNE NEALE AND NEIL WHEELER

Introduction

A cohort is a population group that is defined by a shared characteristic or experience (Friis and Sellers, 2004: 254–5; Bailey et al., 2005: 64–5). Common examples include people born in the same year, living in a defined geographical area, having the same occupation, or receiving a particular drug or medical intervention. In a cohort study, these individuals are followed up and monitored over time in order to identify salient events and changes in their lives (Lilienfeld and Stolley, 1994: 199; Bailey et al., 2005: 65). Findings can then be compared with information about the broader population from which the cohort is drawn or with information about members of another cohort that is similar except in respect of the characteristic or experience that the first cohort shared. Subgroups within the cohort (for example, men and women or different age categories) can also be compared with each other.

Cohort studies are a form of longitudinal research and are sometimes referred to as 'incidence studies' or 'follow-up studies' (Lilienfeld and Stolley, 1994: 199). Their approach is observational rather than experimental. This means that they record or observe what is happening to individuals, often over many years, without attempting to modify or intervene in their lives or environments[1] (Elwood, 2007). This observation can be done 'prospectively' (the researchers identify a cohort and monitor individuals forwards in time) or 'retrospectively' (the researchers identify a cohort and follow individuals backwards in time) (Bailey et al., 2005: 65). Within medicine and related disciplines, cohort studies commonly record instances of disease and seek to identify the likely predictors (or risk factors) of those diseases. Within the social sciences, outcomes of interest tend to include broader factors such as income, employment status, housing circumstances, and social attitudes.

Historical Context

The term 'cohort' is said to originate from the Latin *cohors*, meaning a group of soldiers who marched together (Cummings et al., 2001: 96). The very earliest cohort studies were epidemiological and retrospective in nature. For example, Weinberg's

(1913) German study of 18,212 children whose fathers and mothers had died of tuberculosis between 1873 and 1902 and Andvord's examination of the outcome of tuberculosis in successive generations in Norway (Andvord, 1930). It is, however, Wade Hampton Frost who is generally credited with introducing the expression 'cohort study' into epidemiology in 1933. Frost's work was conducted in Massachusetts, USA, and involved arranging tuberculosis mortality rates in a table,[2] with age on one axis and year of death on the other. This was done separately for males and females and meant that the incidence[3] of tuberculosis in cohorts of either sex born at different times could easily be compared (Frost, 1933).

It was not until several years later that these early 'retrospective' studies were complemented by the emergence of 'prospective' epidemiological cohort studies. One of the first and most famous of these is the Framingham Heart Study of coronary heart disease. This began in 1948 and involved more than 5,000 individuals aged between 28 and 62 years who were living in Framingham, Massachusetts. Since then, members of the cohort have been monitored every two years through a variety of methods, including review of routine records, searching hospital admissions data and cardiovascular examinations. Although the main focus of the Framingham Study was on risk factors for cardiovascular disease, the research has produced important information on many other health problems (see also Friedman, 1994).

A further high-profile early prospective cohort study – this time investigating the effects of smoking on British doctors[4] – was initiated by Doll and Hill in 1951. Noting the difficulties of accessing reliable data on smoking retrospectively, Doll and Hill designed a study that sought to provide clearer insights into the relationship between smoking and mortality, especially the association between smoking and lung cancer (Doll and Hill, 1954). An initial questionnaire was sent to over 60,000 doctors and more than 40,000 provided sufficient data for their smoking status to be determined. Follow-up of these individuals still continues and the findings have provided vital evidence of the health hazards related to tobacco.

Since the 1950s, there have been many examples of both retrospective and prospective cohort studies within epidemiology. Retrospective studies have investigated a wide range of topics, such as mortality among radiologists (Seltser and Sartwell, 1965); bacterial meningitis associated with lumbar drains (Coplin et al., 1999); atypical antipsychotic drugs and risk of ischaemic stroke (Gill et al., 2005); and long-term mortality after gastric bypass surgery (Adams et al., 2007). Prospective studies have explored issues as diverse as the effects of therapeutic irradiation (Court-Brown and Doll, 1957); longevity of atomic bomb survivors (Cologne and Preston, 2000); lung cancer and dust exposure among male Viennese workers (Moshammer and Neuberger, 2004); and the influence of maternal nutrition on the outcome of pregnancy (Mathews et al., 1999).

Cohort studies are not, however, confined to epidemiology and medicine. There is also a long tradition of cohort research within the social sciences and this is illustrated by some very influential national birth cohort studies. These involve children born over a limited period of time who are followed up periodically throughout their lives. Birth cohorts provide evidence of the processes of growing up and enable the changing nature of the life course to be charted. They are also valuable sources of data for informing policy development. In the UK, the first national birth cohort study involved 4,454 people born during a single week (3–9 March 1946) in England, Scotland and Wales. Known as the 1946 National Birth Cohort, this was designed to address a range of policy and scientific questions, particularly relating to the introduction of the National Health Service and the 1944 Education Act (Longview, 2007).

Since then, other UK birth cohort studies have included the 1958 National Child Development Study (NCDS), the 1970 British Cohort Study (BCS70) and the Millennium Cohort Study. In addition, the birth cohort model has been adopted in other countries including Finland (the North Finnish Birth Cohorts); Denmark (the Danish National Birth Cohort); Norway (the Norwegian Mother and Child Cohort Study); and Jamaica (the Jamaican Birth Cohort Study). Studies are also planned elsewhere, including France (Étude Longitudinale Française depuis l'Enfance); the US (National Children's Study); and Canada (the Canadian National Birth Cohort). Outside the UK, these birth cohort studies have mainly focused on answering epidemiological rather than social science questions. Nonetheless, the simultaneous collection of socio-economic, behavioural and environmental data – alongside health and biomedical measures – means that they also have the potential to be of great value to social scientists and policy-makers (Longview, 2007).

Two further developments in the history of cohort studies warrant mention here. First, there is the initiation – in 2006 – of the UK Biobank Project (http://www.ukbiobank.ac.uk/). This is a major medical research project designed to improve the prevention, diagnosis and treatment of a wide range of illnesses (such as cancer, heart disease, diabetes, dementia and joint problems) and to promote health throughout society. To this end, people aged between 40 and 69 years from across the UK are being invited to local assessment centres to answer questions, give samples of blood and urine, and provide some standard health measurements. Follow-up data will then be collected through routine medical and other health-related records, as well as further assessments. It is hoped that 500,000 people will participate, and analyses will provide vital new information on how health is affected by lifestyle, environment and genetic inheritance.

The second development relates to the emergence of qualitative longitudinal research, including qualitative cohort studies (Corden and Millar, 2007). As a predominantly quantitative approach, cohort studies have historically overlooked the fact that individuals' attitudes and actions are context specific. Qualitative cohort studies can, however, enable researchers to understand how and why people think and behave as they do and how and why this might change over time. This knowledge can then be used to modify behaviour and improve service provision. For example, a recent qualitative cohort study conducted in Ireland used baseline and follow-up life history interviews with 40 homeless young people to enhance understanding of their trajectories into, through and out of homelessness and to identify structural and psychological barriers to their service access and utilisation (Maycock and Vekic, 2006).

Current Use

As Doll (2001) has argued, cohort studies have changed and developed over time and there is now wide variation in the way the method is defined and understood. Since it is not possible to explore all types of cohort study within the confines of this chapter, we shall from this point onwards focus largely on the use of the technique in epidemiological research. Here cohort studies have two primary purposes. The first of these is descriptive (that is, to describe the incidence of disease outcomes over time) and the second is analytic (that is, to analyse associations between a range of potential risk factors and those disease outcomes). In so doing, cohort studies can help to establish correlation[5] between a particular risk exposure and a disease occurrence, as well as the temporal order of events (Cummings et al., 2001).

As already indicated, cohort studies can be both prospective (also known as concurrent) and retrospective (also known as historical). Since prospective studies follow cohort members into the future, it is possible to collect data specifically for a study and with full anticipation of what is needed. This increases the completeness and accuracy of the information that is collected and thereby improves the quality of the findings (Fletcher and Fletcher, 2005). In contrast, retrospective cohort studies identify groups on the basis of exposure at some point in the past and then follow them through to the present to establish the outcomes of interest retrospectively. This tends to facilitate quicker and cheaper data access than a prospective study, but the information collected is likely to be less tailored and less accurate (Katz, 2001).

A further type of cohort study is the historical prospective cohort study (also known as an ambispective cohort study) in which data are collected both retrospectively and prospectively (Friis and Sellers, 2004). In addition, it is possible to conduct a case-control study nested within a prospective or retrospective cohort study. Here, the investigator waits until the end of the data collection before identifying all of the individuals in the cohort who developed an outcome of interest (the cases). These individuals are then compared with a sample of subjects who were also part of the cohort but did not develop the outcome of interest (the controls). The nested case control design is particularly useful when predictor variables are expensive to measure and can easily be assessed at the end of the study (Cummings et al., 2001).

Because the success of a cohort study is highly dependent on being able to access good information from cohort members over a lengthy period of time, it is common for researchers to target particular groups of people for participation. For example, healthcare professionals have often been used as their knowledge of disease and interest in health issues mean that they are likely to cooperate with the research and report health problems reliably. People with health and life insurance also make good cohort members since detailed medical information about them is routinely recorded. Similarly, pregnant women have generated valuable information on pregnancy and pregnancy outcomes because they commonly use the same service provider from prenatal care through to delivery.

Additionally, some groups of individuals (such as survivors of atomic detonations or people exposed to radiation in the course of their job) have been researched because of the unusual exposures they have already experienced (Koepsell and Weiss, 2003; Friis and Sellers, 2004).

BOX 10.1

Types of Question Addressed by Epidemiological Cohort Studies

- Cohort studies can describe the incidence of disease outcomes over time. For example:

  - What is the incidence of deep vein thrombosis among women using oral contraceptives?

  - What is the increased risk of developing cancers among individuals using cellular telephones?

- Cohort studies can also analyse associations between potential risk factors and disease outcomes. For example:

  - How do the mortality rates of current smokers compare with those who have never smoked and with ex-smokers?

  - Is there a relationship between weight at birth and subsequent risk of non-insulin-dependent diabetes?

Main Strengths of Cohort Studies

Cohort studies constitute a very robust observational study design (Friedman, 1994). Importantly, they permit the collection of comprehensive quality-controlled data on a range of exposures and outcomes of interest. If this information is sufficiently detailed, it can also be used to study dose–response relationships between exposures and outcomes (Bailey et al., 2005). This means that researchers can identify the level of risk factors associated with particular diseases (not just whether their presence or absence is related). In addition, good data can be gathered on potential confounding factors,[6] so enabling investigators to control for them in their analyses (Bailey et al., 2005). Beyond this, the collection of information on exposure prior to disease onset means that cohort studies provide valuable information on the temporal sequence of exposure and health outcomes (Cummings et al., 2001; Bailey et al., 2005). This gives cohort studies more predictive power than a simple cross-sectional design, such as a survey (see Chapter 9).

A further strength of cohort studies relates to their flexibility. As indicated above, they can be conducted in a variety of ways, including retrospectively and prospectively and with opportunities for nested case control studies. Additionally, they can be undertaken using both new data collected specifically for the study (primary data) and data collected by people outwith the research team for other purposes (secondary data). Cohort studies also permit multiple outcomes related to a specific exposure to be studied simultaneously (Katz, 2001; Bailey et al., 2005). For example, the associations between exposure to radiation and various kinds of cancer as well as other diseases could be investigated within one study. Furthermore, outcomes that were not anticipated at the start of the study can still be investigated as data about them can be collected and analysed later on (Bailey et al., 2005).

Finally, cohort studies have some important practical and ethical advantages over many other study designs. Clearly, it is unethical either to subject individuals to potentially dangerous exposures (such as smoking or radiation) or to withhold from them treatments or interventions that are known to be effective. Likewise, it can be difficult to persuade individuals to participate in a study that is trialling something new, such as a drug. Cohort studies bypass these problems since the researchers simply observe and monitor participants and do not intervene in their lives at all except through the collection of data from them (Elwood, 2007). Additionally, cohort studies can be useful for investigating relatively rare exposures, such as occupational or clinical hazards. This is because participants can be deliberately selected on the basis of their exposure at the start of the study, thus ensuring that sufficient numbers of exposed individuals are included for later analyses (Gerstman, 1998; Bailey et al., 2005) – although also see below on very rare diseases.

Main Weaknesses of Cohort Studies

Like all research methods, cohort studies are not without limitations. For example, they tend to be large and involve many participants. This presents complex challenges in terms of collecting and managing the data, often across many different sites (Friis and Sellers, 2004). The size of cohort studies also creates difficulties in terms of the investment of resources they require. Collecting and analysing large amounts of data can prove very expensive, especially in staff costs (Friedman, 1994; Friis and Sellers, 2004). This is because multi-disciplinary teams – including clinicians, interviewers, researchers, and statisticians – generally have to be employed over many months and often years.

Furthermore, it can prove difficult for researchers to retain contact with large numbers of participants. High levels of attrition can, however, bias the findings as those who drop out of the research may differ in important ways from those who continue to be involved[7] (Bailey et al., 2005). During the course of the research, large numbers of people may also remain at risk because the associations between disease and exposure take a long time to be clearly demonstrated (Cummings et al., 2001). Equally, patterns of exposure or treatments may change over the course of the study in unexpected ways, so rendering the results irrelevant. Such problems are particularly problematic in the study of diseases with long latency periods (Lilienfeld and Stolley, 1994; Bailey et al., 2005).

Cohort studies can additionally be limited when studying rare diseases as prohibitively large numbers of participants may be required to ensure that sufficient cases are found (Cummings et al., 2001; Bailey et al., 2005: Fletcher and Fletcher, 2005). Beyond this, it is generally not possible to ascertain the effect that involvement in the study has on participants' behaviour or what information they should be given about their disease status or how to reduce disease risks. Thus, involvement in a study relating to nutrition might cause individuals to reflect on their diet and then modify their eating habits. Moreover, if people are found to have poor dietary habits, it might be construed as unethical not to give them information on how to eat better. Such information might then change their behaviour, so biasing the results.

Finally, it is important to remember that cohort studies are generally not able to demonstrate that a risk factor causes a particular outcome; they can only show correlation and the temporal ordering of events. This is because cohort studies can never be truly free of confounding or bias (Fletcher and Fletcher, 2005). During the course of a cohort study, participants will inevitably be subject to factors which the investigators are not measuring, either because they have not thought of them or because they are not able to record or monitor them. Ultimately, an experimental design such as a randomised controlled trial (see Chapter 11) remains the most superior methodology in terms of demonstrating causality.

MAIN STRENGTHS AND WEAKNESSES
... OF COHORT STUDIES

Strengths

- Cohort studies permit the collection of robust data on a range of exposures, outcomes and potential confounding factors.

- Cohort studies provide useful evidence of the temporal sequence of exposure and health outcomes.

- Cohort studies can be undertaken flexibly, using a range of data sources.

- Multiple outcomes/diseases related to a specific exposure can be investigated in one study.

- Because cohort studies only observe and monitor participants, they bypass many of the practical and ethical problems involved in more interventionist study designs.

- Cohort studies can be useful for investigating relatively rare exposures.

Weaknesses

- Because of their large size, cohort studies are costly to undertake and can be challenging in terms of data collection and management.

- Prospective cohort studies can take many years to complete, often leading to high levels of attrition that might bias the results.

- Cohort studies can be problematic when investigating diseases with long latency periods.

- Cohort studies are not suited to studying very rare diseases as prohibitively large numbers of participants may be required to ensure that sufficient cases are identified.

- Involvement in the study can affect participants' behaviour in unknown ways and this might affect disease outcome.

- There are ethical issues in deciding how much information should be given to participants about their disease status and how to manage risks.

- Cohort studies can never be truly free of confounding or bias and are consequently unable to demonstrate causality.

Conducting a Cohort Study

In this section, we outline some of the key stages in conducting an epidemiological cohort study.

Justify the use of the method

Since cohort studies require a major investment of time and resources, it is very important to have a clear rationale for using a cohort design rather than any other approach. The desire to examine multiple outcomes at the level of the individual within a single study is usually the strongest justification. Even so, a cohort study should not be undertaken without at least some prior research evidence that there is likely to be an association between the exposures and diseases being investigated (Friis and Sellers, 2004).

Select the study population

Cohort participants should be selected so that they are representative of the population to which the study results will be generalised.[8] In addition, they should be available for follow-up, otherwise attrition will be high and sample representativeness will deteriorate (Cummings et al., 2001). If the exposure of interest is rare, the study sample should be selected on the basis of exposure to ensure that enough exposed individuals are included to make the study viable. If the exposure of interest is commonplace, the study population can be selected before individuals are classified as either exposed or unexposed, and information on exposure can be collected later (Bailey et al., 2005). Sometimes, however, nearly all members of a cohort will have been exposed to the factor of interest. In this situation, a similar unexposed or 'comparison' group is required (Elwood, 2007).

At the outset, participants should be thoroughly briefed on what their participation in the study will likely entail. Additionally, they should give their informed consent prior to any data collection, and usually prior to each follow-up stage. At the time of the exposure of interest, the disease outcome should also not have happened so an initial assessment may be required to identify and exclude any individuals who are already diseased (Friedman, 1994). Finally, sufficient numbers of participants should be recruited to ensure that the findings generated are scientifically robust. This can be determined by the statistical power considered appropriate to detect stated increases in risk, traditionally at the 95% confidence level. Calculations for this (known as 'power calculations') can now be undertaken with freely available computer software (Silman and Macfarlane, 2002).

Collect data

To minimise the likelihood of bias, exposure, outcome and any potential confounding variables must be measured thoroughly, accurately and consistently for all study participants. To achieve this, various data collection strategies can be employed. These include conducting interviews with cohort members, asking them to complete questionnaires, collecting biological samples from them, consulting their medical or occupational records, and scrutinising other forms of routine and vital data. Initial data collection should additionally seek reliable information that will enable individuals to be traced later on. This might include contact details of participants, their relatives, close friends, employees and general practitioners, as well as their insurance or health service/hospital numbers. Follow-up data collection will often repeat earlier measurements so that disease development can be studied in relation to both initial characteristics and changes in those characteristics (Friedman, 1994).

Follow-up participants

As should by now be clear, participants must be followed up (retrospectively or prospectively) in order to identify the relationship between particular exposures and disease outcomes of interest. Follow-up can be both active and passive. When active, the researchers make direct contact with the study participants, for example by letter, phone call, or home visits in order to collect more data. When passive, the researchers do not directly contact the participants. Instead, they collect information on the measures of interest via databases maintained by other organisations – a process which is sometimes possible by record linkage between these external databases and the cohort study database (Friis and Sellers, 2004).

In prospective studies, strategies can also be adopted to help maintain a high follow-up rate. These might include periodic general contact with participants (by emails, letters, telephone calls or birthday cards) and the distribution of items at each follow-up stage that might remind individuals of their involvement in the study (for example stationery with a clear study logo). The actual duration of follow-up will be determined primarily by the number of disease cases needed to provide statistically robust answers to the study questions – a process that might take a few weeks, but more commonly requires many years. Drop-out rates should be calculated and reviewed at the end of each follow-up stage to ensure that those who remain in the study are representative of the original study sample and attrition is not going to bias the results.

Analyse the data

In order to describe the incidence of disease outcomes over time, the entire study population should be divided according to the variables presumed related to the disease. The incidence of disease in each group is then measured. If all participants have been followed up for approximately the same period of time, the incidence can be expressed in terms of the 'incidence risk'. That is, the number of new diseased individuals divided by the size of the population at risk. If follow-up times differ between participants (perhaps because many died or moved away before all of the data collection stages were complete), the 'incidence rate' is usually preferred. This is expressed as the number of new diseased individuals per person-years (or person-months or person-days and so on) of observation[9] (Friedman, 1994).

By comparing the incidence of disease (or mortality) of groups exposed to different levels of risk, associations between risk factors and disease outcomes can be assessed. Such comparisons can be calculated and expressed in different ways, but two common examples are the *relative risk* (the number of times more likely exposed people are to become diseased relative to non-exposed people) and the *attributable risk* (the difference between the disease incidence of the exposed group and the non-exposed groups). If the whole study population has been exposed to a particular risk factor, the incidence of disease or death in the cohort should be compared to those in a similar non-exposed cohort or to standardised morbidity or mortality ratios for the general population (Bailey et al., 2005).

When analysing incidence data, it is also important to consider how chance[10] and confounding might have affected the results. The role of chance can be measured by a *P*-value given by a statistical test, such as a chi-square or *t*-test. The role of confounding can be ascertained by two common techniques. First, the controls can be matched to the exposed subjects so that they have a similar pattern of exposure to the confounder. Second, statistical techniques can be used to model the risk of developing the disease, adjusted for the effects of the possible confounding factors (Lilienfeld and Stolley, 1994). Today, the widespread availability of computer software means that such modelling is relatively easy to undertake, although some statistical knowledge is required in order to ensure appropriate interpretation of the results.

An Example of a Cohort Study

An interesting example of the analysis of data from a national birth cohort study is provided by Jefferis et al. (2005). Their research: 'Adolescent drinking level and adult binge drinking in a national birth cohort' was published in the international journal, *Addiction*. The authors were based in the Centre for Paediatric Epidemiology and Biostatistics at the Institute of Child Health, London, UK and the School of Public Health and Community Medicine at The Hebrew University, Hadassah Medical Organization, Jerusalem, Israel. No specific funding was secured for the study, but the lead author of the paper (Jefferis) was supported by a UK Medical Research Council and Department of Health Special Training Fellowship. Ethical approval for the broader study on which the analyses were based had been obtained previously from a UK Multi-centre Research Ethics Committee.

Alcohol use in the UK is a major public health concern and young people who binge drink (consume large quantities of alcoholic beverages in a single session) have been the focus of much recent government policy and media attention. However, there has been little large-scale longitudinal research exploring binge drinking from youth into mid-adulthood. Using data from a nationally representative British birth cohort study (the 1958 birth cohort), the research had two aims. These were to assess:

● continuities in binge drinking across adulthood and

● the association between adolescent drinking level and adult binge drinking.

The cohort included all individuals born in England, Scotland and Wales in one week in March 1958. Two aspects of alcohol consumption (frequency of drinking and amount of drinking) were recorded at 16, 23 and 42 years. The 8,520 cohort members with complete alcohol data at all four time points were included in the analyses. Binge drinkers were identified by dividing the number of units of alcohol consumed in the last week by usual drinking frequency. Statistical models were then used to assess, *inter alia*, changes in the prevalence of binge drinking at 23, 33 and 42 years; associations between binge drinking at 23, 33 and 42 years; the effect of adolescent drinking level on adult binge drinking at each age; and adolescent drinking as a predictor of adult binge drinking across the three ages.

Prevalences of binge drinking at 23, 33 and 42 years were 37%, 28% and 31% among men and 18%, 13% and 14% among women. Although there was considerable change in binge drinking behaviour during adulthood (only 8% of men and 1% of women were binge drinkers at all three adult time points), binge drinkers at one time point were more likely to binge drink at another time point. In addition, women who rarely or never drank when aged 16 years were less likely than light drinkers to binge drink as adults, and men who were heavier drinkers at 16 years were more likely than light drinkers to binge drink throughout adulthood. The effect of adolescent drinking on adult binge drinking was similar across ages 23, 33 and 42 for men, but for women there was a stronger effect of adolescent drinking on adult binge drinking at age 42 than at ages 23 or 33.

The findings confirmed that binge drinking is common among British men and women throughout adulthood with continuities between the 20s and 40s. Men were more likely than women to be identified as binge drinkers at any age in adulthood and also at more than one age in adulthood. Additionally, teenage alcohol consumption was related to whether individuals went on to binge drink in adulthood – although the overall association was modest. The authors note that whilst binge drinking is widely recognised as a problem among young people, it is less often considered a problem among adults. Nonetheless, binge drinking is clearly common among those in their 40s, with a significant minority of men reporting sustained binge drinking throughout adulthood. The authors conclude that policies addressing binge drinking need to be directed at adults in mid-life as well as adolescents and younger adults.

Further Reading

Fletcher, R.H. and Fletcher, S.W. (2005) *Clinical Epidemiology: The Essentials,* **4th edn (Philadelphia, PA: Lippincott Williams and Wilkins).**

Fletcher and Fletcher provide a good introduction to epidemiology for medical, nursing, and other health and social care students. Chapter 5 is essentially about risk, but provides a clear explanation of how to carry out cohort studies, including an overview of some of their advantages and disadvantages. A useful table on 'cohorts and their purposes' succinctly illustrates how different types of cohort might be used in clinical research.

Friis, R.H. and Sellers, T.A. (2004) *Epidemiology for Public Health Practice,* **3rd edn (Boston, MA: Jones and Bartlett Publishers).**

This is a very simple and well-written epidemiology text, primarily aimed at public health students. Each chapter begins with clear learning objectives and an outline of what is to follow, then ends with study questions and exercises. The chapter on cohort studies (Chapter 7) enables the reader to differentiate between cohort studies and other epidemiologic study designs; list the main characteristics, advantages and disadvantages of cohort studies; and calculate and interpret a relative risk. It also contains some useful examples and summaries of major cohort studies that have taken place over the years.

Mann, C.J. (2003) 'Observational research methods. Research design II: Cohort, cross-sectional, and case-control studies', *Emergency Medical Journal*, **20**, 54–60.

Dr. Mann's paper is part of a research series, freely available from http://emj.bmj.com/. It presents observational research methods (cohort, cross-sectional and case-control studies) in a simple and concise way. Cohort studies are described as the most reliable form of observational research, and particularly valuable when randomised controlled trials are unethical. The article contains a useful section on how to run a cohort study, with some helpful box inserts and a simple diagram demonstrating cohort study design. The paper is ideal for anyone wanting a quick overview of, and guide to, observational research methods including cohort studies.

Silman, A.J. and Macfarlane, G.J. (2002) *Epidemiological Studies: A Practical Guide*, 2nd edn (Cambridge: Cambridge University Press).

This book serves as a valuable introduction for those training in epidemiology and public health, as well as others involved in medical research. Cohort studies are discussed at various points throughout the text, so the reader is advised to read or scan the book as a whole in order to understand cohort studies within their broader context. The selection of cohort study participants is clearly discussed in Chapter 9 and the analysis of cohort study data receives detailed attention in Chapter 17. In addition, the book contains many useful examples and practice exercises to guide the reader.

References

Adams, T.D., Gress, R.E., Smith, S.C., Chad Halverson, R., Simper, S.C., Rosamond, W.D., LaMonte, M.J., Stroup, A.M. and Hunt, S.C. (2007) 'Long-term mortality after gastric bypass surgery', *The New England Journal of Medicine*, **357**, 753–61.

Andvord, K.F. (1930) 'What can we learn by studying tuberculosis by generations?', *Norsk Mag Laegevidensk*, **91**, 642–60.

Bailey, L., Vardulaki, K., Langham, J. and Chandramohan, D. (2005) *Introduction to Epidemiology* (Maidenhead: Open University Press).

Cologne, J. and Preston, D. (2000) 'Longevity of atomic-bomb survivors', *The Lancet*, **356**, 303–7.

Coplin, W.M., Avellino, A.M., Kim, D.K., Winn, H.R. and Grady, M.S. (1999) 'Bacterial meningitis associated with lumbar drains: A retrospective cohort study', *Journal of Neurology, Neurosurgery and Psychiatry*, **67**, 468–73.

Corden, A. and Millar, J. (2007) 'Qualitative longitudinal research for social policy: Introduction to themed section', *Social Policy and Society*, **6**, 529–32.

Court-Brown, W.M. and Doll, R. (1957) *Leukaemia and aplastic anaemia in patients irradiated for ankylosing spondylitis* (London: Medical Research Council).

Cummings, S.R., Newman, T.B. and Hulley, S.B. (2001) 'Designing an observational study: Cohort studies'. In Hulley, S.B., Cummings, S.R., Browner, W.S., Grady, D., Hearst, N. and Newman, T.B., *Designing Clinical Research*, 2nd edn (Philadelphia, PA: Lippincott Williams and Wilkins).

Doll, R. (2001) 'Cohort studies', *Soz Preventivmed*, **46**, 75–86.

Doll, R. and Hill, A.B. (1954) 'The mortality of doctors in relation to their smoking habits: A preliminary report', *British Medical Journal*, **228**(i): 1451–5.

Elwood, M. (2007) *Critical Appraisal of Epidemiological Studies and Clinical Trials*, 3rd edn (Oxford: Oxford University Press).

Fletcher, R.H. and Fletcher, S.W. (2005) *Clinical Epidemiology: The Essentials*, 4th edn (Philadelphia, PA: Lippincott Williams and Wilkins).

Friedman, G.D. (1994) *Primer of Epidemiology*, 4th edn (New York: McGraw-Hill).

Friis, R.H. and Sellers, T.A. (2004) *Epidemiology for Public Health Practice*, 3rd edn (Boston, MA: Jones and Bartlett Publishers).

Frost, W. (1933) 'Risk of persons in familial contact with pulmonary tuberculosis', *American Journal of Public Health*, **23**, 426–32.

Gerstman, B.B. (1998). *Epidemiology Kept Simple: An Introduction to Classic and Modern Epidemiology* (New York: John Wiley and Sons).

Gill, S.S., Rochon P.A., Herrmann, N., Lee, P.E., Sykora, K., Gunraj, N., Normand, S-L.T., Gurwitz, J.H., Marras, C., Wodchis, W.P. and Mamdani, M. (2005) 'Atypical antipsychotic drugs and risk of ischemic stroke: Population-based, retrospective cohort study', *British Medical Journal*, **330**, 445.

Jefferis, B.J.M.H., Power, C. and Manor, O. (2005) 'Adolescent drinking level and adult binge drinking in a national birth cohort', *Addiction*, **100**, 543–9.

Katz, D.L. (2001) *Clinical Epidemiology and Evidence-Based Medicine: Fundamental Principles of Clinical Reasoning and Research* (Thousand Oaks, CA: Sage Publications).

Koepsell, T.D. and Weiss, N.S. (2003) *Epidemiologic Methods: Studying the Occurrence of Illness* (Oxford: Oxford University Press).

Lilienfeld, D.E. and Stolley, P.D. (1994) *Foundations of Epidemiology*, 3rd edn (Oxford: Oxford University Press).

Longview (2007) *Scientific Case for a New Birth Cohort Study*, draft report to the Research Resources Board of the Economic and Social Research Council. http://www.longviewuk.com/pages/documents/MicrosoftWord-Longviewconsolidateddraftreport_000.pdf (accessed 10 October, 2007).

Mathews, F., Yudkin, P. and Neil, A. (1999) 'Influence of maternal nutrition on outcome of pregnancy: Prospective cohort study', *British Medical Journal*, **319**, 339–43.

Maycock, P. and Vekic, K. (2006) *Understanding Youth Homelessness in Dublin City: Key Findings from the First Phase of a Longitudinal Cohort Study* (Dublin: The Stationary Office).

Moshammer, H. and Neuberger, M. (2004) 'Lung cancer and dust exposure: Results of a prospective cohort study following 3260 workers for 50 years', *Occupational and Environmental Medicine*, **61**, 157–62.

Seltser, R. and Sartwell, P.E. (1965) 'The influence of occupational exposure to radiation on the mortality of American radiologists and other medical specialists', *American Journal of Epidemiology*, **81**, 2.

Silman, A.J. and Macfarlane, G.J. (2002) *Epidemiological Studies: A Practical Guide*, 2nd edn (Cambridge: Cambridge University Press).

Weinberg, W. (1913) *Die Kinder der Tuberkuloesen* (Leipzig, Germany: S. Hirzel).

Notes

1 Panel studies are a similar form of longitudinal observational research. However, panel studies follow a broad cross section of the population over time, whereas cohort studies involve a group of individuals chosen because they share a particular characteristic or experience.

2 Known as an 'actuarial life table'.

3 The number of new cases occurring in a given population over a certain period of time.

4 Doctors were selected for the research because they could easily be followed up via their annual registration procedures and because they were considered very likely to cooperate – not because their patterns of smoking were unusual.

5 Correlation is the degree to which two factors are related or move together. For example, if risk factor X increases at the same time that disease Y increases, the two can be described as positively correlated. If one factor decreases as the other increases, they can be described as negatively correlated.

6 A confounding factor is a variable that is an independent risk factor for the outcome (disease) under study as well as being associated with the exposure under study. For example, alcohol consumption may be a confounding factor when exploring the relationship between smoking and coronary heart disease. This is because alcohol consumption is linked to both cigarette smoking and heart disease. If confounding factors are not measured and considered in the analyses, bias can result.

7 For example, they may be too ill to want to participate in the study or, conversely, they may be a very healthy group of individuals who do not see the point of being personally involved.

8 Thus, findings from a cohort study of young males cannot necessarily be generalised to older women.

9 But note that this assumes that the disease risk remains relatively constant over time. The measure would be unsuitable if the risk of disease increased or decreased sharply over time.

10 Chance is more likely to be a problem if the sample size is small.

11 Randomised Controlled Trials

LESLEY SMITH AND TERENCE J. RYAN

Introduction

A randomised controlled trial (RCT) is an experimental study in which participants are allocated at random (by chance, like the toss of a coin) to receive one of two or more possible interventions and the effects on a given outcome are assessed. There are various accepted ways of designing an RCT, but the simplest design is a 'two-arm parallel-group trial'. In this type of trial, one group receives an intervention and the other group receives a control. An intervention might be a new treatment, such as a new type of dressing for leg ulcers, and it is compared with a control: either an existing standard treatment or a placebo (a pill or procedure that does not include active ingredients).

In an RCT, participants are allocated by means of a formal process that guarantees that they all have an equal chance of being assigned to the intervention or to the control group. This ensures that the groups being compared are as similar as possible with respect to age and any other factor that might influence the effects of the intervention on the outcome(s). As a result, any differences in the outcome between groups can be attributed to the intervention and not to differences in other factors. RCTs are prospective studies, meaning that data are collected forwards in time from the start of the study. They are the most rigorous way of determining whether an intervention is responsible for causing a particular outcome; that is, whether a cause–effect relationship exists.

Historical Context

In what is often considered to be the first controlled trial, in 1747, James Lind compared six different interventions in 12 sailors with scurvy (Lind, 1753). He selected sailors 'as similar as I could have them', and all 12 consumed the same basic diet. For two weeks, five groups of two patients each received cider, elixir of vitriol, vinegar, salt water or a mixture of garlic, mustard, horseradish, balsam and gum myrrh; the remaining group of two people received two oranges and one lemon daily for six days only, due to limited supplies. Two weeks later, the sailors in the 'oranges and lemon' group compared very favourably with the other five groups. One of the 'oranges and lemon' group was fit enough to return to work, and the other was appointed as a nurse to the remaining sick sailors. Although the results appeared conclusive, it was still 50 years before the British Navy supplied lemon juice to its ships. A delay in applying trial evidence to current practice and policy is not uncommon even today.

Over the next 100 years, there was increasing recognition of the importance of quantitative approaches for the evaluation of different therapies. Therapeutic evaluation became more common in the British Army and Navy, in particular. One of the earliest accounts of so-called 'alternate allocation' to generate groups for comparison was described in the Edinburgh doctoral thesis of Alexander Hamilton (Hamilton, 1816). Hamilton, together with two colleagues, evaluated the practice of blood-letting. The trial involved 366 sick soldiers 'admitted alternately in such a manner that each of us had one third of the whole. The sick were indiscriminately received, but [were] attended as nearly as possible with the same care and accommodated with the same comforts ... neither Mr. Anderson nor I once employed the lancet. He lost two, I four cases: whilst out of the other third [treated with blood-letting by the third surgeon] thirty-five soldiers died'. Despite being considered one of the most advanced methodological steps achieved at that time, the study was little known outside the circles of Edinburgh and the Army Medical Corps.

R.A. Fisher is regarded as a key figure in introducing the concept of randomisation, rather than simple alternate allocation, in agriculture studies in the 1920s (Fisher, 1926). Reports of trials of the whooping cough vaccine in the USA and UK from the 1930s established the language of the 'well-controlled' trial. However, it was the work of Sir Austin Bradford Hill that was the driving force behind the development and use of RCTs for the British Medical Research Council (MRC). The first clinical trial with a properly randomised control group compared the allocation of streptomycin and bed rest with bed rest alone for the treatment of pulmonary tuberculosis in 1948 (Medical Research Council, 1948). After 6 months, 4 deaths were reported for 55 patients treated with streptomycin and bed rest, compared with 15 deaths in 52 patients receiving bed rest alone.

With the advent of the National Health Service (NHS) in the UK in 1948, there were no limits to prescribing medications for different conditions. This led to questions about over-generous prescribing, as well as about the side effects of many medications. In 1972, Archie Cochrane, an influential medical researcher and former director of the MRC, expressed anxiety about this state of affairs (Cochrane, 1972). In his statement, he singled out Sir Austin Bradford Hill's experience that, with statistics, proof of the effectiveness of given interventions is possible. Moreover, what was once opinion could be upgraded to 'I know because there is good evidence based on measurement' (Cochrane, 1972). Such proof has subsequently become an expectation of best practice. Over the past 50 years, RCTs have continued to provide reliable answers to many important clinical and social questions.

Current Use

Even the most well-intentioned practitioners may do their patients more harm than good if they prescribe the wrong therapy. Practitioners, therefore, have a responsibility to choose the most appropriate treatment for their patients. Nonetheless, an RCT is only required if a practitioner or researcher is genuinely in doubt about which intervention is the most efficacious and safe.

The MRC CRASH Trial in 2004 was a landmark RCT that led to an important life-saving change (CRASH Trial Collaborators, 2004). For decades, intravenous corticosteroids had been given to reduce brain irritation and swelling after head injury. The MRC CRASH RCT enrolled 10,000 patients and showed that the death rate was significantly higher in those treated with corticosteroids (25.7%) compared with those treated with placebo (22.3%); relative risk 1.15 (95% confidence interval: 1.07, 1.24; $p = 0.0001$). This provided clear evidence that treatment with corticosteroids following head injury affords no benefit and should not routinely be used.

The principles of evidence-based medicine require studies that have minimised bias in order to guide clinical decision-making. RCTs provide the most robust evidence when it comes to evaluating the effectiveness of different interventions. Many clinical practice guidelines are based on the results of high-quality RCTs, and policy-makers increasingly look to evidence derived from RCTs to guide decision-making. RCTs have been widely employed in healthcare, and are increasingly being used in other fields, such as education, criminal justice and social care. RCTs are also required by regulatory bodies as proof of efficacy and safety before licensing all new medicines (see http://www.fda.gov/ and http://www.mhra.gov.uk/home/).

Reflecting their greater ability to detect cause–effect relationships, RCTs have on a number of occasions overturned the results of less robust study designs.[1] One such example relates to hormone replacement therapy (HRT) and cardiovascular disease. The best-quality cohort studies (see Chapter 10) consistently demonstrated that women taking HRT showed a 50% lower risk of cardiovascular disease than women not taking HRT (Stampfer and Colditz, 1991). In contrast, RCTs failed to show such a benefit (Hulley et al., 1998; Rossouw et al., 2002; Lawlor and Smith, 2006). The protective effect of HRT found in the cohort studies has since been attributed to the fact that the women who were given HRT differed in important ways from the women who were not given HRT, and the investigators were either unaware of these differences or did not measure them. The technical term for this problem is 'residual confounding'.[2]

One should not, however, automatically discount the effects of interventions which have not been subjected to the rigour of an RCT. Penicillin, for example, did not require an RCT to prove its effectiveness. Indeed, penicillin's efficacy was demonstrated using very few patients. Nonetheless, examples like this are rare, and a lack of randomisation will often produce misleading results (Pocock and Elbourne, 2000). RCTs are often reserved for mature research questions, when other levels of evidence have suggested that a particular intervention may be promising and that it needs further investigation using a more robust design.

BOX 11.1

Types of Question Addressed by RCTs

- Is aspirin more effective than placebo for the treatment of acute dental pain?

- Does adding fluoride to public water supplies prevent dental caries in the general population?

- Is an individual placement and support programme more effective than usual vocational services for helping people who have severe mental illness to gain competitive employment?

- Does a monetary incentive increase the rate of return of a postal health and development questionnaire?

Main Strengths of RCTs

An RCT is a powerful experimental method for evaluating the effectiveness of an intervention. The most important strength of RCTs is the reduction of confounding (see above) and selection bias.[3] Selection bias may be introduced if the investigator presumes that one treatment is more effective than another and, therefore, preferentially allocates a participant to a particular group. It can also be introduced unintentionally. RCTs ensure that, as far as possible at the start of the study, the groups are similar with respect to the number of participants, age, sex, disease status and other factors that might influence the intended effect of the intervention under investigation. This reduction of selection and confounding bias allows strong inferences about causality to be made and helps to ensure that a study has high internal validity.[4]

Another major advantage of RCTs is that they facilitate so-called 'double blinding'. Double blinding is when both investigators and participants are unaware of the group to which participants are assigned, so they will not be influenced by that knowledge. For example, in a placebo-controlled study, an investigator who knows which participants have received a placebo may provide support to these participants in addition to the placebo, which the intervention group does not receive. Double blinding prevents any such unequal provision of care. Equally, double blinding prevents knowledge of group assignment influencing the outcome assessment. This is particularly important when the outcomes are subjective, such as pain.[5] Indeed, studies with no or inadequate double blinding may overestimate treatment effects by as much as 17% (Schulz et al., 1995; Juni et al., 2001).

An additional strength of RCTs is that they permit the analysis of outcome results by what is known as intention-to-treat (ITT). In ITT analyses, outcomes are compared for all participants according to their group assignment, regardless of the participants' degree of compliance with the intervention. An ITT analysis prevents bias resulting from loss of participants, and preserves the balance achieved by the randomisation process. An alternative to ITT is to analyse participants who comply with the intervention or participants who complete the study. However, the danger of these alternative approaches is that participants who withdraw from a study may be different from those who complete the study. For example, in one trial, 153 parents were randomly assigned to a parenting programme called 'Sure Start' or to a waiting list control group (Hutchings et al., 2007). Of those parents assigned to 'Sure Start', 18/104 (17%) were lost to follow-up six months later, compared with only 2/49 (4%) in the control group. If parents who were lost to follow-up were eliminated from the analysis, meaning that only study completers were analysed, the effectiveness of the intervention would have been overestimated. An ITT analysis provides the benefit of a more conservative estimate of the effectiveness of an intervention in the real world.

A further strength, although one not confined to RCTs, is that their prospective design allows more control over measurement and ensures that data collection is consistent and more complete than studies where data are collected retrospectively (see also Chapter 10, Cohort Studies).

Main Weaknesses of RCTs

The most common criticism of RCTs is that participants are often not typical of those seen in clinical practice. For example, in venous ulcer management trials, patients with any of the following common problems are typically ineligible for RCTs: arterial disease, diabetes, rheumatoid arthritis, active infection of the ulcer bed or inability to comply with therapy due to dementia or immobility. Because of this, critics say that RCTs lack external validity.[6]

Another important limitation is the fact that RCTs are not ideal, or even feasible, for answering many important clinical and social questions. This is often the case when researching disorders that are rare or that have a long latent period (such as determining the risk factors for a rare skin disorder, or the incidence of brain tumours with mobile phone use). RCTs are also limited by ethical concerns. It would be unethical, for example, to conduct an RCT to determine birth defects caused by alcohol exposure in pregnancy. Furthermore, exposing patients to an intervention that is believed to be inferior to current treatment is often considered unethical.

A third limiting factor is that RCTs are generally time-consuming and can be expensive. This is due to the need for large numbers of participants and adequate monitoring of the trial conduct and data collection. In poorer countries, it may be considered that the money required to conduct an RCT would be better spent in other ways. In addition, another study design, such as a case-control study, may be more appropriate if answers to an important research question are required quickly.

A final weakness, though one that is not limited to RCTs, is that, in practice, many trials are statistically underpowered and fail to detect important differences between interventions. This sometimes results in effective interventions not being recognised and used as soon as they should be (Antman et al., 1992). It can even lead to ineffective interventions being used (Petrosino et al., 2002; CRASH Trial Collaborators, 2004).

MAIN STRENGTHS AND WEAKNESSES
... OF RCTs

Strengths

- Random allocation ensures that there are no systematic differences between groups, so that a cause–effect relationship can be inferred (high internal validity).

- Double blinding in RCTs ensures that the preconceived views of participants and investigators do not systematically bias assessment of the outcome.

- Intention-to-treat (ITT) analyses in RCTs preserve the balance achieved by randomisation, which can be lost if participants withdraw because of treatment-related reasons.

- The prospective design of RCTs permits more accurate data collection than is possible in studies using a retrospective design.

Weaknesses

- The use of restrictive eligibility criteria in RCTs may limit the extrapolation of results to a broader population group.

- RCTs are limited by ethical concerns and issues relating to feasibility.

- RCTs are generally more costly and time-consuming than other research designs.

- Many RCTS have too few participants to detect clinically meaningful effects.

Conducting an RCT

Although the 'two-arm parallel-group' model is the most common RCT model, there are others too, such as factorial, crossover, cluster, multi-arm and n-of-one trials. For a thorough description of alternative trial designs, see Pocock (1983) and Friedman et al. (1998). These other models raise complex issues in their design and analysis due to the multiplicity of comparisons that can be made. In this section, we cover issues relating to the two-arm parallel-group trial only.

Defining the question

A clearly defined study question is of paramount importance and needs to consider: which participants are eligible, what is the intervention and with what will it be compared, and which outcomes will be assessed? The PICO framework described in Chapter 5 is of use here.

Eligibility criteria – who are the participants?

Having defined the question to be answered, the next step is to define the eligibility criteria. Participants in the trial should be representative of those people to whom the study findings may be applicable in the future. Additionally, it is important to optimise the expected effectiveness of the intervention being studied by recruiting participants most likely to benefit. For example, in a trial investigating the effect of a drug on migraine head-aches, investigators would not want to recruit people who rarely get migraines, as the likelihood of detecting a decrease in the frequency of head-aches would be limited. Instead, investigators would recruit participants who frequently suffer from migraine headaches. Further goals of eligibility criteria are to optimise participant compliance with the protocol and recruitment. For outcomes that occur rarely, such as hip fracture, it is necessary to recruit participants at high risk of the outcome in order to minimise both the number of participants required and the length of follow-up. However, this in turn reduces the generalisability of the study and, as fewer people are eligible, makes recruitment more difficult.

Some exclusion criteria are sensible. For example, it would be unethical to recruit a particular patient group for whom the study treatment would be harmful. Often, exclusion is of the very young or very old, women of child-bearing potential or already pregnant, or those with common diseases, such as diabetes or severe hypertension. Whilst this may be desirable in terms of limiting risk to the participants, it does have an adverse impact on generalisability and potential recruitment to the trial.

Choice of intervention and control groups

Having recruited participants to the RCT, the next stage is to choose the intervention and control groups. In an RCT, the intervention of interest is assessed against either a placebo or against another intervention, or the intervention is compared at different dosages, intensities or frequencies. If a placebo control is to be used, it must mimic all aspects of the real intervention except those that have beneficial effects (Hammerschlag and Zwickey, 2006). If the way the intervention works is unknown, it will not be possible to design an appropriate placebo.

Choice of outcome

In designing an RCT, there should always be a single predefined primary outcome that answers the question posed by the investigators, and for which the sample size is calculated (see below). Secondary outcomes may also be assessed but are afforded less attention. Any outcome should be of clinical and social relevance – all too often, investigators measure what is measurable rather than what is important. The outcome(s) should be evaluated using valid and reliable tools (see Chapter 13 for more details). Adapting an existing measurement scale without demonstrating that it is sensitive to what it sets out to measure lacks credibility. Consideration should also be given to evaluating any unintended effects of the intervention. Friedman et al. (1998) provide a thorough discussion of outcome measures.

Randomisation

Adequate randomisation requires that the procedure used to generate the randomisation schedule is truly unpredictable and that the assignment schedule is tamper-proof (Schulz and Grimes, 2002a; Schultz and Grimes, 2002b). Typically, a computer-generated code is used, but methods such as tossing a coin, drawing lots or rolling a die are also adequate for generating a random sequence. It is important to ensure that the code cannot be tampered with or deciphered, so that the schedule of assignments is concealed from investigators. Schedules based on random numbers are more likely to remain concealed than schedules based on hospital numbers or dates of birth. Concealment protects the study from bias up to and including the point of randomisation (Schultz and Grimes, 2002b).

Simple randomisation may not achieve equally balanced groups if the sample size is small, so stratified randomisation[7] may be used. For example, in a trial of women with breast cancer, it may be important to have similar numbers of pre- and post-menopausal women in each comparison group. To achieve this, women are first divided into subgroups based on menopausal status, and then each subgroup is randomised using a separate allocation schedule.

Double blinding

Although an important facet of an RCT, double blinding can be difficult to achieve. For example, it may not always be possible, as with Chinese herbal mixtures, to prepare identical placebo mixtures, or it may be that it is too expensive to manufacture a placebo. In addition, double blinding may not be feasible for interventions such as physiotherapy regimens or acupuncture where participants tend to know that they have received an intervention – although some RCTs have attempted to double blind participants by using sham or mock treatments (Smith et al., 2000; Carroll et al., 2001; Leibing et al., 2002) or by employing a third-party observer who is unaware of treatment assignment to conduct the outcome assessment (Burns et al., 2007; Haake et al., 2007).

Sample size and power calculations

One of the most important parts of designing an RCT is estimating the number of participants required to detect the expected effect of the intervention. The smaller the expected effect, the larger the sample size required to infer, with adequate statistical power,[8] that the effect is unlikely to be due to chance. For example, we may wish to compare the morbidity rate in participants assigned to a new intervention compared with participants assigned to existing therapy, where we expect the new intervention to reduce morbidity by 10%. To be able to detect a difference of 10% with a probability of 80% (power), we need 80 participants in each group. If the expected difference is increased to 20%, we would need 40 participants. Conversely, if the expected reduction in morbidity was as little as 1%, about 8,000 participants would be required.

One of the challenges in calculating an adequate sample size is to choose the size of the effect that would ideally be detected, or that is of clinical or social importance. An informed guess about a likely difference can be made from reviewing existing studies. In their absence, a small pilot study may be a helpful method to gather this information.

Trials with too few participants to detect meaningful differences are wasteful and may produce misleading results (Williams and Seed, 1993). One example of an inadequately sized trial is a study of 19 children with atopic eczema (of whom 4 were later withdrawn) which compared once-daily hydrocortisone ointment and wet wraps treatment with twice-daily hydrocortisone with no wraps (Sladden et al., 2005). The authors correctly stated that a significant difference between the two treatment regimens was not shown, but then concluded that there was no difference (that is, they were equally effective) and that the added inconvenience of wet wrapping was not justified. The lack of statistical power in this study downgraded what may in fact be a useful regimen.

Subgroup analysis

It is tempting, when an RCT has shown that an intervention (such as a new drug) has no advantage, to seek some advantage in subgroup analyses (comparisons between randomised groups in a subset of the study sample). However, this is often problematic because sample sizes in subgroups are frequently small and therefore lack statistical power. They are also prone to Type I errors (attributing a difference to an intervention when chance is a more likely explanation) as a result of conducting multiple statistical comparisons. Nonetheless, with due care, subgroup analyses can contribute useful information. In order to preserve the benefit of randomisation, subgroups should be defined a priori, and should ideally be based on a stratified factor – for example, comparing the effect of an intervention in pre-menopausal and post-menopausal women separately.

Publication of results

Once completed, the RCT should be published, even if the outcome is not what was expected, and it should be written up in accordance with the CONSORT[9] statement (Moher et al., 2001). Registration of the trial protocol with a clinical trials register, such as that administered by the UK Cochrane Centre, ensures that the trial will be tracked for full and unbiased reporting of the results for public benefit (Abaid et al., 2007).

An Example of an RCT

One interesting example of a simple trial addressing a clinically relevant question is provided by Heggie et al. (2002). An RCT was conducted by a team of research nurses at the Queensland Radium Institute (QRI), Brisbane, Australia, in order to determine if topical aloe vera gel would be more beneficial than aqueous cream in reducing skin reactions in women undergoing post-operative radiotherapy to the breast. Additional aims of the RCT were to evaluate the effects of other factors thought to influence the severity of skin reactions due to radiotherapy. The aloe vera gel was supplied by Aloe Vera Industries, but no further funding for the study was provided.

Standard care advice for patients undergoing radiotherapy at the QRI, Brisbane, included avoiding use of soaps, creams or powders in the affected area. Anecdotal evidence and a small pilot study suggested that topical aloe vera gel may be more beneficial than either aqueous cream or no cream in reducing skin irritation in women following radiotherapy to the breast after surgery.

Women were eligible for the RCT if they were over 18 years of age, and if they had undergone a lumpectomy or partial mastectomy for breast cancer and received radiotherapy. Eligible women were randomised to either topical 98% aloe vera gel or topical aqueous cream to be applied to the irradiated breast three times daily throughout, and for two further weeks after radiotherapy. In addition to the topical applications, routine skin care advice was given to all women by nursing staff. The irradiated area was inspected by a research nurse weekly during radiotherapy and two weeks after the final treatment. Outcomes assessed were: redness, extent of treatment area affected by dry or moist desquamation (shedding of outer layers of the skin), and women's subjective rating of pain and itching.

Randomisation in this RCT was achieved using a computer-generated code, which was concealed from the researchers. Women were stratified by bra size, history of post-operative lymphocele[10] drainage and smoking status. The study was described as double blind, but the gel and cream were of different appearance and consistency, so participants may have guessed which preparation they received (however, the women were asked not to disclose this to the researchers). If moist desquamation occurred, study preparation was discontinued and dressings were applied until healed; weekly skin assessments continued.

A total of 225 women were randomised, and 17 were excluded from the analysis (9 from the aqueous and 8 from the aloe vera group). Of the 17 excluded participants, 2 refused to continue to participate, 12 were ineligible and 3 developed an allergic reaction to the assigned preparation: 2 in the aloe vera group and 1 in the aqueous cream group. Thus, 208 women were included in the analyses: 107 in the aloe vera group and 101 in the aqueous cream group. The median age of the women studied in the RCT was 57.5 years (range 28–89 years).

At follow-up, no significant difference was found between aloe vera gel and aqueous cream for itching, redness or moist desquamation. However, aqueous cream was significantly better than aloe vera for reducing the incidence of any dry desquamation and moderate or more pain related to treatment. For important predictors of radiation skin reactions, few significant differences were found in subgroup analyses. Women who had undergone lymphocele drainage experienced significantly less pain with aqueous cream than with aloe vera gel, and women with a bra size greater than D cup experienced more redness than women with smaller bra sizes, regardless of their treatment group.

Findings did not therefore support the hypothesis suggested by anecdotal evidence or the pilot study. The authors concluded that aqueous cream is superior to aloe vera gel in reducing acute radiation skin reactions, dry desquamation and pain. Based on these findings, clinical guidelines for the QRI recommended that aqueous cream or a similar mild moisturising agent is sufficient for use on skin during post-operative radiation treatment.

Further Reading

Friedman, L.M., Furberg, C.D. and DeMets, D.L. (1996) *Fundamentals of Clinical Trials*, **3rd edn (New York: Springer).**

This book is intended for the clinical researcher interested in developing a protocol and designing a trial. Prior understanding of statistics, whilst useful, is not essential in order to understand the text. The book is also of value for healthcare researchers and practitioners who are interested in the critical appraisal of published clinical trials. The book covers the development of a protocol; randomisation procedures; outcome assessment; sample size calculation; trial management procedures, such as interim analysis and data monitoring; and statistical analysis.

Jadad, A.R. and Enkin, M.W. (2007) *Randomised Controlled Trials: Questions, Answers and Musings*, **2nd edn (Oxford: Blackwell BMJ Books).**

This book presents a clear and accessible account of the basic principles and procedures of RCTs and their role in healthcare. Each chapter is structured in a highly readable format covering issues of design, conduct, analysis and interpretation. At the end of each chapter, the authors highlight their personal thoughts and experiences of trials in healthcare decision-making. This second edition provides broad coverage of the ethics of RCTs and challenges the overreliance on trials in modern healthcare. The authors debate the strengths and weaknesses of RCTs and discuss their optimal use.

Pocock, S.J. (1983) *Clinical Trials: A Practical Approach* **(Toronto, ON: John Wiley and Sons).**

Although published 25 years ago, this accessible book is essential reading for anyone wishing to acquire a good understanding of clinical trials. It is a comprehensive text which covers the principles and practice of clinical trials, giving a detailed account of how to conduct trials and also providing a general perspective on their historical development, current status and future strategy. It covers all stages of clinical trial design, analysis and interpretation, and is written in a non-technical manner using examples of actual trials. Statistical methods are clearly explained for the non-statistician. The book will be of value to those starting out in the field of clinical trials, but also to the more experienced researcher or clinician.

References

Abaid, L.N., Grimes, D.A. and Schulz, K.F. (2007) 'Reducing publication bias through trial registration', *Obstetrics and Gynecology*, **109**, 1434–7.

Antman, E.M., Lau, J., Kupelnick, B., Mosteller, F. and Chalmers, T.C. (1992) 'A comparison of results of meta-analyses of randomized control trials and recommendations of clinical experts. Treatments for myocardial infarction', *Journal of the American Medical Association*, **268**, 240–8.

Burns, E., Zobbi, V., Panzeri, D., Oskrochi, R. and Regalia, A. (2007) 'Aromatherapy in childbirth: A pilot randomised controlled trial', *British Journal of Obstetrics and Gynaecology*, **114**, 838–44.

Carroll, D., Moore, R.A., McQuay, H.J., Fairman, F., Tramer, M. and Leijon, G. (2001) 'Transcutaneous electrical nerve stimulation (TENS) for chronic pain', *Cochrane Database Systematic Reviews*, CD003222.

Cochrane, A.L. (1972) *Effectiveness and Efficiency: Random Reflections on Health Services* (Oxford: Nuffield Provincial Hospitals Trust).

CRASH Trial Collaborators (2004) 'Effect of intravenous corticosteroids on death within 14 days in 10,008 adults with clinically significant head injury (MRC CRASH trial)', *The Lancet*, **364**, 1321–8.

Fisher, R.A. (1926) 'The arrangement of field experiments', *Journal of Ministry of Agriculture of Great Britain*, **33**, 503–13.

Friedman, L.M., Furberg, C.D. and DeMets, D.L. (1998) *Fundamentals of Clinical Trials*, 3rd edn (New York: Springer).

Haake, M., Muller, H.H., Schade-Brittinger, C., Basler, H.D., Schafer, H., Maier, C., Endres, H.G., Trampisch, H.J. and Molsberger, A. (2007) 'German acupuncture trials (GERAC) for chronic low back pain: Randomized, multicenter, blinded, parallel-group trial with 3 groups', *Archives of Internal Medicine*, **167**, 1892–8.

Hamilton, A.L. (1816) *Dissertatio Medica Inauguralis De Synocho Castrensi* (Edinburgh: J Ballantyne).

Hammerschlag, R. and Zwickey, H. (2006) 'Evidence-based complementary and alternative medicine: Back to basics', *Journal of Alternative and Complementary Medicine*, **12**, 349–50.

Heggie, S., Bryant, G.P., Tripcony, L., Keller, J., Rose, P., Glendenning, M. and Heath, J. (2002) 'A Phase III study on the efficacy of topical aloe vera gel on irradiated breast tissue', *Cancer Nursing*, **25**, 442–51.

Hulley, S., Grady, D., Bush, T., Furberg, C., Herrington, D., Riggs, B. and Vittinghoff, E. (1998) 'Randomized trial of estrogen plus progestin for secondary prevention of coronary heart disease in postmenopausal women' *Journal of the American Medical Association*, **280**, 605–13.

Hutchings, J., Gardner, F., Bywater, T., Daley, D., Whitaker, C., Jones, K., Eames, C. and Edwards, R.T. (2007) 'Parenting intervention in Sure Start services for children at risk of developing conduct disorder: Pragmatic randomised controlled trial', *British Medical Journal*, **334**, 678.

Juni, P., Altman, D.G. and Egger, M. (2001) 'Systematic reviews in health care: Assessing the quality of controlled clinical trials', *British Medical Journal*, **323**, 42–6.

Lawlor, D.A. and Smith, G.D. (2006) 'Cardiovascular risk and hormone replacement therapy', *Current Opinion in Obstetrics and Gynecology*, **18**, 658–65.

Leibing, E., Leonhardt, U., Koster, G., Goerlitz, A., Rosenfeldt, J.A., Hilgers, R. and Ramadori, G. (2002) 'Acupuncture treatment of chronic low-back pain – a randomized, blinded, placebo-controlled trial with 9-month follow-up', *Pain*, **96**, 189–96.

Lind, J. (1753) *A Treatise of the Scurvey: In Three Parts. Containing an Inquiry into the Nature, Causes and Cure of that Disease. Together with a Critical and Chronological View of what has been Published on the Subject* (Edinburgh: Kincaid and Donaldson).

Medical Research Council (1948) 'Streptomycin treatment of pulmonary tuberculosis', *British Medical Journal*, **ii**, 769–82.

Moher, D., Schulz, K.F. and Altman, D.G. (2001) 'The CONSORT statement: Revised recommendations for improving the quality of reports of parallel-group randomised trials', *The Lancet*, **357**, 1191–4.

Petrosino, A., Turpin-Petrosino, C. and Buehler, J. (2002) '"Scared Straight"and other juvenile awareness programs for preventing juvenile delinquency', *Cochrane Database Systematic Reviews*, CD002796.

Pocock, S.J. (1983) *Clinical Trials: A Practical Approach* (Toronto, ON: John Wiley and Sons).

Pocock, S.J. and Elbourne, D.R. (2000) 'Randomized trials or observational tribulations?', *New England Journal of Medicine*, **342**, 1907–9.

Rossouw, J.E., Anderson, G.L., Prentice, R.L., LaCroix, A.Z., Kooperberg, C., Stefanick, M.L., Jackson, R.D., Beresford, S.A., Howard, B.V., Johnson, K.C., Kotchen, J.M. and Ockene, J. (2002) 'Risks and benefits of estrogen plus progestin in healthy postmenopausal women: Principal results from the Women's Health Initiative randomized controlled trial', *Journal of the American Medical Association*, **288**, 321–33.

Schulz, K.F. and Grimes, D.A. (2002a) 'Generation of allocation sequences in randomised trials: Chance, not choice', *The Lancet*, **359**, 515–19.

Schulz, K.F. and Grimes, D.A. (2002b) 'Allocation concealment in randomised trials: Defending against deciphering', *The Lancet*, **359**, 614–18.

Schulz, K.F., Chalmers, I., Hayes, R.J. and Altman, D.G. (1995) 'Empirical evidence of bias. Dimensions of methodological quality associated with estimates of treatment effects in controlled trials', *Journal of the American Medical Association*, **273**, 408–12.

Sladden, M.J., Mortimer, N.J. and Milligan, A.M. (2005) 'Wet wraps in atopic eczema: The dangers of inadequately sized "negative" clinical trials', *Clinical and Experimental Dermatology*, **30**, 454–6.

Smith, L.A., Oldman, A.D., McQuay, H.J. and Moore, R.A. (2000) 'Teasing apart quality and validity in systematic reviews: An example from acupuncture trials in chronic neck and back pain', *Pain*, **86**, 119–32.

Stampfer M.J. and Colditz G.A. (1991) 'Estrogen replacement therapy and coronary heart disease: A quantitative assessment of the epidemiologic evidence', *Preventive Medicine*, **20**, 47–63.

Williams H.C. and Seed P. (1993) 'Inadequate size of "negative" clinical trials in dermatology', *British Journal of Dermatology*, **128**, 317–26.

Notes

1 Although other study designs can detect the relationship between an intervention and an outcome, they do not rule out the possibility that the observed relationship was caused by some other third factor.

2 The measure of the effect of an intervention is distorted due to the association of the intervention with some other factor(s) that influences the outcome under investigation.

3 Systematic differences between the groups being compared in prognosis or in responsiveness to treatment.

4 The extent to which systematic error (bias) is minimised in clinical trials.

5 Objective outcomes (such as birth and death) or biochemical measurements (such as drug metabolites present in urine) leave little room for bias.

6 The extent to which the results of trials provide a correct basis for generalisation to other circumstances.

7 Stratified randomisation is used to ensure that equal numbers of participants with a characteristic thought to affect prognosis or response to the intervention will be allocated to each comparison group.

8 Power is a measure of the certainty of avoiding a false negative conclusion that an intervention is not effective when in truth it is effective.

9 Consolidated Standards of Reporting Trials – this statement provides guidance to researchers on how best to report a trial.

10 A mass surrounded by an abnormal sac that contains lymph (fluid that is collected from tissues throughout the body).

12 Economic Evaluations

DAVID R. FOXCROFT AND HAMED A. ADETUNJI

Introduction

Health and social care decision-makers and policy-makers need to make choices about how limited resources and budgets are to be distributed between competing interventions and services. Because there is never enough money to cover all of society's needs at all times, either in developed or developing countries, it is helpful if good evidence is available on the costs and benefits of services and interventions. Economic evaluation provides a logical and explicit framework which enables decision-makers, government and society to make choices regarding the best use of resources. It comprises a clear and detailed listing of the costs and outcomes, or consequences, of specific interventions or services.

Within economic evaluation, the concept of economic efficiency is central. Economic efficiency means making choices that maximise the benefit from the limited or scarce resources available to the community. It involves the appraisal of alternative services or interventions by calculating the amount by which the benefits derived exceed the costs expended. In other words, economic efficiency requires that a specific intervention cannot be preferred to any other simply because it is more beneficial or less costly, but only if the choice is based on both relative benefits and relative costs.

Historical Context

Health economic evaluation techniques have evolved out of decision theory. Decision theory was initially developed in relation to military and oil industry contexts in the 1950s and can be defined as the *'use of systematic methods for assessing the relative values of outcomes'* (Pettiti, 1995). Decision analysis was first introduced to healthcare settings, in the form of cost-effectiveness analysis in relation to the development of diagnostic and treatment pathways, in the 1960s (Locket, 1996). In the 1970s, Weinstein and Stasson (1977) introduced economic evaluation techniques to clinicians and this led to more recent interest in using costs to determine the relative values of health and social care outcomes.

The arrival of economic evaluation techniques in the health field has not, however, been without controversy. For example, a letter to the *New England Journal of Medicine* in 1980 expressed disdain for cost-effectiveness analysis, stating that any clinician who changes their practice because of cost rather than purely clinical considerations has embarked on a *'slippery slope of compromised ethics and waffled priorities'* (Loewy, 1980). Although such sentiments were fairly typical at the time, clinicians have since gradually developed a better understanding of the role of health economic evaluation in society. As Eisenberg has commented:

> For physicians and patients to retain the autonomy intrinsic to their professional relationship, social responsibilities must be incorporated into clinical decisions. Almost all clinicians would agree that, at some point, the extra money spent for tiny improvements in clinical outcomes is not worthwhile and represents inappropriate practice. The money thus mis-spent could have been devoted to medical care that would achieve greater benefit, or to some other meaningful social purpose. (Eisenberg, 1989: 2879)

In the 1990s, a number of countries began to introduce guidelines for the economic evaluation of health technologies, typically pharmaceuticals. Australia was the first to develop and implement such guidelines in 1990. Canada followed soon after, with guidelines issued in Ontario in 1991. In the mid 1990s, The National Institute for Health and Clinical Excellence (NICE) was set up in England and Wales to appraise the cost-effectiveness of medical technologies and to provide guidance to health services. NICE is now seen as a model of good practice by many other countries.

Over the past 20 years, the field of economic evaluation in health and social care has expanded considerably, with a rapid rise in the number of published studies and wider recognition of their use in decision-making. Indeed, a number of countries (such as the UK, Canada, Australia, Sweden, Norway and Germany) now have national bodies providing guidance on the cost-effectiveness and implementation of healthcare technologies.

Current Use

The four types of economic evaluation techniques that are mainly used in health and social care are cost-minimisation analysis, cost-effectiveness analysis, cost–benefit analysis and cost–utility analysis.

Cost-minimisation analysis (CMA)

Cost-minimisation analysis searches for the lowest cost alternative. This technique is used when the two alternatives being considered are known to or can be assumed to produce identical outcomes. For example, it might be necessary to ascertain which of two alternative minor operations – day surgery or two-day hospitalisation for inguinal hernia – costs less. It can be assumed that the operations in both options are successful so the alternatives have the same outcome: in both the hernias are repaired. What is left is the difference in the cost between the two types of surgery, which is the cost per surgical procedure (Drummond et al., 2005).

Cost-effectiveness analysis (CEA)

In cost-effectiveness analysis, alternative interventions are compared in terms of the cost of delivering each intervention *and also* the effectiveness of the intervention in achieving a defined outcome. Importantly, in comparing alternative interventions in cost-effectiveness analysis, the costs and the consequences must be measured in the same way for both alternatives. This is usually the financial costs of delivering the intervention and a reliable and valid measure of the consequences. Typical outcomes in cost-effectiveness analysis are mortality rates, years of life lost to illness and severity of illness measures.

For example, an existing drug treatment programme might cost £20,000 to deliver to 100 problem drug users over a year, compared with a cost of £30,000 per 100 problem drug users for a new, alternative drug treatment programme. Consequences might then be measured by counting the number of problem drug users in each treatment programme not using drugs at the end of the year. If 50 out of the 100 individuals in the existing drug treatment programme are abstinent, but 70 out of the 100 individuals in the more expensive programme are abstinent, it would appear that the new intervention is more expensive but more effective. As a result, it would be difficult to determine which intervention is best and a cost-effectiveness analysis would be helpful.

Obviously, a cost-effeciveness analysis is not always required. For example, a new intervention might be more effective and cheaper. It is then regarded as dominant over the existing intervention and should be adopted. Conversely, if it is less effective and more expensive, it can be regarded as indefensible and consequently should not be adopted. In those situations when cost-effectiveness analysis is relevant, a cost-effectiveness ratio is usually calculated. This is sometimes known as the 'incremental cost-effectiveness ratio' (ICER) and is expressed as:

$$\text{ICER} = \frac{\text{cost}_{\text{new intervention}} - \text{cost}_{\text{existing intervention}}}{\text{effect}_{\text{new intervention}} - \text{effect}_{\text{existing intervention}}}$$

Taking the above drug treatment example, we would calculate the cost-effectiveness ratio as:

$$\text{ICER} = (30,0000 - 20,0000)/(70 - 50)$$
$$= 10,000/20$$
$$= 500$$

This ICER result can be considered as the 'price' of one additional problem drug user being abstinent at one year by switching drug treatment services from the existing programme to the new treatment programme: essentially, £500 per treated drug user. The question for policy-makers and service planners then becomes, is that price worth paying? This requires a value judgement – some people might think that it is a price worth paying whereas others might not.

Cost–utility analysis (CUA)

Developed from cost-effectiveness analysis (CEA), cost–utility analysis (CUA) is used when it is desirable to express the effectiveness of an intervention in a more comprehensive way. Cost–utility analysis combines the effects of an intervention on survival with the effects on an individual's quality of life, converting both into a common measurement scale. The term 'utility' is used to show the preferences that individuals or society can have for a given set of health outcomes or for a particular health state. For example, individuals or society are likely to give a higher utility score to living with a bad back than to living with both legs paralysed. Higher utility scores are associated with better health, and lower utility scores with poorer health: a score of '1' represents perfect health and '0' represents death.

Usually in cost–utility analysis, the utility score for a particular health state is combined with the number of years an individual would live with that health state. Combining 'utilities' with 'life years' provides the measure most typically used in cost–utility analysis, the quality adjusted life year or QALY. QALYs measure the 'usefulness' or utility of a particular health state and the length of life lived under that state. The result of a cost–utility analysis is usually expressed as the net monetary cost (or savings) per QALY gained from a particular intervention.

Cost–benefit analysis (CBA)

In the cost-effectiveness analysis explained above, the consequences for alternative interventions need to use the same measure of effect. However, this is not always practical. Moreover, cost-effectiveness analysis tends to be limited to single consequences rather than the multiple outcomes that are often important in health and social care.

In cost–benefit analysis, outcomes or consequences are measured in monetary terms (for example £, € or $), which are then compared with programme costs, measured in the same monetary units. The results of such a comparative analysis can be stated either in the form of a ratio of money costs to money benefits or as a simple sum (positive or negative) representing the net benefit or loss of one intervention over another.

Cost perspectives

Since economic evaluations are often used to look at the relative efficiency of alternative medical or healthcare interventions, costs can be considered from various cost perspectives. One cost perspective is that of the health service. This means that only those costs that are incurred by the health service are used in analysis, and only health outcomes are considered as consequences. However, health economics is often concerned with costs and benefits to society as a whole, and health economists generally recommend that a societal perspective is used in analysis.

From the societal perspective, the cost elements to consider include: the costs of delivering the intervention (that is, the costs incurred by the health service in terms of staffing, equipment, buildings, infrastructure, services and so on) plus the costs incurred by the patient (for example time lost from work due to treatment or illness), by industry (for example lost productivity costs) and by the state (for example welfare costs). When a societal cost perspective is adopted, the most appropriate economic evaluation technique is cost–benefit analysis (CBA).

BOX 12.1

Types of Question Addressed by Economic Evaluations

- What is the cheapest option out of acupuncture or physiotherapy for low back pain, both of which are similarly effective?

- What does it cost to prevent one death from malaria by distributing mosquito nets, and how does this compare with the cost of preventing one death by distributing anti-malarial drugs?

- What are the societal cost savings associated with the prevention of drug addiction, and is prevention worthwhile?

- Does a new anti-obesity drug improve mortality and morbidity rates in people who are at higher risk for obesity when compared with dietary advice alone?

- How should patients and treatments be prioritised when there are limited resources and difficult choices to be made between patient groups competing for medical care? For example, should a Health Authority increase spending on hip replacements or on coronary artery bypass grafts?

Main Strengths of Economic Evaluations

Economic evaluation is a pragmatic approach that generates important information for those involved in health and social service policy, organisation and delivery. Today's focus on purchasing and providing as a framework for organising health and social care, debates about rationing in health services, and the growing emphasis on economic evaluation in research have all highlighted the need for greater understanding of the principles and methods of economics. Those who have a grasp of economic issues will be better prepared for the decisions and choices that have to be made in the health and social care sectors.

Economic evaluation is also an ethical approach. Since health and social care resources are limited, wasting them by inefficiency is wrong as it reduces the ability to provide the best possible care to patients and clients. It therefore seems unethical not to consider the economics of a health or social intervention.

An additional strength of economic evaluation relates to its ability to capture important concepts for decision-making, particularly opportunity cost and marginal costs and benefits. Opportunity cost represents the benefits that are lost in one area when a resource is used for something else. The concept of opportunity cost is helpful in considering where resources should be directed to get the best possible value out of those resources. The notion of marginal costs and benefits is important for incremental analysis, which is where the costs and benefits of a new intervention are compared with standard care. In incremental analysis, only those costs and benefits that reflect the difference between the new and the old should be considered – in other words the added, or marginal, value of the new over the old.

Another advantage of economic evaluation is its ability to move beyond disease status to consider quality of life issues and the societal impact of health and social care interventions. For example, a cost–utility analysis focuses on symptoms and general health state, not just medical outcomes such as death or infection rates. Meanwhile, a cost–benefit analysis can incorporate the indirect costs of illness, such as those costs attributable to absence from work and lost productivity. By including an analysis of these broader factors, economic evaluation can offer a comprehensive assessment of the consequences of health and social care interventions for individuals, the health service and society more generally.

Main Weaknesses of Economic Evaluations

Economic evaluation is not without its limitations. Health economics is a young discipline and the science and methods of economic evaluations are still developing and being tested. Moreover, confidence in the method is weakened by its complexity, which can make evaluations difficult to understand. In addition, aspects of the methods are academically and practically controversial. For example, bias from measurement errors and poor estimates can easily creep into analyses.

Beyond this, the lack of information on the effects of interventions – as a result of scarce randomised controlled trials (see Chapter 11) or epidemiological studies – means that the information base for economic evaluations is often inadequate or poor. This is especially challenging in developing countries. Sometimes measures of intermediate outcomes of programmes can be used as proxies of effects; for example in evaluating a hepatitis B immunisation programme, the number of fully immunised children – rather than the number of cases or deaths prevented – can be used as a proxy for effectiveness. Nonetheless, this is effectively an indicator and not a true measure of intervention outcomes.

There are also weaknesses associated with the information requirements for the different techniques described in this chapter, most notably cost–benefit analysis. In practical terms, cost–benefit analyses can only be used to compare interventions or policies where both costs and benefits can easily be reduced to monetary terms. However, this is not always straightforward, especially when consequences are not easily given a monetary value – for example mortality, or loss of a limb or arthritic pain. This is one reason why cost–benefit analysis is not a common technique in economic evaluations of health and social care.

In addition, economic evaluations cannot replace decision-making; they simply inform it. Decision-makers still need to make controversial value judgements about which options should be funded, even if they have better information on which to base these decisions. Deciding what constitutes an acceptable threshold for supporting an intervention is one such value judgement. Even the existence of a threshold in itself is controversial. For example, does a value of £30,000 for cost/QALY gained represent good value for money? Should it be £50,000, or £20,000? Should there be a threshold at all? Is it actually possible to put a monetary value on health gain?

Finally, a major challenge for decision-makers and service planners is how to implement any decisions made on the basis of economic evaluations. No matter how good an economic evaluation study is and how cost-effective a new intervention seems to be compared with existing care, it may not be possible to achieve its potential benefits. This might be because of inertia in health and social services – due to existing budget constraints, cumbersome management structures or intransigence by health and social care professionals – or because the new intervention is simply too expensive for health and social care organisations with limited budgets.

MAIN STRENGTHS AND WEAKNESSES
... OF ECONOMIC EVALUATIONS

Strengths

- Economic evaluations are pragmatic techniques that provide important information for decision-makers.

- There are good ethical reasons for the use of economic evaluation as a tool for decision-makers.

- Important concepts – such as opportunity cost and marginal costs and benefits – can usefully be incorporated into economic evaluations.

- Economic evaluations can consider quality of life issues and the societal impact of health and social care interventions, as well as disease status.

Weaknesses

- The complexity of the method can make economic evaluations difficult to understand.
- Bias from measurement errors and poor estimates can easily creep into economic evaluations.
- The lack of information on the effects of interventions can reduce the validity of economic models and results.
- It is not always straightforward to agree what information should be used in economic analysis – for example what is the monetary value of loss of life or sight?
- Decision-makers still need to make controversial value judgements about which interventions should be funded.
- Implementing the decisions made following economic evaluations is often difficult.

Conducting an Economic Evaluation

Although most studies that require economic evaluations will employ an economist to undertake this work, it is useful to get a feel for the steps involved.

Step 1: Decide which two (or more) interventions should be assessed and compared

An economic evaluation should not assess an intervention in isolation. Equally, a new intervention should usually only be compared with alternative interventions that are already of proven benefit or that appear to offer the most potential benefit. In this regard, economic evaluations are similar to RCTs (see Chapter 11). Thus, just as there is typically a 'no treatment' control group in RCTs, so a 'do nothing' alternative is often considered in health economic evaluations.

Step 2: Decide on an objective and perspective for the evaluation

If an analysis is undertaken to help maximise the efficiency of a treatment (technical efficiency), then cost-minimisation or cost-effectiveness techniques are appropriate. If the analysis is undertaken to inform how resources should be allocated, then cost–utility or cost–benefit techniques are likely to prove more useful. If the analysis is to help decide on the allocation of resources in different structural domains, for example the total cost to treat a disease versus a new road building programme, then cost–benefit analysis is the only option. In addition to specifying the objective of an analysis, it is necessary to decide whose perspective the analysis will take (that is, whose costs are of interest). Clearly, the costs of a health intervention to patients and carers will differ from the costs to the health service or the costs to society more generally. Indeed, it is sometimes most appropriate to undertake an evaluation from a range of perspectives.

Step 3: Identify, measure and value resource use

The costs of an intervention are usually classified into three types: direct, indirect and intangible. Direct costs are those associated with treatment, for example the cost of a surgeon, nursing staff and hospital beds. Indirect costs are related to an intervention but usually fall outside the health service, for example a patient's time or travel costs. Intangible costs include the costs that are difficult to estimate, such as the cost of pain and depression. Decisions also need to be made regarding whether to focus on opportunity costs (the value of the alternative use for a resource) or on market costs (the actual financial cost of paying for the resource).[1] Once these have been clarified, researchers will often track patients receiving specific interventions through the healthcare system in order to record the resources that are provided to them. A monetary cost can then be ascribed to these resources.

Step 4: Identify, measure and value benefits

In order to measure benefits, the beneficiaries of an intervention need to be identified. These will depend on the perspective taken, but might include the direct recipient of an intervention, their carer and their employer. Measuring the impact of an intervention also depends on the type of outcomes identified for the alternative interventions being considered. If two alternative interventions have the same outcome (for example mortality rates or drug abstinence), then the outcomes from the two interventions can be compared directly providing they are measured in a reliable and valid way. If alternative interventions do not result in the same type of outcomes, then the benefits need to be translated into measures that are directly comparable, for example QALYs or the monetary value of benefits.

Step 5: Decide how time effects should be incorporated into valuing costs and benefits

Often the costs of an intervention are immediate, but the benefits will not be realised until some time in the future. It can then be desirable to adjust the value of the benefits to reflect the fact that they are not going to be experienced for some time. This is known as 'discounting' and is used in economic evaluations because people generally prefer to have benefits sooner and to defer costs until later. That is, they give a higher value to benefits that are closer in time or to costs that are delayed. Discounting adjusts any future benefits and any delayed costs so that they are equivalent to present day values. The challenge of discounting, however, is in deciding what rates should be applied to make these adjustments. Economists tend to use a range of values that are proposed by the Government or that have been used in other studies and these typically range between 2% and 8%.

Step 6: Analyse data and interpret results

Different economic evaluation techniques require different calculations and provide results in different ways. Cost-minimisation analysis provides a straight-forward comparison of costs, enabling interpretation regarding the cheapest alternative. Cost-effectiveness analysis, as long as an alternative intervention is neither indefensible nor dominant, will provide an incremental cost-effectiveness ratio (ICER) that can be interpreted as the cost of achieving a certain health gain. Cost–utility analysis will typically provide results as cost per QALY gained. Meanwhile, cost–benefit analysis generates the monetary value of benefits compared with the monetary value invested in the intervention, so a ratio of benefits to costs can be presented.

Step 7: Check the results to see how sensitive they are to assumptions and estimates

Sensitivity analysis should be carried out in all economic evaluations to check whether varying the values used in the analysis changes the results markedly. For example, the cost of delivering an intervention might be based on a number of estimates obtained from a range of sources, some more reliable than others. It is therefore sensible to check how a range of other reasonable values affects the overall results. A similar principle applies to the values used for assessing the benefits, and it is good practice to vary all these estimates in various combina-tions to check the robustness of the results. If a sensitivity analysis does not significantly change the initial result, the sensitivity is low. If the level of sensi-tivity is high, this needs to be made clear when presenting the results and it may be necessary to look for alternative sources of information to tighten up the estimates for the data used in the analysis.

An Example of an Economic Evaluation Study

Foxcroft, a health services researcher with a background in general nursing, psychology and research methods, has looked at the cost-effectiveness of a new anti-obesity drug – orlistat – in two separate studies: the first for the NHS in England and the second for the makers of the drug (Foxcroft and Milne, 2000; Foxcroft, 2005). These studies were both written up as papers and, after scientific peer review, were published in the academic journal *Obesity Reviews*. The most recent study is described below.

Orlistat is a medicine developed for the treatment of obesity. Although there are regulatory licensed indications for its use, NICE has provided further guidance because of uncertainties regarding the costs and benefits of orlistat treatment. The NICE guidance specified the prescription of orlistat to those patients who conformed to the licensed indication but also met a number of more restrictive additional criteria for continued use of orlistat (>2.5 kg weight loss pre-treatment; >5% weight loss at 3 months; >10% weight loss at 6 months). Those patients who did not meet these additional criteria would have their orlistat prescriptions stopped. A health economic evaluation study was undertaken in 2004 to assess the costs and benefits of orlistat treatment according to its use under the NICE guidance. The health economic evaluation question was 'What are the costs and benefits of orlistat for the treatment of obesity when used according to NICE guidance?'. This study is described below according to the steps for health economic evaluation set out in the previous section.

Step 1: Decide which two (or more) interventions should be assessed and compared

Effectiveness data for this health economic evaluation were taken from three RCTs of orlistat treatment for people whose body mass index (BMI) defined them as obese. In each trial, the comparison was between orlistat treatment and a diet-only control group (with placebo[2] orlistat). Information from the three trials was pooled for the economic evaluation.

Step 2: Decide on an objective and perspective for the evaluation

As NICE is a body set up to provide guidance on the allocation of resources within the health service, it uses cost–utility analysis as its standard approach to health economic evaluation. The orlistat analysis therefore followed this approach. Similarly, as NICE is concerned with the allocation of resources within the health service according to patient benefit, the perspective chosen for the health economic study was the health service for costs and patient health outcomes for consequences.

Step 3: Identify, measure and value resource use

At the time of the study, prescription costs for orlistat were £45 per month for each person treated, and the overall prescription cost was calculated according to the proportion of patients who responded to treatment and therefore continued with prescriptions over a 12-month period. General Practitioner (GP) consultation costs were £27 per visit and it was estimated that five GP visits would be required: one initial consultation, one at the start of treatment, one at three months, one at six months, and one at 12 months. These cost data were taken from publicly available health service and prescription cost datasets for the NHS.

Step 4: Identify, measure and value benefits

The pooled RCTs provided good information on how much weight loss was achieved in the orlistat group and also the control group over a 12-month period, and this was recorded as average weight loss for those who met the NICE guidance criteria as well as those who did not. Only 12.8% of patients in the orlistat group managed to meet the NICE criteria for continued orlistat treatment, and they achieved an average weight loss of 18.91kg at 12 months. This compares, however, with a much lower figure of only 5.3% meeting similar criteria in the diet-only placebo control group, with an average weight loss of 17.31kg at 12 months. Thus, whilst there was not much difference in average weight loss between the groups, there were over twice as many people able to lose this amount of weight with orlistat treatment compared with the controls.

As the objective was to undertake a cost–utility analysis, the health economic evaluation translated the figures for weight loss into an estimate of quality of life gains, that is, for every unit decrease in body mass index (BMI) what would be the corresponding increase in quality of life? Previous research helpfully provided a figure of a 0.017 (1.7%) increase in health utility (quality of life) achieved for every unit decrease in BMI (remember that health utility is measured along a scale of 0 to 1, with 0 representing death and 1 representing perfect health). For the 12.8% of patients who met the NICE criteria for continued use of orlistat, and who lost an average of 18.91kg over a year, the associated gain in health utility, or increased quality of life, was 0.117 or 11.7% (based on the average weight loss expressed as a decrease in BMI).

Step 5: Decide how time effects should be incorporated into valuing costs and benefits

Although the risk of future mortality and morbidity is higher with obesity, the economic evaluation did not project forward the costs and benefits of orlistat treatment into future years. This was because orlistat, according to NICE guidance, should not normally be used for more than one year and, also, because other studies have shown that there is a possibility of rebound weight gain once treatment is stopped. Therefore any longer term benefits of orlistat treatment in terms of weight loss, reduced BMI and increased quality of life could not be guaranteed – the longer term effects of short-term weight loss are not clear. The time perspective in this evaluation was thus one year, with no discounting of costs or benefits.

Step 6: Analyse data and interpret results

A computer model was developed containing values for the various costs and effects and combining them using an algorithm to provide an overall estimate of the cost per quality adjusted life year gained with orlistat treatment. The result was an estimate that orlistat may cost £24,431 for each QALY gained. Given that a cost/QALY gained of under £30,000 is seen to be reasonable (Raftery, 2001), this result seems to support the use of orlistat according to NICE guidance.

Step 7: Check the results to see how sensitive they are to assumptions and estimates

Although the figure of £24,431 for each QALY gained is often seen as the headline result, it is only part of the picture. A sensitivity analysis varies the assumptions made about the values used in the health economic model and in this particular analysis the sensitivity analysis varied the cost assumptions according to the number of GP visits that might be required (either fewer or more visits) and also varied the estimated utility gains associated with weight loss (either higher or lower). This provided a more detailed result, with a sensitivity analysis range from £10,856 to £77,197 per QALY gained. This suggests that the economic analysis is quite sensitive to varying assumptions, and in this analysis the result was particularly sensitive to variation in utility gains associated with weight loss.

Further Reading

Drummond, M.F., Sculpher, M., Torrance, G.W., O'Brien, B. and Stoddart, G.L. (2005) *Methods for Economic Evaluation of Health Care Programmes*, **3rd edn (Oxford: Oxford University Press).**

This is probably the standard textbook in this field worldwide. It should be required reading for anyone commissioning, undertaking or using economic evaluations in health or social care, and will be useful to health and social service professionals, health economists, and health and social care decision-makers. The key methodological principles are outlined using a critical appraisal checklist that can be applied to any published study. The methodological features of the basic forms of analysis (cost-minimisation analysis, cost-effectiveness analysis, cost–utility analysis, and cost–benefit analysis) are then explained in more detail. In the third edition, there is new material on collecting and analysing data, and presenting and using economic evaluation results. This comprehensive textbook will have something useful for undergraduates, postgraduates, and both novice and more experienced researchers.

Gold, M.R., Siegel, J.E., Russell, L.B. and Weinstein, M.C. (1996) *Cost-effectiveness in Health and Medicine* (Oxford: Oxford University Press).

This is a unique, in-depth discussion of the uses and conduct of health economic evaluation techniques as decision-making aids in the health and medical fields. Exploring economic evaluation techniques in the context of societal decision-making for resource allocation purposes, the authors propose that analysts include a reference case (the 'best guess' scenario) in all analyses designed to inform resource allocation. Important theoretical and practical issues encountered in measuring costs and effectiveness, evaluating outcomes, discounting and dealing with uncertainty are examined in separate chapters. This is a more advanced book that will be useful for health economists, health technologists and decision analysts.

Lockett, T. (1996) *Health Economics for the Uninitiated* (Oxford: Radcliffe Medical Press).

Designed as a general introduction and assuming no prior knowledge of the field, this short book is written in a clear and straightforward manner. It explains general economic principles and shows how they are used in practice. The book is a practical guide to understanding health economic issues, and to examining articles and other literature 'without terror'. It is suited to undergraduates, postgraduates and novice researchers with little or no knowledge or experience of the discipline of health economics.

Raftery, J. (1998) 'Economics notes. Economic evaluation: An introduction', *British Medical Journal*, **316**, 1013–4.

This is the first in a series of brief and informative articles on health economics that have been published in the British Medical Journal (BMJ) and are now available on the BMJ website (www.bmj.com).[3] The articles in the series do not seek to provide a comprehensive overview of economic evaluation, but rather aim to discuss issues which have arisen in the course of designing and carrying out health economic evaluations. The series provides a useful read for those struggling with the terminology of health economic evaluation, offering useful definitions and clarifications. Although aimed at the medical practitioner, all the articles are clearly written and accessible to a wider audience of clinicians and novice researchers.

References

Drummond, M.F., Sculpher, M., Torrance, G.W., O'Brien, B. and Stoddart, G.L. (2005) *Methods for Economic Evaluation of Health Care Programmes*, 3rd edn (Oxford: Oxford University Press).

Eisenberg, J.M. (1989) 'Clinical economics: A guide to the economic analysis of clinical practice', *Journal of the American Medical Association*, **262**, 2879–86.

Foxcroft, D.R. (2005) 'Orlistat for the treatment of obesity: Cost utility model', *Obesity Reviews*, **6**, 323–8.

Foxcroft, D.R. and Milne, R. (2000) 'Orlistat for the treatment of obesity: Rapid review and cost-effectiveness model', *Obesity Reviews*, **1**, 121–6.

Lockett, T. (1996) *Health Economics for the Uninitiated* (Oxford: Radcliffe Medical Press).

Loewy, E.H. (1980) 'Cost should not be a factor in medical care', *New England Journal of Medicine*, **302**, 697.

Pettiti, D.B. (1995) *Meta-analysis, decision analysis and cost-effectiveness analysis* (Oxford: Oxford University Press).

Raftery, J. (2001) 'NICE: Faster access to modern treatments? Analysis of guidance on health technologies', *British Medical Journal*, **323**, 1300–3.

Weinstein, M.C. and Stasson, W.B. (1977) 'Foundations of cost-effectiveness analysis for health and medical practice', *New England Journal of Medicine*, **296**, 716–21.

Notes

1 In practice, many studies focus on market costs because of difficulties in determining the value of opportunity costs.

2 Dummy or inactive.

3 A search for 'economics notes' will bring up a list of all the articles.

Measuring Health Status

13

JILL DAWSON

Introduction

Healthcare staff use a variety of technologies and techniques to investigate the symptoms and signs of illness, measure the severity of disease processes, gauge patients' recovery, and evaluate healthcare interventions. Common examples of these technologies and techniques include thermometers, blood tests, X-rays, imaging machines, endoscopy (looking inside the body with a special viewing instrument), palpation (feeling with the hands during a physical examination), and auscultation (listening to the body, normally with a stethoscope). None of these methods of assessing health status is totally free from measurement error and subjective judgement is frequently involved in their interpretation. Nonetheless, such methods tend to be referred to as 'objective'.

Over the past two decades, attempts have been made to devise ways of systematically measuring subjective health status. This has involved collecting information directly from patients using health status questionnaires – also known as 'instruments', 'assessment tools' or 'patient-reported questionnaires'. Some health status questionnaires seek to measure patients' views of their general (or 'generic') health. For example, the Short-Form 36 (SF-36) assesses self-perceived health status via 36 questions (or 'items') relating to eight broad areas (or 'domains') of physical and psychological health. Other instruments assess subjective health status in relation to specific diseases or conditions. For example, the Arthritis Impact Measurement Scales (AIMS) assess the health of individuals who suffer from a joint disease via 45 questions. Meanwhile, the VF-14 is a highly specific questionnaire that uses 14 questions to measure various aspects of visual function affected by cataracts.

Today, health status questionnaires are commonly used (with or without blood tests, X-rays or other more 'objective' measures) to assess the health of individuals following a medical or psychosocial intervention. To this end, health status questionnaires are most often employed in clinical trials (see Chapter 11) and other studies to compare the outcomes of care across different patient groups. Occasionally, however, they may be used for other purposes, including monitoring individual patients within a clinical setting.

Historical Context

In 1948, the World Health Organization (WHO) defined health as 'a state of complete physical, mental and social well-being and not merely the absence of disease' (World Health Organization, 1948). This was an important statement since it emphasised that health is a multidimensional construct which involves subjective as well as objective dimensions. At around the same time (1947), the Karnofsky Performance Scale was devised. This is a simple scale that allows healthcare professionals to assess patients by giving them a score ranging from 0–100, where 0 represents dead and 100 represents 'normal, no complaints, no evidence of disease'. The Karnofsky Performance Scale was one of the first standardised questionnaires that permitted patients' functional impairment (and not merely their physical condition) to be measured within the clinical setting. Subsequently, other questionnaires began to measure aspects of functional ability and 'activities of daily living' (ADL), although patients' subjective well-being was still not considered.

From the late 1970s, a convergence of factors spurred a growing interest in patients' views of their own health status – that is, patient-reported outcome measures or PROMs. For example, there was an increasing acceptance that much healthcare (including surgery, medicines, nursing care, physiotherapy and occupational therapy) should be directed towards improving the *quality*, rather than merely the *quantity*, of people's lives. It was also recognised that therapeutic interventions often prolonged life without necessarily curing the underlying condition and could even produce detrimental side effects (as in the case of treatments for various cancers). Additionally, governments and health authorities were experiencing problems in funding healthcare and thus demanded greater evidence of the benefits of treatments relative to their costs. As a result of such factors, myriad questionnaires, interview schedules, rating scales and assessment forms emerged to assess the impact of healthcare interventions from the patient's point of view (Epstein, 1990; Garratt et al., 2002).

The methodology needed to assess people's subjective health status obviously required a firm scientific foundation and those working in healthcare were fortunate in being able to look to other disciplines for this. During the first half of the twentieth century, psychologists and educators had been devising and applying methods to measure educational achievement, intelligence, personality differences and so on. These methods – termed psychometrics – assessed subjective states in a manner that was both reproducible (produced similar results when repeated in similar circumstances) and valid (appeared to measure what was intended to be measured). By the late 1980s and early 1990s, a well-described psychometric methodology for developing health status questionnaires that were applicable to clinical situations had been developed (Streiner and Norman, 1989). This methodology continues to evolve, but its core components now constitute accepted practice and are described further below.

Current Use

Patient-reported outcome measures are primarily used to evaluate the outcomes of healthcare interventions, most obviously in randomised controlled trials (RCTs) (Fitzpatrick et al., 1998, and see Chapter 11). In RCTs, the objective is to detect differences – if they exist – between groups receiving different interventions. For results to be meaningful in this context, psychometrically validated measures (that is, measures that have been confirmed by rigorous scientific examination) must be used. Moreover, these measures must cover areas (or 'domains') appropriate to the study in question (for example pain, physical function or mental health) and should ideally be quite specific in their focus (for example knee pain, walking ability or anxiety). While health status measures may be used in a research study with a non-randomised design (such as a cohort study – see Chapter 10), the interpretation of results is more complex here since it is difficult to control for all the possible factors that may be influencing outcomes.

A further somewhat controversial use of health status questionnaires is in studies relating to cost containment and prioritisation, generally termed 'cost–utility studies' (see Chapter 12). In cost–utility studies, outcome measures are obtained in order to generate a single figure that can then be used to rank-order treatments or patients. The most widely known summary value of this type is the quality adjusted life year (or QALY) (Torrance et al., 1995). The QALY is designed to combine the quantity and quality of life into a single measure which can then form the basis of resource allocation decisions where difficult choices have to be made between patient groups competing for medical care. Usually, the involvement and expertise of a health economist is essential in such studies.

Patient-reported questionnaires have also been used in comparing the health of populations or sub-samples within populations. For example, the World Health Organization Quality of Life Assessment (WHOQOL) and the International Quality of Life Assessment (IQOLA) groups are collaborations seeking to compare the health status of people in different countries. Historically, international comparisons of health were undertaken by using simple measures of mortality and morbidity that focused on illness and failed to capture broader health experiences. The development of health status questionnaires has enabled information about the impact of disease and its treatment on functioning and well-being to be monitored around the world. Indeed, versions of the WHOQOL have now been administered to people in over 40 countries (WHOQOL, 2007).

In addition, patient-reported measures are increasingly being used in service audit (see Chapter 8) and in the routine evaluation of healthcare. The collection of outcomes data through routine systems has already been successfully demonstrated (Bardsley and Coles, 1992; Lansky et al., 1992) and the recent establishment of UK clinical effectiveness committees and yearly appraisals for hospital consultants suggest an imminent extension of audit as part of general clinical governance. This could result in treatment outcomes being audited throughout all hospital specialties (McDonald, 2000). Where such audits are concerned with the amount of change (or improvement) in patient condition that occurs following a clinical intervention, PROMs could potentially be used – although this form of application remains largely unevaluated.

One final application of health status questionnaires is by clinicians in screening individual patients for health problems that might not otherwise be revealed or in selecting patients for treatment (such as for surgery). Although this application may be questionable (see below), PROMs data can still complement the standard clinical interview and may be helpful in informing clinical practitioners of the well-being of individual patients in their care. The Dartmouth Primary Cooperative Research Network (or COOP) Charts are a rare example of a questionnaire that was designed with this purpose in mind (Nelson et al., 1990). The COOP charts are used to assess the full range of patient needs and the degree to which these needs will be addressed by the healthcare system, ultimately improving care practices.

BOX 13.1

Types of Question Addressed by Health Status Measures

- In randomised controlled trials or other clinical studies, how does health status differ between groups of patients receiving different interventions for a similar condition?

- In cost–utility studies, how should patients and treatments be prioritised when there are limited resources and difficult choices to be made between patient groups competing for medical care?

- In international research, how does the health status of populations and sub-samples within populations compare?

- In audit, how does actual clinical practice compare with best clinical practice? (Although this application is currently relatively unevaluated).

- In a clinical setting, which individuals have particular health problems or might be suitable for treatment? (Although this application requires a cautious approach as the reliability of PROMs is less good for assessing individuals than for comparing group scores).

Main Strengths of Health Status Measures

Perhaps the most important benefit of using patient-reported questionnaires is that the method gives prominence to the patient's – rather than the clinician's – perspective. Whilst this seems reasonable in itself, there are other reasons for utilising measures that are independent of those providing the care. For example, research shows that assessments of health status made by healthcare professionals can differ from those made by patients (Jenkinson, 1994). Additionally, patients and clinicians may disagree about the relative importance of different aspects of the outcome of an intervention. This may be because those who provide care do not have first-hand experience of the health problem in question and/or (wittingly or unwittingly) present a biased assessment. In this situation, the patient's perspective is likely to provide a better indication of satisfaction with treatment.

A second strength of health status questionnaires is their convenience. A questionnaire can be completed anywhere, including in the patient's home. It can be delivered in person, by post or electronically (by email or internet). Such flexibility can avoid much of the inconvenience and cost – to all parties – that is associated with having to deliver an assessment within a busy clinical setting. This can in turn make large-scale studies more attractive and feasible.

Thirdly, health status questionnaires that have been validated have robust scientific credibility. The process of validation involves applying psychometric methodology to test that the questionnaire used in the assessment and any measurement scales used within the questionnaire meet certain (minimum) standards (Fitzpatrick et al., 1998). Findings should then be presented in a peer-reviewed journal. This process of validation is discussed in more detail below.

A final strength of using subjective health status questionnaires is that there are now many validated measures available. The broad range of content and general applicability of generic questionnaires mean that they can be applied to a wide range of health problems. This is useful if no disease or condition-specific instrument exists in a particular area. In contrast, highly specific questionnaires avoid the danger of other non-related medical conditions affecting the measurement of the condition of interest (for example, poor eyesight affecting scores relating to a hip condition). The appropriate instrument will be the one that is most acceptable to patients and will address research questions with the greatest degree of precision.

Main Weaknesses of Health Status Measures

Inevitably, PROMs have their limitations. Most obviously, the perfect questionnaire does not exist and there is generally no obvious 'gold standard' against which measures of health status can be compared.[1] Furthermore, choosing the most appropriate instrument for a particular purpose can be challenging, given that there may be a number of questionnaires from which to choose, or alternatively none may seem entirely appropriate. This may occur if individual questions (or items) appear irrelevant to the study sample. For instance, a questionnaire that includes items about sports participation may not suit a study focusing on elderly people. Equally, some people may find it difficult or impossible to complete a questionnaire – for example, individuals with dementia or patients who are unconscious.

Due to their increased availability and apparent ease of use, there is also a danger that PROMs are used inappropriately (or too readily) by people with limited expertise. Indeed, those conducting clinical trials (see Chapter 11) have sometimes used measures that have not been psychometrically validated or measures that covered an inadequate range of health dimensions for their area of investigation.

Difficulties can additionally arise when using instruments that have been translated into other languages. This is because the meaning of questions can change or be interpreted differently. Compounding this, it is not always easy to determine what constitutes a 'clinically relevant' or 'meaningful' difference – as distinct from a 'statistically significant' difference – when comparing outcome measures for different groups of patients. Thus, a study may show that individuals receiving a particular intervention have significantly better life satisfaction than those not receiving the intervention. If, however, life satisfaction was not a problem for either group initially, the actual clinical impact of the intervention may not be very important.

Finally, some applications of health status measures require further evaluation and are still currently best used with caution. For instance, the value, feasibility and costs (in the broadest sense) of setting up and maintaining long-term systems for auditing clinical outcomes using PROMs remain largely unevaluated. Additionally, there are concerns regarding the assessment and screening of 'individuals' in the clinical setting since measurement error is much greater here than when comparing 'groups of individuals' in a large-scale clinical trial (Fitzpatrick et al., 1992).

MAIN STRENGTHS AND WEAKNESSES
... OF HEALTH STATUS MEASURES

Strengths

- Health status questionnaires give prominence to the patient's – rather than the clinician's – perspective on the outcome of healthcare.

- Health status questionnaires are very convenient. A questionnaire can be completed anywhere, including in the patient's home, which avoids the inconvenience and costs associated with being assessed at a hospital.

- Health status questionnaires developed using psychometric methodology have robust scientific credibility.

Weaknesses

- The perfect questionnaire does not exist and some people cannot complete a questionnaire (for all sorts of reasons).

- Due to their increased availability and apparent ease of use, questionnaires may be used inappropriately (or too readily) by people with limited expertise.

- The interpretation of PROMs can be complex.

- Some applications of PROMs may be ill-advised – for example, in assessing or screening individual patients.

Developing a Health Status Measure

Although people using health status questionnaires are very unlikely to be involved in developing new measures, it is useful to understand how instruments are designed and validated. This is because a basic appreciation of the robust scientific processes and complex statistical analyses behind what often present as very straightforward and easy-to-administer tools can help to ensure that those using patient-reported methods select measures carefully and administer and interpret them appropriately.

The development of a new health status questionnaire will generally either begin with discussions between relevant experts in the field or, preferably, relatively unstructured interviews conducted with a relevant range of patients. If the questionnaire is intended to measure outcomes of a particular intervention (such as medication or surgery), it is important to interview patients who have already received the intervention as well as patients who are at the pre-intervention stage. The aim of both the clinical expert discussion and patient interviews is to identify the main themes that exemplify the particular condition to be measured. In the case of arthritis of the hand, this might include pain affecting the joints, perceptions concerning joint deformity, range of joint movement, and perceived dependency on others.

Once the main themes have been identified, the next stage is to devise candidate questions or statements (items that may or may not ultimately be used). Each candidate item will also be given a response category. Often this will be in a Likert scale format, such as 'strongly disagree', 'disagree,' 'undecided', 'agree', or 'strongly agree' (Bowling, 1997). Alternatively, a visual analogue scale (VAS) might be used. This takes the form of a continuous line (generally measuring 10 or 15 cm) on which patients are asked to mark their response as a point somewhere between two stated extremes, such as 'no pain' and 'unbearable pain'. At this point, it can also be useful to look at a range of existing validated questionnaires to assist with producing the precise wording of candidate items. In order to further standardise the way in which people respond, all candidate items need to be associated with a particular time period (for example 'today', 'in the last week', or 'in the last month') and these need to make sense in relation to the condition/intervention under study.

Although the final questionnaire should be relatively short,[2] it is sensible to begin with a longer list of candidate questions and statements since some will likely prove unsatisfactory and have to be rejected. These candidate items and their response options should then be piloted on a small sample of relevant patients, with amendments made to items in response to the patients' written or verbal feedback. This process can then be repeated until patients are generally answering items satisfactorily with no one item appearing to cause serious difficulty and with no new major themes being raised.

Ultimately, each item will generate an item score (for example 'strongly disagree' = 0; 'disagree' = 1'; 'undecided' = 2; 'agree' = 3; 'strongly agree' = 4). Individual item scores will then be summed (or transformed) to produce one or more dimension scores (that is, a score for each of the scales included in the questionnaire). The final questionnaire content will be decided by testing candidate questionnaire items and overall scale properties on an adequate and representative sample of patients within a relevant context. This should ideally be done by undertaking a prospective study with participants being assessed at baseline and then again at one or more follow-ups (if possible, pre- and post-intervention).

Although there is little theoretical basis for deciding (and no general agreement on) the appropriate sample size of any such prospective study, well-respected authors in the field state that somewhere between two and ten times as many respondents as questionnaire items are required. On the whole, it is probably best to aim for a reasonably large sample size given that some individuals will inevitably drop out of the study or be lost to follow up (Fayers and Machin, 2000).

Baseline measurements should include some descriptive information (such as participants' age, sex, level of education and socio-economic class) in addition to their responses to the candidate questionnaire items. Additionally, participants should complete any other assessments which purport to measure similar aspects of health-related quality of life, such as a relevant standard clinical assessment, relevant biomedical measures (for example radiographic scoring system or blood test) and one or two other generic or disease-specific measures. If possible, participants should also complete the candidate questionnaire items again, fairly soon (ideally between 48 hours and one week) after the first completion.

Statistical techniques are then used to compare participants' responses to the questionnaire items (once their scores are combined to form scales) against the various other measures collected. This is the process of validating the questionnaire and will help to ensure that the final questionnaire is both acceptable to patients and produces results that are, *inter alia*, reliable (remain consistent over repeated tests of the same subject under identical conditions); valid (measure what they purport to measure); and responsive to change (detect changes over time). More recently, Rasch analysis – a specialised and stringent statistical assessment of underlying scale structure and dimensionality derived from item-response theory – is increasingly being used (Andrich, 1988).[3]

Once validated, health status questionnaires should be used carefully. It is important to choose the right measure for the condition and research questions to be addressed. Moreover, the questionnaire must be completed in accordance with any instructions provided and missing information needs to be minimised. This requires good methods for following up patients, high levels of participant cooperation, and accurate questionnaire completion. In order to gauge whether or not an intervention has resulted in any change in health status, the questionnaire should be completed on at least two occasions: once shortly before the intervention and then again at some predetermined time following intervention (preferably within the context of an RCT). Analyses will, meanwhile, require suitable statistical software and appropriate statistical techniques. Lastly, the results should be interpreted carefully and precisely so that false or misleading conclusions are not drawn.

An Example of a Health Status Measure

In 1996, Dawson, Fitzpatrick and Carr – of the Departments of Public Health and Orthopaedic Surgery at the University of Oxford and the Nuffield Orthopaedic Centre in Oxford – published a paper on the development and validation of the Oxford Shoulder Score (OSS) for evaluating shoulder surgery. They were funded by a grant from the Oxford Regional Health Authority and their work was undertaken between March 1994 and June 1995.

The initial draft of the OSS questionnaire was informed by interviews conducted with 20 patients attending an outpatient clinic for shoulder problems. This resulted in 22 candidate items. Three cycles of piloting were then undertaken before the final 12-item OSS questionnaire was derived. The current recommended scoring system (rather than the one employed in the original publication) is used in this chapter. In the current system, each item is scored from 4 (least difficulty) to 0 (most difficulty) and item scores are summed to produce a single score with a range from 48 (least difficulties) to 0 (most difficulties).[4]

Once the 12-item questionnaire had been formed, a prospective study was conducted to examine the measurement properties of the OSS. For this, 111 consecutive patients receiving shoulder surgery (excluding instability problems) completed a variety of assessments when attending a pre-admission clinic and then again in an outpatient clinic six months after shoulder surgery. Their pre- and post-operative scores for all 12 OSS items are shown in Table 13.1.

Table 13.1 Pre- and post-operative scores obtained on the 12-item Oxford Shoulder Score questionnaire

Item	Scoring categories	Pre-op N = 111 No. (%)		Post-op n = 56 No. (%)	
During the past 4 weeks ...					
1. How would you describe the *worst* pain you had from your shoulder?	4 None	0	(0.0)	6	(10.7)
	3 Mild	3	(2.7)	19	(33.9)
	2 Moderate	31	(27.9)	20	(35.7)
	1 Severe	56	(50.5)	7	(12.5)
	0 Unbearable	21	(18.9)	4	(7.1)
2. Have you had any trouble dressing yourself because of your shoulder?	4 No trouble at all	11	(9.9)	25	(44.6)
	3 A little bit of trouble	37	(33.3)	20	(35.7)
	2 Moderate trouble	47	(42.3)	9	(16.1)
	1 Extreme difficulty	15	(13.5)	2	(3.6)
	0 Impossible to do	1	(0.9)	0	(0)
3. Have you had any trouble getting in and out of a car or using public transport (whichever you tend to use) because of your shoulder?	4 No trouble at all	41	(36.9)	38	(67.9)
	3 A little bit of trouble	36	(32.4)	12	(21.4)
	2 Moderate trouble	25	(22.5)	4	(7.1)
	1 Extreme difficulty	8	(7.2)	2	(3.6)
	0 Impossible to do	1	(0.9)	0	(0)
4. Have you been able to use a knife and fork – at the same time?	4 Yes, easily	62	(55.9)	43	(76.8)
	3 With little difficulty	26	(23.4)	7	(12.5)
	2 With moderate difficulty	16	(14.4)	2	(3.6)
	1 With extreme difficulty	4	(3.6)	0	(0)
	0 No, impossible	3	(2.7)	4	(7.1)

Item	Scoring categories	Pre-op N = 111 No. (%)	Post-op n = 56 No. (%)
5. Could you do the household shopping on your own?	4 Yes, easily	26 (23.4)	22 (39.3)
	3 With little difficulty	26 (23.4)	18 (32.1)
	2 With moderate difficulty	22 (19.8)	3 (5.4)
	1 With extreme difficulty	16 (14.4)	2 (3.6)
	0 No, impossible	21 (18.9)	11 (19.6)
6. Could you carry a tray containing a plate of food across a room?	4 Yes, easily	35 (31.5)	29 (51.8)
	3 With little difficulty	29 (26.1)	13 (23.2)
	2 With moderate difficulty	21 (18.9)	5 (8.9)
	1 With extreme difficulty	9 (8.1)	3 (5.4)
	0 No, impossible	17 (15.3)	6 (10.7)
7. Could you brush/comb your hair with the affected arm?	4 Yes, easily	7 (6.3)	19 (33.9)
	3 With little difficulty	17 (15.3)	18 (32.1)
	2 With moderate difficulty	40 (36.0)	5 (8.9)
	1 With extreme difficulty	22 (19.8)	5 (8.9)
	0 No, impossible	25 (22.5)	9 (16.1)
8. How would you describe the pain you usually had from your shoulder?	4 None	1 (0.9)	9 (16.1)
	3 Very mild	2 (1.8)	18 (32.1)
	2 Mild	25 (22.5)	8 (14.3)
	1 Moderate	67 (60.4)	17 (30.4)
	0 Severe	16 (14.4)	4 (7.1)
9. Could you hang your clothes up in a wardrobe – using the affected arm?	4 Yes, easily	9 (8.1)	19 (33.9)
	3 With little difficulty	16 (14.4)	18 (32.1)
	2 With moderate difficulty	37 (33.3)	7 (12.5)
	1 With great difficulty	20 (18.0)	3 (5.4)
	0 No, impossible	29 (26.1)	9 (16.1)
10. Have you been able to wash a dry yourself under both arms?	4 Yes, easily	31 (27.9)	33 (58.9)
	3 With little difficulty	22 (19.8)	11 (19.6)
	2 With moderate difficulty	27 (24.3)	5 (8.9)
	1 With great difficulty	19 (17.1)	1 (1.8)
	0 No, impossible	12 (10.8)	6 (10.7)
11. How much has pain from your shoulder interfered with your usual work (including housework)?	4 Not at all	2 (1.8)	17 (30.4)
	3 A little bit	6 (5.4)	16 (28.6)
	2 Moderately	36 (32.4)	12 (21.4)
	1 Greatly	53 (47.7)	8 (14.3)
	0 Totally	14 (12.6)	3 (5.4)
12. Have you been troubled by pain from your shoulder in bed at night?	4 No nights	5 (4.5)	25 (44.6)
	3 Only 1 or 2 nights	7 (6.3)	8 (14.3)
	2 Some nights	30 (27.0)	9 (16.1)
	1 Most nights	31 (27.9)	4 (7.1)
	0 Every night	38 (34.2)	10 (17.9)

Source: Dawson, J., Fitzpatrick, R. and Carr, A. (1996) Questionnaire on the perceptions of patients about shoulder surgery. *Journal of Bone and Joint Surgery* [Br]; **78-B**: 593–600. (Table I)

Measurement properties examined in this prospective study were: internal consistency; test–retest reliability; construct validity; and sensitivity to change over time:

● *Internal consistency* measures how consistently individuals respond to the items within a scale (that is, the inter-item correlations of all items on a scale). This was tested using Cronbach's alpha (Cronbach, 1951). Values of Cronbach's alpha range from 0.0–1.0, with values of 0.7 or more indicating internal consistency. Cronbach's alpha for the OSS was 0.89 pre-surgery and 0.92 at six month follow-up.

● *Test–retest reliability* shows how reliable the questionnaire is in duplicating similar responses over time. In order to examine test–retest reliability, 60 patients completed the OSS for a second time, 24 hours after first completion. The two sets of scores were then compared with the coefficient of reliability (Bland and Altman, 1986). The coefficient of reliability was calculated as 6.8, with 95% of score differences falling between 0 ± 6.8 and 83% of score differences falling between 0 ± 4 points.

● *Construct validity* seeks evidence that the questionnaire measures the concept(s) it purports to measure. This was examined using Pearson correlation coefficients between the total score of the OSS and other related measures obtained at the same assessment. These other related measures were:

  ● the Constant shoulder score assessed by a clinician;
  ● the SF-36 general health status questionnaire; and
  ● the Stanford Health Assessment Questionnaire (HAQ).

The OSS correlated well (r >0.5) with the Constant scores and at least moderately with the SF-36 and HAQ scales, particularly those of physical function and pain.

● *Sensitivity to change* measures how good the questionnaire is in detecting changes in health status over time. This was examined by comparing changes between pre- and post-operative scores when compared with the SF-36 and the HAQ. Effect sizes were also compared. Effect sizes calculate the extent of change measured by an instrument in a standardised way that allows direct comparison between instruments (Kazis et al., 1989). The OSS clearly distinguished between patients who rated the most positive change in their shoulder following surgery and those who said that change had been only slightly better or worse. In each case, the level of significance for the OSS was superior to that for any of the relevant domains in either the SF-36 or the HAQ. Effect sizes were also larger for the OSS than for all scales of the SF-36 or HAQ, thus further indicating the superior sensitivity of the OSS.

The OSS was developed at a time when PROMs were almost never used in orthopaedics. It is one of the few validated shoulder scores to have been developed with input (interviews) from patients. Providing a measure of outcome for shoulder surgery that is short, practical, reliable, valid and sensitive to clinically important changes over time, the OSS was kept very simple in order to encourage usage in outcome studies on shoulder patients. It has consistently performed well in comparison to clinician-based scores and general health status measures (Dawson et al., 2002), and has superior measurement properties to other shoulder measures (Kirkley et al., 2003). Acceptance of new measures takes time. The OSS has now been translated into German and has recently been adopted as the primary outcome measure in a 5-year randomised controlled trial (the UKUFF Trial, funded from 2007) of interventions for rotator cuff tears.

Further Reading

Bowling, A. (2001) *Measuring Disease: A Review of Disease-specific Quality of Life Measurement Scales*, 2nd edn (Buckingham: Open University Press).

This is a very readable and valuable source book, covering a large number of examples of health status measures representing varying degrees of specificity. Following a general first chapter on the meaning, use and measurement of health-related quality of life, subsequent chapters explore the measurement of health status in relation to a wide range of health conditions (including cancers, psychiatric conditions and psychological morbidity, respiratory conditions, neurological conditions, rheumatological conditions and cardiovascular diseases). The book provides many examples of widely used and 'classic' instruments and this makes it particularly useful for anyone needing to choose a relevant and appropriate disease-specific measure with which to assess outcomes of care.

Fayers, P.M. and Machin, D. (2000) *Quality of Life – Assessment, Analysis and Interpretation* (Chichester: John Wiley and Sons).

This book is divided into four sections covering: an introduction to key concepts; developing and testing questionnaires; the analysis of quality of life data; and practical aspects and clinical interpretation. Examples of health status measures of varying degrees of specificity are given and used in worked examples. The book is a great companion to Streiner and Norman (2003) (see below) since it covers some similar topics in greater detail (such as item-response theory and clinical interpretation of health status scores), some similar topics in a different way, and some extra topics. It is also more sociological and applied than Streiner and Norman. The book is suitable for people at all levels of study, both medical and non-medical readers.

Munro, B.H. (2005) *Statistical Methods for Health Care Research*, 5th edn (Philadelphia, PA: Lippincott Williams & Wilkins).

Health status measurement is applied in many different types of studies and contexts, so a book covering – in detail – the most usual forms of analysis and statistics used in healthcare research is essential. This text is particularly accessible. Worked examples (using the SPSS – www.spss.com – data analysis programme) are presented clearly. There is also an accompanying CD and mathematical equations are kept to an absolute minimum. The book is particularly useful for people studying at Masters level and beyond.

Streiner, D.L. and Norman, G.R. (2003) *Health Measurement Scales: A Practical Guide to their Development and Use* (Oxford: Oxford University Press).

Anyone with a serious interest in health status measurement should have this book on their bookshelf. Generally quite readable (although demanding in places), it describes the first principles that underpin the methodology of health status measurement and scale development. Chapters include devising the items, scaling responses, selecting the items, reliability, validity, measuring change, and ethical considerations. The book is suitable for clinicians and people at all levels of study.

References

Andrich, D. (1988) *Rasch Models for Measurement* (London: Sage Publications).

Bardsley, M. and Coles, J. (1992) 'Practical experiences in auditing patient outcomes', *Quality in Health Care*, **1**, 124–30.

Bland, J.M. and Altman, D.G. (1986) 'Statistical methods for assessing agreement between two methods of clinical measurement', *Lancet*, **1**, 8476, 307–10.

Bowling, A. (1997) *Research Methods in Health* (Philadelphia, PA: Open University Press).

Cronbach, L. (1951) 'Coefficient alpha and the internal structure of tests', *Psychometrica*, **16**, 297–334.

Dawson, J., Fitzpatrick, R. and Carr, A. (1996) 'Questionnaire on the perceptions of patients about shoulder surgery', *Journal of Bone and Joint Surgery [Br]*, **78**, 593–600.

Dawson, J., Hill, G., Fitzpatrick, R. and Carr, A. (2002) 'Comparison of clinical and patient-based measures to assess medium-term outcomes following shoulder surgery for disorders of the rotator cuff', *Arthritis and Rheumatism*, **47**, 513–19.

Epstein, A.M. (1990) 'The outcomes movement – will it get us where we want to go?', *New England Journal of Medicine*, **323**, 266–70.

Fayers, P.M. and Machin, D. (2000) *Quality of Life – Assessment, Analysis and Interpretation* (Chichester: John Wiley and Sons).

Fitzpatrick, R., Davey, C., Buxton, M.J. and Jones, D.R. (1998) 'Evaluating patient-based outcome measures for use in clinical trials', *Health Technology Assessment*, **2**, i–74.

Fitzpatrick, R., Fletcher, A., Gore, S., Jones, D., Spiegelhalter, D. and Cox, D. (1992) 'Quality of life measures in health care. I: Applications and issues in assessment', *British Medical Journal*, **305**, 1074–7.

Garratt, A., Schmidt, L., Mackintosh, A. and Fitzpatrick, R. (2002) 'Quality of life measurement: Bibliographic study of patient assessed health outcome measures', *British Medical Journal*, **324**, 1417.

Jenkinson, C. (1994) 'Measuring health and medical outcomes: An overview'. In Jenkinson, C. (ed.), *Measuring Health and Medical Outcomes* (London: UCL Press) pp. 1–6.

Kazis, L.E., Anderson, J.J. and Meenan, R.F. (1989) 'Effect sizes for interpreting changes in health status', *Medical Care*, **27**, 3, S178–S189.

Kirkley, A., Griffin, S. and Dainty, K. (2003) 'Shoulder systems for the functional assessment of the shoulder', *Arthroscopy*, **19**, 1109–20.

Lansky, D., Butler, J.B.V. and Frederick, W.T. (1992) 'Using health status measures in the hospital setting: From acute care to "outcomes management"', *Medical Care*, **30**, MS57–MS73.

McDonald, I.G. (2000) 'Quality assurance and technology assessment: Pieces of a larger puzzle', *Journal of Quality in Clinical Practice*, **20**, 87–94.

Nelson, E.C., Landgraf, J.M., Hays, R.D., Wasson, J.H. and Kirk, J.W. (1990) 'The functional status of patients. How can it be measured in physicians' offices?', *Medical Care*, **28**, 1111–26.

Streiner, D.L. and Norman, G.R. (1989) *Health Measurement Scales: A Practical Guide to their Development and Use* (New York: Oxford University Press).

Torrance, G.W., Furlong, W., Feeny, D.H. and Boyle, M. (1995) 'Multi-attribute preference functions: Health Utilities Index', *PharmacoEconomics*, **7**, 758–62.

WHOQOL (2007) http://www.bath.ac.uk/whoqol/questionnaires/info.cfm (accessed 22 April, 2007).

World Health Organization (1948) *Constitution of the World Health Organization* (Geneva: WHO Basic Documents).

Notes

1   A gold standard could theoretically include changes in 'the condition of interest' that could accurately be measured from radiographs or blood tests and were very closely correlated with patients' reports of symptoms and other aspects of quality of life.

2   Anecdotally, many people find the SF-36 – with 36 items – quite long enough. Indeed, the longer the questionnaire, the greater the risk of obtaining missing responses.

3   Further useful information on Rasch models is provided in Fitzpatrick et al. (1998).

4   The original method scored each item from 1 to 5, from least to most difficulty or severity. Items were summed to produce a single score with a range from 12 (least difficulties) to 60 (most difficulties). This method of scoring changed recently, because clinicians have found the original scoring system unintuitive.

Part 4

Qualitative Research

In-depth Interviews

14

LINDSEY COOMBES, DEBBY ALLEN, DEBORAH HUMPHREY
AND JOANNE NEALE

Introduction

The in-depth interview (also referred to as the 'depth', 'open-ended', 'informal', 'personal' or 'qualitative' interview) is a generic term used to describe the type of data collection that commonly takes place in qualitative research. In-depth interviewing essentially involves a verbal interaction between a researcher, who has a research topic or research question that they want to investigate, and an interviewee (sometimes referred to as a participant, respondent or informant), who has been selected because of their experience or knowledge of the issues being explored. Usually, the in-depth interview involves only one researcher and one interviewee[1] and the aim is primarily to gather opinions, facts and stories that will shed light on the research topic or question from the viewpoint of an expert 'insider'.

In-depth interviews are most commonly conducted in person (face-to-face), but can also be undertaken by telephone. In the future, it seems likely that more in-depth interviewing might be carried out via video-conferencing or email. The format of the in-depth interview is often described as unstructured or semi-structured.[2] In the former, the interviewer conducts the interview with no preconceived view of the content or flow of the information to be gathered. In the latter, the interviewer has a broad set of questions that they want to ask, but encourages the interviewee to develop and expand upon issues that they deem important and lets the questioning flow naturally dependent on how the interviewee responds.

Historical Context

The history of in-depth interviewing lies within the broader development of social research methods and particularly ethnography (see Chapter 17). The businessman and social commentator Charles Booth is generally credited with being the first person to undertake a study relying on interviewing (Converse, 1987). In 1886, Booth investigated the economic and social conditions of people living in London. This involved interviews with Londoners from all walks of life which were recorded in notebooks and used as a basis for a monumental 17-volume report *Life and Labour of the People in London*.

Throughout the twentieth century, interest in understanding the lives of groups and individuals from their own perspective (known as an interpretive approach to data collection and analysis) increased. Within this tradition, a further important study conducted in the 1920s used a life history approach to produce a detailed account of the experiences of Polish immigrants (Thomas and Znaniecki, 1996). Rather than exploring Polish immigration from the perspective of the wider society looking in at the Polish immigrant community, a rich cultural understanding of this group was produced by allowing community members to document their own stories and speak for themselves. This was achieved through the analysis of documentary materials – such as personal letters, autobiographies, and diaries – but also oral information.

The work of Thomas and Znaniecki was subsequently influential in inspiring other major studies of urban and city life within the Chicago School at the University of Chicago in the USA. These studies made important contributions to the field of ethnography and involved combinations of observation, analyses of personal documents and informal interviews conducted with members of deviant and marginalised groups. They included Anderson's classic study of homeless workers (Anderson, 1923); Whyte's research into urban young men in an Italian neighbourhood in Boston (Whyte, 1943); and Shaw's case study of a delinquent boy called Stanley whose petty crime resulted in him being sent to a Chicago correctional facility (Shaw, 1930).

In the 1950s and 1960s, interviewing lost some of its qualitative flavour as the social survey (see Chapter 9) – with its emphasis on closed questioning and the quantification of data – came into prominence. Despite this, qualitative interviewing continued, particularly within the broader context of American ethnographic research and still often focusing on marginalised communities. For example, Preble and Casey (1969) conducted interviews with, and observations of, the lives of heroin users in the streets of New York City and Warren (1974) adopted interviews and other ethnographic methods in her study of a Southern California gay community. In addition, some researchers reacted against the rise of more structured interviewing formats and advocated very creative forms of interviewing – such as interviews that lasted for one or more days, emphasised free expression and facilitated deep disclosure (Douglas, 1985).

In the UK, qualitative interviewing took longer to establish than in the USA. Nonetheless, it formed part of seminal ethnographies such as Young and Willmott's (1957) study of family life and kinship in East London and Paul Willis's (1977) research into working-class boys and their relationships to school and work. Feminists also began to use in-depth interviewing as a means of exploring the lives of women. In so doing, they questioned various assumptions built into in-depth interviewing techniques – for example, that the interviewer was male; the interview was a one-way process in which the researcher did not disclose any information; the interviewee was simply a source of data and not part of a human interaction; and the interviewee was somehow subordinate to the researcher. They then adapted the interviewing process to make it more egalitarian. Studies within this tradition focused on issues as diverse as the role of the housewife (Oakley, 1974), women's access to general practitioners (Barrett and Roberts, 1978) and female drug use (Taylor, 1993).

More recently, attention has turned to the importance of race, social status and age (as well as gender) in interviewing processes (Seidman, 1991). Furthermore, the basic techniques of in-depth interviewing have developed and changed quite markedly. Thus, whilst the earliest researchers wrote up their notes once their interviews were over, today's researchers almost always audio record (and sometimes video) their interviews. Likewise, the development of computer software packages (such as MAXqda2, Atlas.ti, Nud*ist, NVivo, HyperRESEARCH, and Qualrus) have enabled the processes of sorting and coding large quantities of in-depth interview data to become more systematic and rigorous.

Current Use

In-depth interviewing is an important method of collecting data within a wide range of qualitative research approaches. Its role in studying groups of people in their own environment (ethnography) and biographical accounts of individuals' lives (life history) have already been identified. However, in-depth interviewing is also a means of collecting data for oral histories (studies concentrating on specific events or periods); phenomenological research (studies of human experience in which considerations of objective reality are not taken into account); and grounded theory research (studies which categorise empirically collected data to build a general theory to fit that data).

Today, in-depth interviewing is used extensively across the social science disciplines, including anthropology, history, sociology, criminology, social policy, politics and urban studies. In addition, it has a strong established presence in health and social care – particularly within nursing and medical sociology. Here it is commonly used to explore the lived experiences of professionals, patients, clients and carers. Sometimes the method is used simply as a means of increasing knowledge in order better to understand health and caring issues – for example Cheung and Hocking's (2004) study of the lived experience of spousal care for people with multiple sclerosis. On other occasions, it is employed as a technique for generating information that will help to change policy and practice and improve people's lives – for example, Fischer et al.'s (2007) study of how best to involve drug users in making decisions about their own treatment.

An innovative example of in-depth interviewing that seeks both to understand health and social care issues and change practice is provided by the Charity DIPEx. The DIPEx research group undertakes in-depth interviews (usually videoed) with individuals affected by various health and social care issues (such as cancer, pregnancy, mental health, living with dying and neurological conditions). The data collected are then systematically analysed and published in peer-reviewed papers. However, extracts of the interviews also appear (with participants' informed consent) on the DIPEx website (http://www.dipex.org/Home.aspx). Here, they provide a valuable resource for others wanting to know more about the various conditions covered, as well as teaching and learning materials for a wide range of professionals seeking to improve their practice.

Despite the increasing use and acceptance of in-depth interviewing in recent years, the extent to which an interview can ever give a researcher straightforward access to experience is a contested issue. Indeed, interesting philosophical debates persist between qualitative researchers regarding how far the knowledge produced through in-depth interviewing is a pre-existing phenomenon or constructed during the interview process itself (Legard et al., 2003). Thus, Kvale (1996) has argued that those adhering to the 'knowledge as a pre-existing phenomenon' position tend to see knowledge as buried metal and the interviewer as a miner whose job is to uncover the metal. In contrast, those who see knowledge as 'constructed during the interview process' perceive knowledge as created and negotiated and the interviewer as someone who travels with the interviewee, leading them to new insights and helping them to interpret their views and experiences.

BOX 14.1

Types of Question Addressed by In-depth Interviews

- What are older people's experiences of moving into a nursing home?

- How do community mental health nurses work with younger women experiencing depression?

- What are health visitors' views of the single assessment process?

- What is the lived experience of young men diagnosed with diabetes?

On a more consensual note, it is widely accepted that in-depth interviewing involves a number of key features. Legard et al. (2003) summarise these as follows:

- First, in-depth interviews combine structure with flexibility. So, even the most unstructured interview will be initiated with at least some sense of the themes that will be explored.

- Second, they are interactive in nature. That is, the researcher and the interviewee inevitably interact with each other in the interviewing process.

- Third, the researcher will use a range of techniques (such as probes and follow-up questions) to encourage the interviewee to reflect and expand on their responses.

- Finally, the interview will be likely to generate at least some new knowledge and ideas as interviewees explore avenues of thought that they have not previously considered.

Main Strengths of In-depth Interviewing

One of the key strengths of qualitative interviewing is the detailed contextual data it produces. The flexibility of the interviewing process encourages the researcher and participant to explore issues in depth and to reflect on feelings, emotions, beliefs and experiences. This helps to enhance the validity of the findings produced since participants can be assisted to understand questions and interviewers can ask for clarifications and probe for further responses if necessary. Furthermore, the production of data as part of a broader narrative reduces the danger that responses are taken out of context and misinterpreted.

A further important strength of in-depth interviewing is the priority given to the participant's perspective. Those who are interviewed are usually selected because they have some direct experience or knowledge of the subject being researched. They are thus able to tell it like it really is from the inside out, rather than as it might appear from the outside looking in. In addition, the focus on the participant's views and experiences permits issues or topics that the researcher may never have considered or deemed important to emerge. The use of direct quotations from participants when writing up in-depth interviews is also a very powerful way of bringing the findings alive and reinforcing their validity.

Beyond this, in-depth interviewing is particularly good at investigating topics about which relatively little is known and where it is therefore difficult to propose a research hypothesis or predefine all of the questions that might need to be asked. As such, in-depth interviewing can be described as 'inductive' rather than 'deductive' in its approach. In other words, it is used to generate new ideas and theory rather than to test existing hypotheses. Because of this, in-depth interviews are sometimes used prior to a quantitative study to help identify and refine the structured questions that will be included. However, they can equally be conducted after a quantitative study to explore possible reasons for unanticipated or interesting findings (see also Chapter 19).

Finally, in-depth interviews are very suited to researching sensitive issues and complex behaviours. This is because the informal atmosphere of the in-depth interview affords the researcher ample time to develop trust and rapport with participants. Furthermore, there are many opportunities to reassure them of the confidentiality of their responses, remind them that anything they say will be anonymised, and reinforce the importance and relevance of their views. All of these factors can help interviewees to feel more engaged with the study, relaxed about participating, and therefore willing to open up and discuss their views at length.

Main Weaknesses of In-depth Interviewing

Because in-depth interviewing is a highly subjective technique, it is often criticised for being susceptible to researcher bias. As previously suggested, the interview may be as much a reflection of the social encounter between the interviewer and the interviewee as it is about the interviewee's personal beliefs. Furthermore, the researcher's own viewpoint on the topic of investigation may have an impact on how they collect, analyse and interpret the data. For example, a researcher who has personally had a negative experience of a particular medical intervention may unwittingly focus more on the negatives than on the positives if interviewing others about the treatment. Such high levels of subjectivity can raise questions about the validity and reliability of qualitative interviewing.

A further weakness is that in-depth interviews can be extremely time-consuming to undertake. Gaining access to participants can be slow, especially if approval has to be gained from one or more ethics or research and development committees (see Chapters 2 and 3). In addition, it is often necessary to travel quite lengthy distances in order to meet potential interviewees at a time and venue that is convenient to them. Moreover, interviewing frail and vulnerable groups brings further challenges in terms of negotiating with carers and professionals who may see the interview as unnecessary or an added burden. Even after the data have been successfully collected, transcribing the interviews can be time-consuming and/or costly.

Further to the above, it is easy for the inexperienced and unskilled researcher to conduct a poor in-depth interview. For example, they may ask leading questions,[3] forget to probe for more depth and detail, talk over the interviewee, digress into their own personal anecdotes or experiences, or simply be unable to keep the interviewee sufficiently focused on the research topic. There is also the danger that recording equipment might fail – or the researcher might forget to turn it on.

Finally, researchers can struggle to know how to analyse the large quantities of unstructured narrative information that in-depth interviewing tends to produce. Remarkably few books or journal articles describe in detail or with any clarity the processes of analysing qualitative data. Instead, there are often vague references to findings 'emerging' and the importance of analysis being 'inductive' or 'grounded'. The lack of clearly formulated procedures and conventions can result in an undisciplined 'anything goes' mentality or as one commentator has argued:

> It is sometimes difficult to know what the researchers actually did during this [analysis] phase and to understand how their findings evolved out of the data ...

In describing their processes some authors use language that accentuates this sense of mystery and magic. For example, they may claim that their conceptual categories 'emerged' from the data – almost as if they left the data out overnight and awoke to find that the data analysis fairies had organised the data into a coherent new structure that explained everything! (Thorne, 2000: 68).

MAIN STRENGTHS AND WEAKNESSES
... OF IN-DEPTH INTERVIEWING

Strengths

- A key strength of in-depth interviewing is the detailed contextual information it produces. This helps the researcher to understand the full meaning of the interviewee's response and enhances the validity of the findings.

- A further important strength of in-depth interviewing is the priority given to the participant's perspective. Participants have direct experience or knowledge of the topic being researched and are thus able to give an insider's perspective.

- In-depth interviewing is suited to investigating topics about which relatively little is known.

- In-depth interviews are valuable when researching sensitive issues and complex behaviours.

Weaknesses

- The subjective nature of in-depth interviewing makes it susceptible to criticisms of bias.

- In-depth interviewing can be extremely time-consuming to undertake.

- It is easy for the inexperienced and unskilled researcher to conduct a poor in-depth interview.

- Researchers can struggle to know how to analyse the large quantities of unstructured narrative data that in-depth interviewing tends to produce and this can result in an unacceptable 'anything goes' mentality.

Conducting In-depth Interviews

In-depth interviewing requires careful thought and planning. As with any research technique, the central aims of the study and the key information required should be established from the outset. It is also important to have a good knowledge of the existing literature. Together, this will help in making decisions about who should be interviewed and the kinds of issues that should be raised. Once this has been decided, an interview guide (also known as an interview schedule or topic guide), an information sheet about the study, and any necessary consent forms can be prepared.

Although interview guides vary in their level of detail, a typical semi-structured guide has three main sections. The first includes some ice-breaking and factual questions. These will help the participant to relax and enable the researcher to understand something of the participant's life (for example, who they live with, whether they are married, what their job is). The second and main part includes a list of open-ended questions and probing follow-ups relating directly to the key issues of interest. These questions and probes provide a framework to ensure that the interviewee keeps to the research topic and there is consistency between interviews. The final part of the guide begins by signalling that there are only a few questions left, invites the interviewee to add any further comments, and ends on a positive note so that the interviewee is not left in a negative frame of mind.

Since the types of topic investigated in semi-structured interviews are often sensitive or difficult, the preparation stage should additionally include thinking through how the researcher will respond if a participant becomes distressed or embarrassed, asks for help with a problem, or discloses criminal or potentially life-threatening behaviour during the interview. Thus, the researcher may need to plan strategies to prevent any interviewee being left feeling vulnerable or exposed and they may need to inform themselves of local sources of support so that details can be provided at the end of the interview to anyone requesting more information. Additionally, the study information sheet and consent form should clarify the kinds of information that may need to be reported to a third party.

Beyond this, researchers should think in advance about the best places and times to conduct interviews, how to dress, and what gender and ethnic combinations in interviewer–interviewee pairs might most likely lead to open exchanges. Because the interviewer and participant need to establish a good rapport, it is wise to conduct an interview at a time and venue to suit the interviewee whilst simultaneously ensuring sufficient opportunity to talk in privacy and uninterrupted. The interviewer should also attempt to dress in a way that makes the participant feel at ease. For example, interviewing a drug user whilst wearing a suit would be as inappropriate as interviewing a hospital consultant whilst wearing shorts and a T-shirt.

Prior to starting the interview, the researcher should record the time, date and place as well as any other notable circumstances. They should also introduce themselves and the study, and allow the participant time to read the information sheet and sign any consent forms.[4] The interview should then be conducted in a conversational manner, using the interview schedule in a flexible way so that the key areas are covered but there is also opportunity to discuss any emergent issues. On balance, the interviewee will do most of the talking. The interviewer must communicate interest in and respect for the interviewee and allow them to reflect prior to responding. They should also avoid making any judgemental comments that will inhibit the interviewee's free expression. Crucially, the interviewer's job is to listen carefully (to both verbal and non-verbal cues) and probe for clarification, depth and detail.

In-depth interviews should always be recorded to avoid any detail being lost. Although this was often done by hand in the past, today it is standard practice to audio record and, increasingly, to use video interviews. At the end of the interview, the researcher must thank the participant for their time and avoid rushing off if the interviewee wants to talk further. Sometimes, a participant will use this as an opportunity to provide additional reflections and the interviewer may request permission to turn the recording equipment back on. Once the interview is definitely over, the interviewer should privately record their own observations, thoughts and feelings about the interview (either on paper or into the recording equipment). All of this information then becomes part of the analysable data.

All recorded material should be transcribed – ideally verbatim. The transcriptions must then be indexed, a process which is increasingly being carried out electronically with the assistance of software packages such as those already identified. Indexing[5] involves reviewing each transcript line by line and assigning segments of text to codes which represent key issues or themes evident in the data. The codes tend to be grouped into categories and the categories collectively comprise a coding frame. For example, in Gagliardi's (1991) grounded theory study of the experiences of families living with a child with Duchenne muscular dystrophy, coding categories included 'relationships', 'feelings', 'events' and 'activity' and individual codes under the 'relationships' category were 'father', 'mother', 'siblings' and 'extended family'.

Indexing helps to sort, order and structure the data ready for analysis. Analysis is a highly personal activity that involves making sense of the information collected (Jones, 1985). Although there is plenty of scope for flexibility, analysis must always be systematic, rigorous and complete and there are various accepted techniques for achieving this. These include thematic analysis, constant comparative method, analytic induction, narrative analysis, grounded theory, deviant cases, content analysis and framework. While it is not possible to examine each of these here, they all share a number of key processes. These include identifying important phrases, patterns and themes; isolating emergent patterns, commonalities and differences; producing a small set of generalisations that cover the consistencies discerned in the data; and confronting those generalisations with a formalised body of knowledge in the form of constructs or theories (Miles and Huberman, 1994).

An Example of an In-depth Interview Study

A study of key worker services for disabled children provides a good example of in-depth interviewing within the field of social care (Greco et al., 2006). The research was published in the journal *Health and Social Care in the Community* and was undertaken by researchers from the Social Policy Research Unit at the University of York, the Department of Educational Studies at the University of York and the Personal Social Services Research Unit at the University of Kent. The investigation was part of a larger project exploring different models of multi-agency key worker services for disabled children and was funded by a range of UK Government Departments (Greco et al., 2005).

Key workers for disabled children and their families have been recommended in the Children's National Service Frameworks for England and Wales. These key workers are the main point of contact for families with disabled children and have a remit to work across health, education and social services. To this end, they require a broad knowledge of disability, the roles of other agencies and professionals, local and national service availability, and key information sources. The aim of the study by Greco et al. (2006) was to investigate the views of staff (key workers, service managers and steering group members) working in key worker services regarding the organisation and management of those services.

Seven services (four from England and three from Wales) were selected from thirty key worker services that had been identified previously in a national survey (Greco and Sloper, 2004). The seven services were chosen to represent variation in terms of models of service and types of locality covered. The intention was to interview all managers, up to ten key workers, and up to eight steering group members in each service. Packages – containing cover letters, information sheets, response forms and postage-paid return envelopes – were sent to the managers of the seven services for distribution to others in their service. Recipients who were willing to participate then provided contact details on the response form, and researchers subsequently contacted them to arrange an interview.

The study was approved by a Multi-Centre Research Ethics Committee and informed consent was obtained from each participant prior to interview. In total, 50 key workers, 7 managers and 32 multi-agency steering group members were interviewed, generating a response rate of 62%. The interview schedules used to guide the data collection differed slightly for each of the respondent groups, but always asked about the role of key workers, the advantages and disadvantages of the service, and suggested improvements. Whilst each of the three interview schedules included lists of questions and possible prompts, interviewing was undertaken flexibly so that the issues raised by the interviewees themselves could be explored. Each interview lasted approximately one hour and was tape-recorded.

Data were systematically analysed following established qualitative analysis procedures (Taylor and Bogdan, 1984). To begin, three researchers read a number of interview transcripts to identify the key emerging themes and, from this, a coding framework was agreed. The interview transcripts were then coded to the framework using the software program MAXqda. Analyses sought to identify and compare the characteristics and views obtained from different models of services. This occurred in two stages. First, separate reports of findings for each service were produced, checked and then sent to the appropriate service manager for further checking. Second, the individual service reports were amalgamated to identify differences and similarities between services.

Findings revealed that basic service aims were similar in all seven services and included: identifying the needs of the child; providing key workers as a main point of contact for the child and family; drawing up and reviewing a multi-agency care plan; working with other professionals providing information to families; providing support for families; and helping families to access services. Despite this, there were evident differences between services in respect of the processes used to achieve these various aims; how positive staff were about the services provided; the problems encountered by staff; understanding of the key worker role; the amount of training key workers received; the availability of supervision; opportunities to meet other key workers; level and stability of funding; and the roles of the service manager and steering group.

Greco et al. (2006) used their findings to make a number of recommendations for future policy and practice in key worker services for disabled children. Thus, they advocated clear, written job descriptions to help clarify the key worker role and structures to support key workers (for example training focused on the key worker role, supervision specific to the role, opportunities for contact with other key workers, and agreement on the time needed for key workers to undertake the role). The importance of dedicated funding – at least for a manager and a training budget – was also highlighted, and it was emphasised that managers on steering groups needed to be senior enough to be able to take decisions and prioritise steering group meetings. Finally, it was recommended that parent representatives on steering groups should have a genuine say in decision-making processes and should not feel powerless when decisions were made.

Recognising the limitations of their research, Greco et al. noted that their study only provided a snapshot in time and aspects of the services involved might already have changed by the time of writing. They also commented that their study was focused on disabled children with complex needs so their findings could not be generalised to key working for other groups of children. Equally, only small proportions of staff in some services were interviewed and this might have restricted the range of viewpoints identified.

Further Reading

Gubrium, J.F. and Holstein, J.A. (eds) (2002) *Handbook of Interview Research* (Thousand Oaks, CA: Sage).

This is an excellent resource which contains a broad collection of essays on various aspects of interview research. The book is divided into six main parts which cover the different types of interviewing; interviewing particular groups of individuals (such as older people, men, women and those who are ill); interviewing in different contexts (such as medical settings, forensic investigations, education and employment); technical issues and the use of technology in interviewing; analytic strategies; and reflection and representation. It comprehensively combines practical and theoretical issues in a manner suitable for students new to research and those who are more experienced.

Hardy, M. and Bryman, A. (eds) (2004) *Handbook of Data Analysis* **(London: Sage).**

This handbook provides a one-stop account of qualitative and quantitative data analysis and is suitable for both postgraduate students and research specialists. Part V deals with qualitative data analysis and includes eight chapters written by experts in the field. Each chapter includes useful examples and key references for further reading. Content analysis, discourse analysis, grounded theory, narrative analysis and postmodern approaches are all covered. The editors successfully present readers with a range of qualitative analytic options so that they can select that which seems most appropriate to their particular study.

Holstein, J.A. and Gubrium, J.F. (1995) *The Active Interview* **(Thousand Oaks, CA: Sage).**

In this book, the differences between the active interview (where interviewers and interviewees are considered equal partners in constructing meaning around an interview) and the traditional interview (where the interviewee is considered the passive conduit through which information is transmitted to the omniscient interviewer) are discussed. Novice researchers are given clear guidance on conducting an interview that is the rich product of both parties.

McCracken, G. (1988) *The Long Interview* **(Newbury Park, CA: Sage).**

This relatively short text provides comprehensive coverage of the key theoretical and methodological issues involved in intensive qualitative interviewing. It begins with a general overview of the nature and purpose of qualitative inquiry before examining a number of key issues, including the investigator as instrument; the obtrusive/unobtrusive balance; and the investigator/respondent relationship. The author outlines the four steps of the long qualitative interview – these being an exhaustive review of the literature; self-examination; developing questions; and analysing data. The reader is provided with information on how to judge quality and write up data, as well as practical advice on commissioning and administering research.

Silverman, D. (2006) *Interpreting Qualitative Data*, **3rd edn (London: Sage).**

This is an invaluable text examining recent developments, methodologies and interpretive strategies in qualitative research. It is particularly suited to students and others embarking on their own qualitative research project for the first time. Chapter 4 is dedicated to interviews and sets itself four objectives. These are, to enable the reader to distinguish between the different kinds of interview; understand the skills used in doing an interview; recognise the various theoretical bases of interview research; and conduct a simple analysis of interview data. Both the uses and pitfalls of interview data are explored, usefully supplemented by worked examples, exercises, 'tips', web links, summaries and recommended reading.

References

Anderson, N. (1923) *The Hobo: The Sociology Of The Homeless Man* (Chicago, IL: Phoenix Books).

Barrett, M. and Roberts, H. (1978) 'Doctors and their patients: The social control of women in general practice'. In Smart, C. and Smart, B. (eds), *Women, Sexuality and Social Control* (London: Routledge & Kegan Paul).

Cheung, J. and Hocking, P. (2004) 'Caring as worrying: The experience of spousal care', *Journal of Advanced Nursing*, **47**, 475–82.

Converse, J.M. (1987) *Survey Research in the United States: Roots and Emergence 1890–1960* (Berkley, CA: University of California Press).

Douglas, J.D. (1985) *Creative Interviewing* (Beverly Hills, CA: Sage).

Fischer, J., Jenkins, N., Bloor, M., Neale, J. and Berney, L. (2007) *Drug User Involvement in Treatment Decisions* (York: Joseph Rowntree Foundation).

Gagliardi, B.A. (1991) 'The family's experience of living with a child with Duchenne muscular dystrophy', *Applied Nursing Research*, **4**, 159–64.

Greco, V. and Sloper, P. (2004) 'Care coordination and key worker schemes for disabled children: Results of a UK-wide survey', *Child: Care, Health, and Development*, **30**, 13–20.

Greco V., Sloper P., Webb R. and Beecham J. (2005) *An Exploration of Different Models of Multi-Agency Key Worker Services for Disabled Children: Effectiveness and Costs* (Nottingham: DfES Publications).

Greco V., Sloper P., Webb R. and Beecham J. (2006) 'Key worker services for disabled children: The views of staff', *Health and Social Care in the Community*, **14**, 445–52.

Jones, S. (1985) 'The analysis of depth interviews'. In Walker, R. (ed.), *Applied Qualitative Research* (Aldershot: Gower) pp. 56–70.

Kvale, S. (1996) *InterViews: An Introduction to Qualitative Research Interviewing* (Thousand Oaks, CA: Sage Publications).

Legard, R., Keegan, J. and Ward, K. (2003) 'In-depth interviews'. In Ritchie, J. and Lewis, J. (eds), *Qualitative Research Practice: A Guide for Social Science Students and Researchers* (London: Sage).

Miles, M.B. and Huberman, A.M. (1994) *Qualitative Data Analysis: An Expanded Source Book*, 2nd edn (London: Sage).

Oakley, A. (1974) *Housewife* (London: Allen Lane).

Preble, E. and Casey, J. (1969) 'Taking care of business: The heroin user's life on the streets', *International Journal of Addiction*, **1**, 1–24.

Seidman, I.E. (1991) *Interviewing as Qualitative Research* (New York: Columbia University, Teachers College Press).

Shaw, C.R. (1930) *The Jack-Roller: A Delinquent Boy's Own Story* (Chicago, IL: University of Chicago Press).

Taylor, A. (1993) *Women Drug-users: An Ethnography of a Female Injecting Community* (Oxford: Clarendon Press).

Taylor, S. and Bogdan, R. (1984) *Introduction to Qualitative Research Methods: The Search for Meaning* (New York: John Wiley and Sons).

Thomas, W. and Znaniecki, F. (ed. Zaretsky, E.) (1996) *The Polish Peasant in Europe and America: A Classic Work in Immigration History* (Urbana, IL: University of Illinois Press).

Thorne, S. (2000) 'Data analysis in qualitative research', *Evidence-Based Nursing*, **3**, 68–70.

Warren, C.A.B (1974) *Identity and Community in the Gay World* (New York: Wiley).

Whyte, W.F. (1943) *Street Corner Society: The Social Structure of an Italian Slum* (Chicago, IL: University of Chicago Press).

Willis, P.E. (1977) *Learning to Labour: How Working Class Kids Get Working Class Jobs* (Farnborough: Saxon House).

Young, M. and Willmott, P. (1957) *Family and Kinship in East London* (London: Routledge).

Notes

1   Occasionally, more than one interviewee may participate – for example, a couple may be interviewed together.

2   Although some would argue that it is better to conceive of the level of structure as a continuum, with most studies falling somewhere between very little or no structure at one end and a very clear structure at the other.

3   That is, a question that leads the interviewee to respond in a certain way. For example, 'Did you feel really terrible when your child was taken into care?' affords the interviewee little opportunity other than to respond with 'Yes, really terrible'.

4   It is often advisable to introduce the study and distribute information sheets and consent forms to potential participants a week or two before the actual interview date, thus allowing them ample time to reflect on their involvement and removing any sense of pressure to participate.

5   Also known as coding.

Focus Groups 15

Julia Foster-Turner

Introduction

Focus groups are a qualitative research technique that is used to collect data through the process of group member interaction and discussion. Groups 'focus' on a topic which is determined by the researcher who is active in the group process (Morgan, 1996; Krueger and Casey, 2000). Members are selected because they have a particular characteristic, need or interest in common. The aim is to promote self-disclosure among group members in order to learn more about how they think and feel, their attitudes and their opinions. The emphasis is on understanding their experiences, behaviours and perspectives; that is, not only *what* they think about an issue, but also *how* they think about it and *why* they think the way that they do (Morgan, 1997).

As with individual interviewing techniques (see Chapter 14), focus groups rely on the researcher (who often acts as the group 'moderator' or 'facilitator') posing questions and group members (commonly known as the 'participants' or 'respondents') giving answers. The defining quality of the focus group process is that it actively encourages interaction, in the form of dialogue, between the group members themselves. This arises when participants question each other or challenge the views that other members hold. In response, those involved in the dialogue expand on their opinions and share the reasons behind their thinking. Thus, focus groups constitute a powerful interactive process for accessing and generating data. Nonetheless, they need a trained and skilled moderator to keep this interaction on track.

Historical Context

In the late 1930s and early 1940s, social researchers began developing non-directive interviewing techniques.[1] These allowed participants take an active role in communicating issues that were a concern and significant to them and required the researcher to use active listening skills to bring out the participants' attitudes and feelings. Central to this approach was the open-ended question, whereby participants were invited to respond in their own words instead of being confined to a predefined list of answers created by the researcher (Kreuger and Casey, 2000). In the Second World War, American social scientists started to use these non-directive interviewing techniques in groups. For example, Merton and Kendall (1946) used them to examine the persuasiveness of wartime propaganda activities and the effectiveness of training materials for soldiers.[2]

At about the same time, market researchers began to recognise the potential of focus groups in helping them to gain a better understanding of consumers and clients. An important contributor to the commercial use of the focus group was the sociologist Paul Lazarsfeld, who had been a colleague of Merton in Columbia, USA. Indeed, it was Lazarsfeld's research into audience responses to radio broadcasts during the 1940s that was said to have first exposed Merton to group interviews (Morgan, 1997). As the head of academic market research centres in both Newark and Columbia, Lazarsfeld had employed focus groups, alongside a wide range of other social science research techniques, to solve problems for a range of clients, including the dairy industry (Morgan, 1997).

With the growth of the economy in the 1950s, commercial market researchers continued to make use of focus groups to inform product development and presentation. One very well-known example from the period (cited by Morgan and Krueger, 1998) related to boxed cake mixes. The American company Betty Crocker had invented a cake mix which simply required the addition of liquid in order to make cake batter. Although this seemed like a perfect convenience product, the company was surprised to find that consumers were not happy. Focus groups with housewives indicated that the cake mix was too simple, leaving consumers with no sense of accomplishment or achievement. As a result, Betty Crocker reformulated the mix so that the user had to add an egg as well as liquid. This generated a product that better simulated homemade cake baking and so better satisfied customers.

During the mid-twentieth century, social scientists preoccupied themselves with quantitative rather than qualitative research methods and the focus group largely disappeared from academia (Morgan, 1997). When it re-emerged in the 1980s, social scientists applied and adapted Merton's original techniques but also drew upon more recent practices from market research (Stewart and Shamdasani, 1990; Krueger and Casey, 2000). The academic application of group interviews slowly expanded as focus groups were increasingly used to explore knowledge, attitudes and practices in a diverse range of areas. These included the prevention of 'battering' during pregnancy (Helton et al., 1987), alcohol-related problems in primary care (Babor et al., 1986) and safety belt use (Merrill and Sleet, 1984).

Focus group research continued to spread in the 1990s, particularly in the areas of programme evaluation, marketing, public policy, advertising and communications (Stewart and Shamdasani, 1990). This growth continues today. As a simple indicator of this expansion, in 2000, a limited search in a single database (psycINFO) yielded less than 1,000 articles on the keyword 'focus group' (Hyden and Bulow, 2003). A similar search on the same keyword in the same database in late 2007 yielded 4,167 articles.

Current Use

Focus groups are often used in the preliminary stage of a larger study in order to test the construction, utility or validity of the data collection instrument – for example, a survey (see Chapter 9) or a health outcome measure (see Chapter 13). Alternatively, they can be undertaken to gain greater insight and understanding of the results emerging from a survey or another research method, particularly if such results are ambiguous, suspect or need further clarification or elaboration (see Chapter 19). In addition, focus groups are of course a valuable 'self-contained' qualitative research method in their own right. As such, they can be used to explore new research areas or to consider research problems from the perspective of diverse groups of research participants (Morgan, 1997).

Within health and social care, the application of focus groups continues to expand, particularly in service development, priority setting, provision and evaluation. For example, Hills and Kitchen (2007) used focus groups to explore patient satisfaction with outpatient physiotherapy services for individuals suffering from acute and chronic musculoskeletal conditions. In Australia, meanwhile, Shrimpton et al. (2007) asked members of the public and professionals to discuss which stakeholders should be involved in healthcare decision-making. Beyond this, focus groups can capture patients' views on the suitability and quality of healthcare products (Garmer et al., 2004) or even the risks and regulations relating to medicines and medical devices (Ipsos MORI, 2006).

Focus groups have also been used to examine the concerns of healthcare workers (for example Jinks and Daniels (1999) used them to identify and explore the workplace health concerns of healthcare workers within an acute UK NHS Trust) and the concerns and needs of specific client/patient groups and their carers (for example Roose and John (2003) used them to investigate young children's understanding of mental health and their views on appropriate services for their age group). In particular, focus groups have been very effective in understanding the needs and experiences of very marginalised social groups, such as Dominican and Puerto Rican mothers living in the Bronx, New York (Guilamo-Ramos et al., 2007), homeless people who feared dying on the streets (Song et al., 2007) and people with learning disabilities (Fraser and Fraser, 2001).

Building on Krueger and Casey's (2000) ideas, focus groups have additionally been employed to research change management in relation to local and national policy and service developments. To this end, they can be undertaken at different strategic points within the cycle of change. For example, *prior to change*, focus groups can be used to assess whether a proposed change is needed and to inform the nature of that change before any implementation activity. *During change*, they can help monitor and evaluate progress, for example by providing interim feedback from the perspective of different key stakeholder groups. Finally, *post change*, focus groups are a useful mechanism for assessing how the change was managed, its outcomes in relation to the initial objectives and any indicators for future actions.

BOX 15.1

Types of Question Addressed by Focus Groups

- What are your views/thoughts/feelings/opinions/experiences/concerns/understanding about ... ?

- How have you used service ... ? What aspects have you found particularly helpful/unhelpful ... and why?

- What are your needs in relation to ... ?

- What help/support would you like in relation to ... ?

- What is most satisfying and most dissatisfying regarding ... and why ... ?

- What influences your decisions regarding ... ?

- What is the impact of ... on your life?

Main Strengths of Focus Groups

One of the key strengths of focus groups lies in the dynamic created by the group interaction. This is because other group members – as well as the researcher – are able to clarify responses, probe for further detail and incorporate follow-up questions. By encouraging the participants to compare and contrast their views and experiences, the researcher is able to gain insights into the consensus and diversity of perspectives (Morgan, 1997). In addition, researchers can check their interpretation of the findings by involving other researchers in observing or participating in the group proceedings.

Beyond this, focus groups can be very valuable in engaging disadvantaged and marginalised groups who may feel inhibited in a one-to-one interview (see Chapter 14) or who may be unable to participate in a survey (see Chapter 9) (Morgan, 1996; Smithson, 2000). For example, they are well suited to gathering data from people who have problems with literacy, such as children or people who have learning disabilities. Those who lack confidence or feel they have nothing to say will often join in a discussion initiated by other group members (Kitzinger, 1995) or become more willing to talk if they discover that they have similar thoughts, feelings or experiences to others (Stewart and Shamdasani, 1990).

A further strength of focus groups is that they can be used across a wide variety of topics, people and settings. Like other qualitative techniques, they are useful for exploring ideas and concepts as well as people's thoughts, feelings and opinions, particularly in respect of sensitive subjects (Morgan, 1996). However, they have the added advantage of being much quicker and cheaper to conduct than one-to-one interviews. Likewise, they require less notice to arrange than a more systematic survey (Stewart and Shamdasani, 1990). Arguably, it is such pragmatic factors that have helped to make them so attractive across the business and market research sectors.

Main Weaknesses of Focus Groups

An important weakness of focus groups is that participants are generally not representative of the broader population that interests the researcher and so the results cannot be generalised. There are various reasons for this. For example, the number of people who participate in a focus group study tends to be small and these individuals are often recruited through convenience rather than systematic sampling strategies.[3] Furthermore, the type of person who is willing to take the time and effort to participate, who is able to travel to the focus group location, and who is prepared to talk publicly about their views and experiences may have characteristics that distinguish them from the wider population of interest (Stewart and Shamdasandi, 1990).

Secondly, the dynamics of focus group interactions can introduce bias into the findings. For example, one or two participants may dominate the discussions whilst other members may refuse to speak (Stewart and Shamdasani, 1990; Kitzinger, 1995). Equally, the group dynamic may have an effect on what people say and how they say it (Morgan, 1997). As a result, some individuals may communicate more extreme views than they would in private. Conversely, conformity within the group may mean that some members withhold things that they may say in private or may agree with things that they would usually dispute (Morgan, 1997). Another risk is that the moderator consciously or unconsciously influences the discussion by the responses or cues that they give (Stewart and Shamdasani, 1990).

MAIN STRENGTHS AND WEAKNESSES

... OF FOCUS GROUPS

Strengths

- Focus groups provide participants with the opportunity to develop and refine their ideas through discussion and interaction with like others.

- The method is valuable in engaging disadvantaged and marginalised groups and those who feel they have nothing to say.

- Focus groups tend to be quicker and cheaper to undertake than many other types of research.

Weaknesses

- Focus group participants are generally not representative of the broader population of interest and so the results cannot be generalised.

- The group dynamics (arising from very dominant or very reticent individuals; group members' desire to conform to the views of others; or the conscious or unconscious views of the moderator) can all bias the discussion and findings.

- A good focus group is difficult to conduct, requiring an experienced moderator with good interpersonal skills as well as sufficient time and analytical competence to ensure that the complex data collected are rigorously summarised, analysed and interpreted.

One further limitation relates to the difficulty of conducting a good focus group and analysing the material appropriately. The widespread use of the technique, often by those with little formal research methods training or those who want a quick answer to a complex problem, means that examples of poor focus group practice are legion. In addition to appropriate training, a focus group moderator must have good rapport-building and facilitative skills. Similarly, a high level of analytical competence, as well as time, is needed to ensure that the large volume of complex open-ended data collected is rigorously summarised, analysed and interpreted (Stewart and Shamdasani, 1990; Mansell et al., 2004).

Conducting a Focus Group

Developing focus group questions

Once a research problem has been identified (see Chapter 2), the researcher can develop the more specific questions that will be used in the group discussions. If the focus group is primarily exploratory (because there is little existing research on the topic and issues are poorly understood), the discussion can be relatively unstructured and only a small number of questions will be needed. If, however, there is a clear research question or aim, more questions and more moderator intervention are required to prevent the participants straying from the key issues.

Focus group questions should be open-ended and straightforward and more general questions need to be asked before more specific ones. It is always advisable to test out ('pilot') questions in advance to ensure that they are clear and will generate useful discussion. If a study requires only one category of participants (for example pregnant women), the same questions should be used with each focus group conducted so that their responses can be compared and contrasted. When focus groups are conducted with different types of participant (for example pregnant women, partners of pregnant women and midwives), it is common to have core questions that are the same across all groups with some additional group-specific questions (Krueger and Casey, 2000).

Sampling participants

In selecting focus group participants, a first consideration is to identify which types of people are likely to produce the desired data (Krueger and Casey, 2000). If this is more than one type of participant, it is advisable to run different groups for each participant category. Beyond this, it might be sensible to further segment groups in relation to age, gender, ethnicity or social class. A key reason for this is to maximise homogeneity within groups, since differences between members can potentially inhibit interaction and communication. Equally, lack of homogeneity within groups can make it more difficult to compare responses across groups during the analyses (Morgan, 1997).

A further issue to consider when selecting participants is whether group members are known to each other or are strangers. Participants who are already acquainted or friends may encourage each other to talk more openly about their experiences. However, such participants may not question or justify an issue within the focus group itself because it falls within a set of assumptions and beliefs that members have already developed within their relationships elsewhere. Meanwhile, strangers may feel more at ease discussing sensitive issues because they are with people whom they will never meet again (Bender and Ewbank, 1994).

Establishing number of groups and group size

Ideally, there should be three to five groups for each participant category in order to ensure that data saturation is reached (that is, the moderator can predict what will be said in the next group and any further groups are unlikely to generate new insights) (Glaser and Strauss, 1967; Morgan, 1997). Traditionally, a group size of six to ten participants is recommended, but groups of four or twelve are common. Smaller groups allow each participant more time to talk and this usually works well when the topic is very familiar (such as experiences of a frequently used service). Larger groups offer less 'talking space' per participant and are more useful when participants are less familiar with the topic (such as the potential implications of a proposed new service or policy).

Planning a group

Good planning includes identifying a suitable date, time and venue for each group. The venue needs to be pleasant, easily accessible to the participants and free from interruptions. Since non-attendance on the day is common, it is wise to build in time for running additional groups if necessary. Equally, participants should be given a reminder call several days before the meeting and, if possible, an incentive to attend (such as book tokens or a small monetary reward). Planning also involves deciding whether there will be one moderator or two, whether a separate note taker is required, and how the group will be recorded. It is usual to audio record sessions and take written notes so that the data collected can be cross-compared. However, video and flipcharts might also be used.

Running the group

Prior to the designated start time of the group, the room should be organised and the equipment checked. As participants arrive, they should be allowed to meet informally, preferably over some refreshments. Following this, the moderator should welcome everyone and introduce themselves, their colleagues and the reason for the group. They must also explain how the group will run, including its content and timing; recording procedures; ground rules relating to confidentiality and respect for others; the uniqueness of each person's experience; the lack of any right or wrong answers; and the value of different viewpoints in providing a basis for exploration and discussion.

Most focus groups last for one-and-a-half to two hours and it is important not to overestimate how many questions can be fully addressed in this time. A typical group will begin with a couple of general opening questions to help participants relax and to start them talking. These will be followed by introductory questions, which clarify the research topic and encourage individuals to think about how they connect to it. After this, the main questions – those that probe for participants' thoughts and feelings on the research issue – are asked. About 15 minutes before the group is due to finish, the moderator should let the participants know that the session is coming to an end, check that each individual's responses have been accurately recorded and invite any final comments. Finally, the participants should be thanked for their help and the next stages of the research outlined.

Throughout the focus group, the moderator must create a supportive and non-judgemental atmosphere so that people feel relaxed and comfortable. In addition, they must probe responses for depth, detail, clarity and examples and encourage dialogue between the group members. If any participants begin their own private discussion, the moderator needs to draw them back into the main group. It may also be necessary to prevent dominant members from speaking for too long and to encourage those who are reticent to speak out. Usually this is done by subtle non-verbal communication, such as eye contact, and the timely use of spoken prompts.

Analysing the data

The initial stage of the analysis involves the researcher coding the recorded material from the focus group discussions. This can be done by hand, by using the 'cut' and 'paste' functions of a word processing package, or with a qualitative data analysis software programme (such as Atlas.ti or NVivo). Essentially, coding involves grouping segments of text[4] from each focus group transcript under the relevant focus group question. All the segments of text under each question are then grouped again into themes.[5] Ideally, this process should be undertaken independently by two or more analysts to test the reliability of the coding and to reduce the risk of subjectivity and bias (Stewart and Shamdasani, 1990).

Once the material has been coded, a descriptive summary of what each participant group said in response to each focus group question can be prepared. Similarities and differences between the various participant groups' responses to each question can then be explored and themes that cut across the questions identified. Key factors for consideration include how often something is said; by how many different people it is said within each group; in how many groups it was discussed; the level of specific detail given; and the amount of energy, enthusiasm and passion with which it was discussed (Kreuger and Casey, 2000).

Ethical considerations

Key ethical issues in conducting a focus group relate to participants' entitlement to opt out at any stage; the need for confidentiality regarding the content of the group discussions; secure data storage; the taking of informed consent from participants; and assurances of anonymity when the data are reported. Researchers must also ensure that individuals are in no way physically or psychologically harmed. To this end, moderators should monitor participants' stress levels during the group and diffuse tension as needed. At the end of the group, it can also be helpful to incorporate a debriefing session and/or hand out topic-orientated educational briefs or other literature for participants to take away (Slaughter et al., 1999).

An Example of a Focus Group Study

As explained above, an important strength of focus groups is that they can be used to access the views and experiences of people with communication problems. In the following example, the aim was to explore the needs that arise when young people with learning difficulties make the transition from adolescence to adulthood. The research was commissioned by the UK Social Care Institute for Excellence (SCIE) and was undertaken by the Norah Fry Research Centre at the University of Bristol, North Somerset People First and the Home Farm Trust. It involved focus groups, a systematic literature review, and a review of extant information resources.

The study ran from October 2003 to March 2004 and produced a number of outputs including an online report: Tarleton, B. (2004) *The Road Ahead: Information for Young People with Learning Difficulties, their Families and Supporters at Transition*. The report was intentionally written in clear and simple language in recognition of the fact that focus groups must refer to, and be inclusive of, their target population from instigation to completion. The focus group component is described below.

Focus groups were conducted with three types of participant: young people with learning difficulties, their parents, and their supporters (for example learning support assistants, volunteers, and sessional staff from an advocacy project). In total, 12 groups were conducted (four with each of the three participant types). The study included 27 young people, 19 parents and 19 supporters.[6] The young people were of varying ages from 13 years upwards; five were black, five were deaf, and one had high support needs. Although there was only one black parent,[7] there were four black supporters who provided some insights into the black parents' views.

Invitations using clear language and visual images to help explain the topic and introduce the research team were sent to the young people along with a consent form. At the same time, similar letters and consent forms were sent to their parents and supporters. Participants were also contacted by the researcher to give further explanation and to negotiate access and venues.[8] In each venue, a contact (such as a teacher) acted as a 'go-between' and, in at least two areas, wrote a covering letter to parents confirming their organisation's support for the research.

The aim was that the young people, their parents and their supporters would arrive at the same venue at the same time, start with drinks or a meal together, and then separate into their own specific focus groups. For the young people's focus groups, the research team had prepared questions, supporting pictures and symbols representing the topics to be discussed, and a chart on which the pictures and symbols could be placed to illustrate their relative importance (close to the centre of the chart if important and further away if less important).[9] The groups were intended to run for a maximum of two hours and began with introductions; explanations regarding confidentiality; clarification of participants' understanding of transition; and asking what the young people wanted to do when they were older or what they had done as they had grown up.

In order to identify their information needs and priorities, the young people were then asked to place the pictures/symbols on the prepared chart. They were also asked how they obtained information, how they would like information to be provided to them, what a website about transition might look like, and the most important thing that they would like to have known two years earlier. The content of the parents' and supporters' groups was designed to parallel that of the young people's meetings in order to facilitate comparison of data across groups. For example, parents and supporters were asked what they thought the young person and supporter/parent would need to know. Data collection was undertaken via note taking.[10]

Initial observations indicated that the pictures often represented something different to the young people than the picture artists had envisaged. Also, the parents and supporters struggled to prioritise the different types of information. Thus, on a few occasions, they deemed all of the information very important. More detailed analyses examined the specific content, emphases, similarities and differences within the responses of the three participant groups, including in relation to the age of the young person. Differences in the parents' and supporters' views were also explored and, when material from the young person, parent and supporter in one 'triangle' was available, differences of perspective in relation to the individual in question were analysed.

Findings revealed that young people did not understand the term 'transition', but they all had clear expectations about what they wanted to do or change as they grew up. Young people, parents and supporters wanted the same information during transition, covering the transition process, their roles within the process and their rights and entitlements. They also wanted to know about the local situation, including accessing person-centred approaches and the support/ services available. The rights and responsibilities of young people as adults – such as information on self-advocacy, empowerment, risk taking and safety – were additionally highlighted. In essence, people wanted to know about all of the choices and changes available.

The report indicated a clear deficit in the content and delivery of information for young people with learning difficulties, their parents and supporters. In response, SCIE launched a web-based resource to enable service providers, advocacy organisations, relatives and other supporters to understand the kind of information needed and how to present it (http://www.scie.org.uk/publications/tra/ index.asp). Information on this website is made more accessible through the use of simple, clear language, images and some audio material. It is also likely that further research regarding the level of impact this has had on young people, their families and supporters will be needed.

Further Reading

Barbour, R. and Kitzinger, J. (eds) (1999) *Developing Focus Group Research: Politics, Theory and Practice* (London: Sage).

This stimulating book examines and critically discusses different ways of designing, running and analysing focus groups and explores how the technique can be combined with other research methods. There are some particularly interesting sections on accessing the views of minority groups, use of focus groups in feminist studies, discourse analysis, software packages, and the epistemological and political underpinnings of research. Both the novice and experienced researcher will find themselves encouraged to question and challenge current thinking in the field.

Krueger, R.A. and Casey, M.A. (2000) *Focus Groups: A Practical Guide for Applied Research*, 3rd edn (Thousand Oaks, CA: Sage).

Krueger and Casey's book offers a detailed but practical step-by-step guide to developing and running focus group studies, including when and when not to use the technique; understanding different styles of focus groups; designing focus group studies; selecting participants; moderating groups; analysing data; and reporting. It is a suitable text for novice researchers or those with limited experience. As this is a largely practical book, less space is given to the theoretical underpinnings of the method.

Morgan, D.L. (1997) *Focus Groups as Qualitative Research*, 2nd edn (London: Sage).

Morgan's seminal text provides detailed discussion on social science approaches to focus groups; debates about their relative merits and weaknesses; some comparisons between focus groups and individual interviews; reflections on self-contained focus groups; and developments in focus group design. The book also offers useful information on developing and running focus groups and analysing and interpreting the data they generate. It is essential reading for both new and more advanced researchers and would be a useful supplementary text for general research methods courses.

Stewart, D.W., Shamdasani, P.N. and Rook, D.W. (2006) *Focus Groups Theory and Practice*, **2nd edn (London: Sage).**

In this book, the design, running and interpretation of focus group data within the context of social science research and theory are examined. Each stage of the focus group process is examined, incorporating some useful discussions on designing the interview guide and the impact of focus group composition. It also considers how to conduct focus groups and the characteristics needed by group moderators. New to the second edition is a discussion on the use of information technology for conducting groups online and by video-conferencing. This is, again, a relevant text for both novice and more experienced researchers and a valuable supplementary text for more general research methods courses.

References

Babor, T.F., Ritson, E.B. and Hodgson, R.J. (1986) 'Alcohol-related problems in the primary health care setting: A review of early intervention strategies', *Addiction*, **81**, 23–46.

Bender, D.E. and Ewbank, D. (1994) 'The focus group as a tool for health research: Issues in design and analysis', *Health Transition Review*, **4**, 63–76.

Fraser, M. and Fraser, A. (2001) 'Are people with learning disabilities able to contribute to focus groups on health promotion?', *Journal of Advanced Nursing*, **33**, 225–33.

Garmer, K., Ylvén, J. and Karlsson, M.A. (2004) 'User participation in requirements elicitation comparing focus group interviews and usability tests for eliciting usability requirements for medical equipment: A case study', *International Journal of Industrial Ergonomics*, **33**, 85–98.

Glaser, B.G. and Strauss, A.L. (1967) *The Discovery of Grounded Theory* (Chicago, IL: Aldine).

Guilamo-Ramos, V., Dittus, P., Jaccard, J., Johansson, M., Bouris, A. and Acosta, N. (2007) 'Parenting practices among Dominican and Puerto Rican mothers', *Social Work*, **52**, 17–30.

Helton, A., McFarlane, J. and Anderson, E. (1987) 'Prevention of battering during pregnancy: Focus on behavioral change', *Public Health Nursing*, **4**, 166–74.

Hills, R. and Kitchen, S. (2007) 'Satisfaction with outpatient physiotherapy: Focus groups to explore the views of patients with acute and chronic musculoskeletal conditions', *Physiotherapy, Theory and Practice*, **23**, 1–20.

Hydén, L.C. and Bülow, P.H. (2003) 'Who's talking: Drawing conclusions from focus groups – some methodological considerations', *International Journal of Social Research Methodology*, **6**, 305–21.

Ipsos MORI (2006) *Risks and Benefits of Medicines and Medical Devices – Perceptions, Communication and Regulation*. Report on Qualitative Research among the General Public. Research Study Conducted for the Medicines and Healthcare Products Regulatory Agency. www.mhra.gov.uk/home/idcplg?IdcService=SS_GET_PAGE&nodeId=1017 (accessed 18 October, 2007).

Jinks, A.M. and Daniels, R. (1999) 'Workplace health concerns: A focus group study', *Journal of Management in Medicine*, **13**, 95–105.

Kitzinger, J. (1995) 'Qualitative research: Introducing focus groups', *British Medical Journal*, **311**, 299–302.

Krueger, R.A. and Casey, M.A. (2000) *Focus Groups: A Practical Guide for Applied Research*, 3rd edn (London: Sage).

Mansell, I., Bennett, G., Northway, R., Mead, D. and Moseley, L. (2004) 'The learning curve: The advantages and disadvantages in the use of focus groups as a method of data collection', *Nurse Researcher,* **11**, 80–8.

Merrill, B.E. and Sleet, D.A. (1984) 'Safety belt use and related health variables in a worksite health promotion program, *Health Education and Behavior,* **11**, 171–9.

Merton, R.K. and Kendall, P.L. (1946) 'The focused interview', *American Journal of Sociology,* **51**, 541–57.

Merton, R.K., Fiske, M. and Kendall, P.L. (1956) *The Focused Interview: A Manual of Problems and Procedures* (Glencoe, IL: Free Press).

Morgan, D.L. (1996) 'Focus groups', *Annual Review of Sociology,* **22**, 129–52.

Morgan, D.L. (1997) *Focus Groups as Qualitative Research,* 2nd edn (London: Sage).

Morgan, D.L and Krueger, R.A. (1998) *The Focus Group Kit* (vols 1–6) (Thousand Oaks, CA: Sage).

Roose, G.A. and John, A.M. (2003) 'A focus group investigation into young children's understanding of mental health and their views on appropriate services for their age group', *Child, Health and Development,* **29**, 545–50.

Shrimpton, B., McKie, J., Hurworth, R. and Richardson, J. (2007) *A Focus Group Study of Health Care Priority Setting at the Individual Patient, Program and Health System Levels,* Research Paper, 17 (Melbourne, VIC: Centre for Health Economics, Monash University).

Slaughter, P., Pinfold. P., Flintoft, V., Gort, E., Thiel, E., Blackstein-Hirsch, P., Axcell, T., Paterson, M., Cameron, C., Easterbookes, C., Mercer, S.L., Goel, V. and Williams, J.I. (1999). *Focus Groups in Health Services Research at the Institute for Clinical Evaluative Sciences,* Technical Report No. 99-02-TR www.ices.on.ca/file/focus%20groups (accessed 15 April, 2007).

Smithson, J. (2000) 'Using and analyzing focus groups: Limitations and possibilities', *International Journal of Social Research Methodology,* **3**, 103–19.

Song, J., Bartels, D.M., Ratner, E.R., Alderton, L., Hudson, B. and Ahluwalia, J.S. (2007) 'Dying on the streets: Homeless persons' concerns and desires about end of life care', *Journal of General Internal Medicine,* **22**, 435–41.

Stewart, D.W. and Shamdasani, P.N. (1990) *Focus Groups, Theory and Practice* (London: Sage).

Tarleton, B. (2004) *The Road Ahead: Information for Young People with Learning Difficulties, their Families and Supporters at Transition* http://www.scie.org.uk/publications/tra/report/index.asp (accessed 13 November, 2007).

Notes

1 As opposed to the more directive or structured interviewing techniques used in surveys (see Chapter 9).

2 Drawing upon this work, Merton, Fiske and Kendall later published the first detailed procedural guide for group interviews (Merton et al., 1956).

3 That is, individuals are chosen because they are relatively easy to access.

4 These are each labelled to show who was speaking and at what point in the focus group they were speaking.

5 See Krueger and Casey (2000) for a more detailed explanation.

6 These were all parents or supporters of the participating young people.

7 This was despite efforts to include the black parents.

8 Three of the venues were in England and one in Wales; they included two special schools and two self-advocacy organisations.

9 These materials had previously been tested in two special schools and subsequently improved.

10 It is not clear whether any form of audio recording was undertaken.

16

Participant Observation

BRIDGET TAYLOR

Introduction

Participant observation is an observational research method, which involves the researcher participating in the activities of the group being studied. It is often described as an oxymoron as it combines two apparently contradictory terms (Savage, 2000), implying 'simultaneous emotional involvement and objective detachment' (Tedlock, 2000: 465). As Grigsby (2001: 334) explains, 'the researcher works to maintain the role of being "inside and outside" the experience simultaneously'.

Participant observation emphasises the part played by the researcher in the production of data, with the researcher and data considered inextricably connected (Melia, 1982). The method involves more than observation; it relies upon the researcher's subjective experiences to gain a better understanding of a social phenomenon (Grigsby, 2001). To this end, participant observation seeks to uncover motives, intentions and interpretations of events from 'the insider's' perspective; to consider what goes on, who is involved, when and where things happen, how they occur and why things happen as they do (Jorgensen, 1989). This insider perspective is also known as the 'emic' perspective.

Participant observation is a type of 'fieldwork' or 'field research' and is one of the techniques used in ethnographic studies (see Chapter 17). It is somewhat misleading to consider participant observation as a single method as it involves a complex blend of different data-collection techniques. These include direct observation, direct participation, formal and informal interviews, and enumerations of salient events and activities.

Historical Context

Following his work in the Trobriand Islands, the British anthropologist Bronislaw Malinowski (1884–1942) is widely credited with developing participant observation as a serious research method. Unlike previous studies in which researchers had simply adopted the role of an observer, Malinowski 'stepped off the veranda' and participated in the lives of the group he was studying. By developing an understanding of the emic perspective, he generated a richness and depth to research data that had previously been missing.

While anthropologists continue to make the most consistent use of participant observation in their ethnographic work, the method also has deep roots in sociology, with studies in areas such as education, medicine, religion and deviance. Goffman's (1961) study of the asylum is a classic example of sociological research that was reliant on participant observation. In order to observe life in a psychiatric institution, Goffman obtained employment there as an assistant athletic director. In his accepted role as a member of staff, he was able to participate in the day-to-day life of the institution, functioning both as a participant and as a researcher. This enabled him to uncover practices that might otherwise have remained hidden. These included patients being force-fed and needing to obtain permission before going to the toilet.

In addition, participant observation studies have sometimes used covert observation techniques. Here, the researcher deliberately sets out to deceive the research participants, entering a setting without telling those around them of their real research intentions. For example, in one American study (Rosenhan, 1973) researchers feigned the characteristics of schizophrenia in order to obtain admission to a psychiatric hospital as patients. Covert studies such as this raise many ethical issues and tend to be disapproved of in the research literature, where today the emphasis is very much on the researcher's moral responsibilities and on gaining participants' informed consent (see Chapter 3).

Participant observation has also been adopted as a research method in a wide range of studies in the field of health and social care and examples of these appear throughout this chapter.

Current Use

Participant observation is particularly useful in the exploratory phase of a study, where the research questions are unclear and little is known about a topic. It is also commonly used in descriptive studies and those that aim to generate theoretical interpretations. Participant observation provides valuable insights into phenomena that are usually hidden from public view (such as deviant, criminal or sexual behaviour) or when insiders and outsiders have different views (it provides opportunities for exploring the emic perspective). Additionally, the method illuminates phenomena that are best understood in the natural setting, such as the relationships between people and events and the socio-cultural contexts of behaviour and processes (Jorgensen, 1989).

Through the development of trusting relationships between the researcher and participants, participant observation uncovers data that would otherwise remain inaccessible. For example, in Muller's (1995) research into the interactions of trainee doctors with dying patients, participants were unusually open about their personal dilemmas, professional struggles and the stresses of their role over time. Participant observation also provides opportunities for gathering quantitative data, such as the incidence of abuse in an institution for those with learning difficulties (Taylor, 1987), and the rate of unplanned discharge from a youth shelter (Grigsby, 1992). The collection of quantitative data in these studies is likely to involve a structured observation schedule such as that used by Edwards (1998) in her study of touch between patients and nurses.

BOX 16.1

Types of Question Addressed by Participant Observation

- What goes on?

- Who is involved?

- When and where do things happen?

- How do they occur?

- Why do things happen as they do?

For example:

- What are participants' intentions?

- Who makes decisions?

- When is information shared?

- How do individuals communicate with each other?

- Why do participants make certain decisions?

Main Strengths of Participant Observation

Grigsby (2001: 337) describes one of the main strengths of participant observation as the 'comprehensive nature of its perspective'. Unlike many other methods, participant observation places great emphasis on the context within which the observed activities and events are embedded. The researcher studies people as they go about their everyday lives and this generates a unique richness in the data produced. Furthermore, the advantage of being with a group of people over a period of time is that the researcher can 'capture the process of change as well as the change itself' (Muller, 1995: 70).

Participant observation is equally a valuable method for researching topics that 'expose the beliefs and social *meanings* held by individuals and groups' (Miller and Brewer, 2003: 223). The participant observer can study what actually takes place, not just what participants say takes place. There are many actions or relationships that participants themselves may be unaware of, or reluctant to disclose, such as deviant behaviour or poor health and social care practices. Indeed, interview and questionnaire data often reveal discrepancies between what people report that they have done, or will do, and the reality (Robson, 2002). Participant observation has clear advantages over these methods since data collection does not rely on participants' honesty, memory or knowledge of events.

A further advantage of participant observation is its flexible research design. This permits the researcher to respond and adapt to changing circumstances, events and situations. Through this flexible approach, participant observation provides opportunities to pursue themes, hunches and working hypotheses that evolve. It also enables the research questions to be modified and refined, during both data collection and analysis.

Main Weaknesses of Participant Observation

Because of its focus on one setting or group, participant observation is often criticised for its limited generalisabilty and lack of objectivity. Inevitably, the researcher's ethnic background, gender, social class, age and professional background will all impact on the relations established, the discussions and observations noted, and the data generated. For example, the researcher's own gender can influence how they perceive others and how others perceive them. Moreover, the personal characteristics or personality of the researcher may facilitate stronger relationships with some participants than with others, limiting their access to certain information and activities and resulting in observer bias (Roper and Shapira, 2000).

The role that the researcher assumes will ultimately enhance opportunities for interactions with one group of individuals, but restrict opportunities with another. Thus, a researcher who adopts the role of a cleaner on a hospital ward will encounter many opportunities for observing and talking to other cleaners and patients, but will probably have limited contact with medical staff. In organisations where there is a strong hierarchical structure, a higher status member may not accept being observed or questioned by a lower status member, and a lower status member may present 'accepted' feelings and behaviour when observed or questioned by a higher status member.

Because of the time it takes to develop relationships, it can be tempting for the researcher to conduct participant observation within a familiar setting, such as their place of work. However, objectivity is likely to be impaired if the researcher is already a 'native' of that setting (Robson, 2002). Over-involvement or 'going native' (Adler and Adler, 1987) is one of the perils faced by researchers conducting participant observation. Overfamiliarisation with language and events may result in the commonplace being overlooked, and can result in valuable data being lost (Kennedy, 1999). For health or social care practitioners studying an aspect of practice, there is also the danger that they may revert to their practitioner role at the expense of observation and objectivity (Kite, 1999). Morse and Lipson (1991: 72) argue that 'nurses are the worst people to do participant observation because they cannot sit in the ward and "do nothing". They have to go and tuck in the bed, take the bedpan, get the water, and before you can turn around, they are working!'

A further disadvantage of participant observation is that it can be very time-consuming and the researcher may observe many irrelevant events while waiting for those in which they are interested to occur. For some researchers, participant observation may also feel too unstructured, flexible and open-ended (Miller and Brewer, 2003). In addition, participant observation requires a very high level of skill in balancing the demands of being both 'insider' and 'outsider'. This involves getting close to the people being studied in order to develop relationships with them, yet retaining objectivity and distance. For many, trying to balance these roles with integrity creates an uneasy compromise (Jarvie, 1982), resulting in role strain.

Two final weaknesses of participant observation relate to vulnerability and risk, for both the researcher and the participants. For the researcher, there can be particular concerns when studying illegal or immoral behaviour. For participants, there is a danger that their identities may be revealed when findings are published – again, a particular worry if research has focused on illegal or immoral behaviour, deviant acts or poor practice. Sluka (1990) and Lee (1995) offer sound, practical advice on how to minimise the hazards of fieldwork in dangerous and violent social contexts. Meanwhile, triangulation of methods – drawing on the experiences of others beyond the research setting – can help to preserve the anonymity of participants in reports and publications (Taylor, 2005).

MAIN STRENGTHS AND WEAKNESSES
... OF PARTICIPANT OBSERVATION

Strengths

- Participant observation is valuable in studying the social contexts of behaviour and processes. This generates a unique richness to the data produced.

- Unlike many other methods, the data collected through participant observation does not rely on the memory or honesty of participants. It may also uncover actions or relationships of which the participants are themselves unaware.

- The flexible research design allows the researcher to respond to changing situations and pursue themes, hunches and working hypotheses that evolve.

Weaknesses

- A major criticism of participant observation is researcher bias, where the researcher's own personality, characteristics and beliefs influence the data collected and the interpretation of these data. On occasions, the researcher can also become over-involved with participants, a situation known as 'going native'.

- Participant observation is potentially very time-consuming.

- The vulnerability of both the researcher and participants should not be overlooked. Some settings may pose risks to the researcher and the participants' identities need to be protected.

Conducting a Participant Observation Study

Participant observation is not a series of mechanical steps; it requires ongoing creativity and flexibility by the researcher (Jorgensen, 1989). Once a research problem requiring participant observation has been identified, some key stages are as follows.

Planning

Prior to entering the field, participant observers need to consider how they will manage situations where they might be exposed to deviance, illegal behaviour or poor practice. They also need to reflect on how they will act if antagonistic views, violence, racism or sexism threaten their values or presence in the research setting. Obtaining pre-study consent from all research participants may well be impossible. Therefore, the researcher will need to think through how they might obtain consent from individuals as the study progresses and how they will spend their time and record data while in the presence of individuals who have not consented to being involved. They should equally prepare for the sense of loss that some participants might feel when the study is over and they leave the field. Such issues should all be discussed in any application to an ethics committee (see Chapters 2 and 3).

Sampling

Clearly, careful thought needs to be given when choosing a research setting. As indicated previously, pre-existing relationships may considerably speed up the process of gaining access. However, objectivity may be compromised in familiar settings (Grbich, 1999) given that the familiar will remain familiar and much may be overlooked. Unlike most other research methods, the sampling of participants in participant observation does not normally occur in advance of a study starting. Rather, the researcher must choose how to spend their time, who and what to observe, and who to question about what on an ongoing basis. Since contact with one participant often opens up access to another, opportunistic and snowball sampling are most commonly adopted and researchers tend to describe their sample after the event (McCall and Simmons, 1969).

Establishing a role

The role and identity that the researcher assumes in the research setting will significantly determine where they can go, with whom they can interact, what they can see, and what they can ask (McCall and Simmons, 1969). The researcher needs to assume a role with 'acceptable incompetence' (Lofland, 1971) that is most strategic for obtaining the relevant information. To study patient care, for example, the researcher could select the role of a nurse, doctor, care assistant, porter, patient, visitor, volunteer, ward clerk, cleaner or administrator. It is important that the researcher does not 'stand out' yet does not 'blend in' to the extent that their dual role is compromised. In some clinical settings, it might be preferable not to wear a nurse's uniform (Turnock and Gibson, 2001). In others, this uniform might give legitimacy to a researcher's presence and enable them to access the 'backstage' (Goffman, 1959) world behind the screens around a patient's bed.

The differing proportions of time the researcher spends in observing and participating are identified by Gold (1958) as constituting four different roles: 'complete observer'; 'observer-as-participant'; 'participant-as-observer'; and 'complete participant'. Many authors describe these four roles as distinctly separate, implying that the researcher adopts one of the roles, perhaps even selecting their chosen role before entering the field. However, it may be more useful to view these four roles as a continuum, with participation at one end and observation at the other. Ideally, the researcher should spend the majority of the time in either the observer-as-participant or the participant-as-observer role. Nonetheless, a good researcher will move flexibly in and out of all four roles throughout the study period.

The 'complete observer' is essentially a passive role that focuses solely on data collection. While it is particularly likely to be adopted during the settling-in period of a study, it can also be used profitably at other times when the researcher is peripheral to the core activities of those under investigation (Richards and Postle, 1998). The 'observer-as-participant' role is, meanwhile, characterised by brief relationships and is most frequently adopted when conducting research of a short duration. In contrast, the 'participant-as-observer' role requires the researcher to immerse themselves into a role that is recognised by other participants, while simultaneously ensuring that those other participants know that the researcher is also present in order to understand and record what is going on as part of a study.

By participating in the activities of the group, the 'participant-as-observer' researcher acquires similar perspectives and experiences to the ordinary members and gains some sense of the subjective nature of events. However, to verify that these perspectives correspond to those of the ordinary members, the researcher also asks questions. Thus, they slip between 'observer-as-participant' and 'participant-as-observer'. As the emphasis on participation rather than observation increases, the risk of 'going native' grows and this is most likely to occur when the researcher becomes a 'complete participant'. Although it is often assumed that complete participation only occurs when observation is covert, it is also possible for the researcher in an overt study to become so highly involved that they lose the perspective of 'detached wonder'. A good example of this is provided in O'Neill's (2001) work with the ambulance service.

Establishing and maintaining relationships

The key to effective participant observation is establishing good relations with participants. To this end, care needs to be taken when explaining the purpose of the research to those in the field. The explanation given needs to be plausible so that participants do not become suspicious of the researcher's motives and restrict what they are willing to share. The researcher therefore needs to ease themselves into the research setting at an appropriate pace, avoiding rebuff by blundering into sensitive situations and topics (McCall and Simmons, 1969). Additionally, they need to explain to participants the kinds of activities in which they will participate, the sorts of information needed, and the purposes for which this information will be used. If this is explained at the outset, participants will be prepared for the researcher's questions and may also volunteer information that they consider relevant.

To avoid being a drain on participants' time, researchers may further need to identify reciprocating favours such as running errands, providing lifts, and offering to make the coffee. They may likewise need to prove their trustworthiness by, for example, participating in 'membership tests' such as smoking in prohibited areas or engaging in illegal activities (Adler and Adler, 1987; Taylor, 1987). Such activities can facilitate entry into the 'back regions' of a research setting, where the researcher is permitted to observe that which would normally remain hidden (Berreman, 1968). However, they can have legal, moral and ethical implications for the researcher and so must be carefully considered.

Data collection

Fieldnotes are the most frequent means of recording data in participant observation. The kinds of data recorded should include the layout of the environment, the characteristics of the participants, the sequence of events, and the goals and feelings of those involved (Robson, 2002). Merriman (1998) suggests that it is useful to structure observations to include descriptions of people, tasks, events, behaviour and conversations (both verbal and non-verbal). The data collected should describe relationships, hierarchies, roles and rules (Bowling, 1997). It is only by capturing *all* of this information that the context is established. Recording what at the time appears to be irrelevant information might later enable the researcher to identify and trace cycles, spirals and sequences, as well as the circumstances surrounding their occurrence (Lofland and Lofland, 1995).

In taking fieldnotes, the researcher inevitably needs to strike a balance between observation and participation. Interestingly, many authors reject overt note taking since this can over-prioritise the observer role and the researcher may miss valuable expressions and actions while writing. In contrast, Bernard (2000) warns against trying to become an inconspicuous participant, only recording notes when unobserved (such as in the toilet). He advises researchers to be clear that they are an observer who wants to participate as much as possible. Following this approach, the goal should be to make brief notes that will prompt more detailed recall later.

Although fieldnotes are the most frequent means of recording data in participant observation, the researcher must not assume that their own experience in the setting holds for others. Thus, fieldnotes need to be verified through informal and in-depth interviews with participants. Reflecting this, Yin (1989) offers three useful principles for data collection. First, the researcher should use multiple sources of evidence, speaking to several participants about the same theme or observation. Second, they should develop a comprehensive database of fieldnotes, documents, quantitative data and narrative accounts. And third, they should construct a 'chain of evidence' throughout their data collection to assist their analysis and increase the reliability of their findings.

Data analysis

Data analysis occurs simultaneously and continuously alongside data collection, beginning with the first observation and continuing iteratively with each subsequent interview and observation. The credibility of the preliminary data analysis is established by searching for rival explanations, explaining negative cases and through member-checking (corroborating information gained from one participant with information obtained from others). Reflexivity is a key component of this process. Defined by Marshall (2002: 176) as a 'perpetual source of questioning and self-revelation', reflexivity increases awareness of one's own feelings, beliefs, values and attitudes, and the potential effect of these on the people and setting being studied (Payne and Payne, 2004). Through a reflexive approach to both fieldwork and analysis, the researcher is aware of the potential for bias and strives to overcome it by seeking both evidence and counter-evidence. Any bias in relationships and interpretation is made explicit in reports and publications so that the reader can weigh up the validity of the findings and determine what is believable and plausible (Koch and Harrington, 1998). Researchers such as Sword (1999), Bland (2002) and Ladino (2002) all clearly demonstrate the importance of reflexivity in data analysis.

An Example of a Participant Observation Study

Unfortunately, research publications rarely present both the results of a participant observation study and an adequate reflexive analysis of the researcher's role. Jan Savage has, however, achieved this through a one-year research project that produced three valuable publications (Savage, 1995; 1997; 2000).

Savage's study considered the emphasis that is placed on 'closeness' when considering the therapeutic potential of nurses' relationships with patients. As nurses' attitudes and beliefs may not always correspond with the realities of their work, participant observation was a valuable method for experiencing, observing and asking about this aspect of practice. In addition to her participant observer role, Savage conducted informal interviews and semi-structured in-depth interviews with nurses, patients and non-nursing staff.

The study was conducted on two medical/surgical gastrointestinal wards in southern England. Not having nursed for many years, Savage assumed the role of a 'research nurse' and identified activities in which she could participate within her limited competence. Thus, she took part in handovers and ward meetings, assisted nurses with bathing patients, fetched and carried, and generally tried 'to make myself useful' (2000: 332).

From the outset, Savage identified her surprise at the changed ethos in nursing since her career break. During her time on the ward, she learnt to use her body in the same way as the other nurses. She found that she adopted a similar stance and began to use touch in a way that she had previously thought was inappropriate (1995). This unconscious adoption of nurses' behaviour led Savage to sense that some of her relationships with patients were becoming similar to those of the nurses, providing some awareness of the nurse–patient interaction, and a focus for some of her subsequent interview questions.

Data analysis occurred simultaneously and continuously throughout the data collection period and was shaped by informants' explicit statements, Savage's own observations and participant experiences, and the pre-existing literature. She found that close interpersonal relationships were developed and sustained by physical proximity and the sharing of common space (2000). Although nurses had difficulty explaining their meaning of 'closeness', they used touch, humour and body posture to both promote and manage closeness with patients. Through participant observation, Savage was able to gain a deeper understanding of the participants' world by placing herself in the same situations as the nurses. By kneeling, sitting and standing when they did at bedside handovers, she describes an 'orchestrated undulation, a kind of Mexican wave' (2000: 332–3) as the nurses moved as one flexible body.

The benefits of the flexible research design in participant observation are evident in Savage's shifting focus from 'closeness', to the use of the body and touch, to the nurses' strategic use of the body as a means of resistance to relations of power (with medical colleagues):

> Developing 'close' relationships with patients was not only regarded as a means of unlocking the therapeutic potential of nursing, but also a political strategy, a sign of nurses' authentic claim to represent the patient that was not available to other groups. (1997: 241).

A disadvantage of participant observation identified by Savage was the opportunistic sample she used. By only talking to nurses who were willing and available, she risked excluding those whose relative inaccessibility might have been meaningful. At times, Savage also encountered a problematic merging of the boundaries between nurse, researcher and individual (1995). For example, some relationships developed into friendships and she needed to make decisions about whether to include information that had been gained through social interactions as data.

Further Reading

Adler, P.A. and Adler, P. (1987) *Membership Roles in Field Research* (London: Sage Publications).

This book provides an overview of the history and epistemology of fieldwork research, and offers an insightful analysis of the characteristics of different membership roles, including those of the peripheral, active and complete member. Using their own studies of drug dealers, as well as other examples of contemporary research in a wide range of settings, the authors describe the distinct stages and features of each role, discussing the processes of becoming a member, factors that assist and hinder membership, and the demands of the different roles. The book is intended for both the novice and the professional field researcher, and successfully reaches its audience by avoiding jargon while providing a comprehensive account. It is a valuable resource in the planning stage of field research, and would be useful to return to during reflexive analysis in order to seek greater understanding of the impact of self on the research process.

Bernard, H. (2000) *Social Research Methods: Qualitative and Quantitative Approaches* (London: Sage Publications).

In this general text, Bernard's chapter on participant observation locates participant observation within the context of ethnographic studies. In the section on the skills of a participant observer (pp. 328–37), he draws on a variety of studies and presents useful, practical examples for the participant observer's skill development. These include learning a new language, building explicit awareness, building memory, maintaining naivety, developing rapport and maintaining objectivity. The recommendations for recording data and differentiating between the jottings, the diary, the log and the notes are useful for the novice, as are the practical exercises designed to develop skills in observation and memory (p. 371).

Lee, R. (1995) *Dangerous Fieldwork* (Thousand Oaks, CA: Sage).

This accessible book explores a range of contexts that pose risks when conducting participant observation. Drawing on the experiences of different researchers, Lee explores violent social conflict, deviant groups, drug-related violence, sexual harassment and assault. In so doing, he differentiates between *ambient dangers*, when the researcher is exposed to otherwise avoidable dangers simply from having to be in a dangerous setting to conduct the research, and *situational dangers*. Situational dangers arise when the researcher's presence or actions evoke hostility, aggression or violence from those being studied. Although the book may alarm the novice researcher, who might wonder why anyone would ever want to conduct participant observation if these are the risks faced, it is sensible for researchers to consider the potential hazards before entering the field. In any case, Lee provides helpful practical advice on managing such problems.

Lofland, J. and Lofland, L. (1995) *Analyzing Social Settings: A Guide to Qualitative Observation and Analysis*, **3rd edn (Belmont, CA: Wadsworth).**

This very readable, practical book is a useful introductory text for those embarking on participant observation research. The main focus is on the simultaneous processes of gathering, focusing and analysing data. There are many practical tips and examples on selecting a site, gaining entry and establishing effective relationships, as well as recording, sorting and ordering data. The practical suggestions for data analysis would be useful to researchers engaged in participant observation as well as other forms of qualitative research.

Spradley, J. (1980) *Participant Observation* **(London: Thomson Learning Wadsworth).**

This book is intended for the inexperienced student wishing to conduct participant observation. Notwithstanding its focus on ethnographic work, it provides a useful discussion of the practical issues and skills required to learn the craft of participant observation. The style is very readable and the points made are illustrated by many everyday examples. The first part of the book is devoted to introducing the concepts of ethnography and culture. The second part contains a step-by-step guide to the stages involved in participant observation. The authors claim that the book contains 'everything that is required to begin research, collect data, analyze what you find and write up your report' (p. v). For this reason, students may consider it the 'bible' of participant observation. However, while valuable, it should not be read in isolation.

References

Adler, P. and Adler, P. (1987) *Membership Roles in Field Research* (London: Sage Publications).

Bernard, H. (2000) *Social Research Methods: Qualitative and Quantitative Approaches* (London: Sage Publications).

Berreman, G. (1968) 'Ethnography: Method and product'. In Clifton, C. (ed.) *Introduction to Cultural Anthropology: Essays in the Scope and Methods of the Science of Man* (Boston, MA: Houghton-Mifflin).

Bland, M. (2002) 'Patient observation nursing home research: Who was that masked woman?', *Contemporary Nurse*, **12**, 42–8.

Bowling, A. (1997) *Research Methods in Health: Investigating Health and Health Services* (Buckingham: Open University Press).

Edwards, S. (1998) 'An anthropological interpretation of nurses' and patients' perceptions of the use of space and touch', *Journal of Advanced Nursing*, **28**, 809–17.

Goffman, I. (1959) *The Presentation of Self in Everyday Life* (London: Penguin Books).

Goffman, I. (1961) *Asylums* (New York: Doubleday).

Gold, R. (1958) 'Roles in sociological field observations', *Social Forces*, **36**, 217–23. Reprinted in McCall, G. and Simmons, J. (eds) (1969) *Issues in Participant Observation. A Text and Reader* (Reading, MA: Addison-Wesley) pp. 30–8.

Grbich, C. (1999) *Qualitative Research in Health: An Introduction* (London: Sage Publications).

Grigsby, R. (1992) 'Mental health consultation at a youth shelter: An ethnographic approach', *Child and Youth Care Forum*, **21**, 247–61.

Grigsby, R. (2001) 'Participant observation'. In Thyer, B. (ed.) *The Handbook of Social Work Research Methods* (London: Sage Publications).

Jarvie, I. (1982) 'The problem of ethical integrity in participant observation'. In Burgess, R. (ed.) *Field Research: A Sourcebook and Field Manual* (New York: Routledge).

Jorgensen, D. (1989) *Participant Observation: A Methodology for Human Studies*. Applied Social Research Methods Series, Vol. 15 (London: Sage Publications).

Kennedy, C. (1999) 'Participant observation as a research tool in a practice-based profession', *Nurse Researcher*, **7**, 56–65.

Kite, K. (1999) 'Participant observation, peripheral observation or apart-icipant observation?', *Nurse Researcher*, **7**, 44–55.

Koch, T. and Harrington, A. (1998) 'Reconceptualizing rigour: The case for reflexivity', *Journal of Advanced Nursing*, **28**, 882–90.

Ladino, C. (2002) 'You make yourself sound so important', *Sociological Research Online*, **7**(4). http://www.socresonline.org.uk/socresonline/7/4/ladino.html

Lee, R. (1995) *Dangerous Fieldwork* (Thousand Oaks, CA: Sage).

Lofland, J. (1971) *Analyzing Social Settings: A Guide to Qualitative Observation and Analysis* (Belmont, CA: Wadsworth).

Lofland, J. and Lofland, L. (1995) *Analyzing Social Settings: A Guide to Qualitative Observation and Analysis*, 3rd edn (Belmont, CA: Wadsworth).

McCall, G. and Simmons, J. (eds) (1969) *Issues in Participant Observation. A Text and Reader* (Reading, MA: Addison-Wesley).

Marshall, J. (2002) 'Borderlands and feminist ethnography'. In Moss, P. (ed.) *Feminist Geography in Practice: Research Methods* (Oxford: Blackwell).

Melia, K. (1982) '"Tell it as it is" – qualitative methodology and nursing research: Understanding the student nurses' world', *Journal of Advanced Nursing*, **7**, 327–35.

Merriman, S. (1998) *Case Study Research in Education: A Qualitative Approach* (San Francisco, CA: Jossey Bass).

Miller, R. and Brewer, J. (2003) *The A–Z of Social Research: A Dictionary of Key Social Science Research Concepts* (London: Sage Publications).

Morse, J. and Lipson, J. (1991) 'Dialogue: On fieldwork in your own setting'. In Morse, J. (ed.) *Qualitative Nursing Research: A Contemporary Dialogue* (London: Sage), p. 72.

Muller, J. (1995) 'Care of the dying by physicians-in-training', *Research on Aging*, **17**, 65–88.

O'Neill, M. (2001) 'Participation or observation? Some practical and ethical dilemmas'. In Gellner, D. and Hirsch, E. (eds) *Inside Organisations: Anthropologists at Work* (Oxford: Berg).

Payne, G. and Payne, J. (2004) *Key Concepts in Social Research* (London: Sage Publications).

Richards, S. and Postle, K. (1998) 'Surviving in the field: An exploration of the challenges of participant observation in social work settings', *Issues in Social Work Education*, **18**, 7–41.

Robson, C. (2002) *Real World Research: A Resource for Social Scientists and Practitioner–researchers*, 2nd edn (Oxford: Blackwell Publishing).

Roper, J. and Shapira, J. (2000) *Ethnography in Nursing Research* (London: Sage Publications).

Rosenhan, D. (1973) 'On being sane in insane places', *Science*, **179**, 250–8.

Savage, J. (1995) *Nursing Intimacy: An Ethnographic Approach to Nurse–Patient Interaction* (London: Scutari Press).

Savage, J. (1997) 'Gestures of resistance: The nurse's body in contested space', *Nursing Inquiry,* **4**, 237–45.

Savage, J. (2000) 'Participative observation: Standing in the shoes of others?', *Qualitative Health Research,* **10**, 324–39.

Sluka, J. (1990) 'Participant observation in violent social contexts', *Human Organization,* **49**, 114–26.

Sword, W. (1999) 'Pearls, pith and provocation. Accounting for presence of self: Reflections on doing qualitative research', *Qualitative Health Research*, **9**, 270–8.

Taylor, B. (2005) 'The experiences of overseas nurses working in the NHS: Results of a qualitative study', *Diversity in Health and Social Care*, **2**, 17–27.

Taylor, S. (1987) 'Observing abuse: Professional ethics and personal morality in field research', *Qualitative Sociology*, **10**, 288–302.

Tedlock, B. (2000) 'Ethnography and ethnographic representation'. In Denzin, N. and Lincoln, Y. (eds) *Handbook of Qualitative Research* (Thousand Oaks, CA: Sage), pp. 455–86.

Turnock, C. and Gibson, V. (2001) 'Validity in action research: A discussion on theoretical and practice issues encountered whilst using observation to collect data', *Journal of Advanced Nursing*, **36**, 471–7.

Yin, R. (1989) *Case Study Research: Design and Methods* (Newbury Park, CA: Sage).

17 Ethnography

Sarah Harper and Jenny La Fontaine

Introduction

Ethnography has been defined as:

> The study of people in naturally occurring settings or fields by means of methods which capture their social meanings and ordinary activities, involving the researcher participating directly in the setting if not also the activities, in order to collect data in a systematic manner but without meaning being imposed on them externally. (Brewer, 2000: 10)

Essentially, ethnography is the study of people within their living and/or working environments, the goal of which is to achieve a rich and detailed understanding of the actions, beliefs, constructions and meanings associated with that group (Jordan and Yeomans, 1995; Pring, 1995). Ethnographic researchers conduct fieldwork – participant observation, interviews and the analysis of documents – over prolonged periods of time in order to learn from the group of people being studied (Edmond, 2005). Their primary method of data collection is participant observation, which requires the researcher to develop a way of being within the setting, incorporating a questioning of self and others and reflecting at every stage on the impact their presence has upon the research (Toren, 1996).

Historical Context

The origins of ethnography have evolved from two largely independent schools of thought within the USA and the UK – although the primary goal of both was cultural description (Brewer, 2000). The most significant development of ethnography within the British School occurred in social anthropology from the 1920s onwards. Here, two of the main proponents were Malinowski and Radcliffe-Brown, who were responsible for the production of detailed first-hand monographs. These monographs were about particular people or cultures, most frequently obtained through long-term participant observation with the researcher spending protracted periods of time living with and among the people being studied. Malinowski's study of the Trobriand Islands and his subsequent publication *Argonauts of the Western Pacific* (1922) are thought to have established fieldwork and, in particular, participant observation as a 'central element of ethnography' (Tedlock, 2000: 457).

The Chicago School developed independently of the British School and took a different focus (Brewer, 2000). The Chicago School emerged from the Sociology Department at the University of Chicago, where key figures – including Park, Burgess and Blumer – developed a rich tradition of studying urban society. These sociologists concentrated on studies of urban life, predominantly within the USA, highlighting groups of people who were often at the margins of society, including homeless people, migrant workers and minority ethnic groups (Deegan, 2001). The Chicago School utilised both quantitative and qualitative data, and also case study research. It was strongly influenced by the theory which came to be known as *symbolic interactionism*. The prolific literature of the Chicago School has shaped the discipline of ethnography from the 1920s to the present day (Deegan, 2001: 19).

Between the end of the Second World War and the late 1960s, ethnography expanded into work, socialisation and complex institutions. This is evidenced, for example, by the seminal works of Erving Goffman on asylums (1961) and stigma (1963). During the early 1970s, however, social anthropology and ethnography underwent a crisis as their orientation towards naturalism – and particularly the belief that a single, objective and truthful account could be gained from in-depth observation – were questioned (Hammersley and Atkinson, 1995). Additionally, feminists began to criticise the masculine bias of ethnographic research (MacDonald, 2001), arguing that existing ethnographic texts had largely ignored women both as the subject of research and as researchers (Deegan, 2001; MacDonald, 2001). In particular, feminists suggested that ethnographic studies had exploited participants and had not addressed the power relationships inherent within research (Hammersley, 1998).

As a result of such challenges, ethnography in the twenty-first century is now informed by a range of epistemologies – such as feminist, phenomenology, critical theory and symbolic interactionism – and advocates a range of perspectives and practices.

Current Use

Today, ethnography is used in many contexts including women's studies, sociology, cultural geography and social psychology. Additionally, it has been implemented successfully in applied areas, such as education, counselling, healthcare, psychology, nursing and social work (Tedlock, 2000). In the fields of health and social care, ethnographic studies have been highly influential in researching professional practice, with key texts including those by R.D. Laing (1960) and

Erving Goffman (1961) (see Bloor, 2001). As Charmaz and Olesen argue, ethnographic work in health and illness has successfully challenged both lay and medical ideas about experiences and meanings of health, illness, care and cure (Charmaz and Olesen, 1997: 482).

The application of ethnography within health and social care has not, though, been without challenge. Within healthcare, in particular, the emphasis has often been on quantitative rather than qualitative approaches in determining what counts as valid research evidence (Bloor, 2001; see also Chapter 1). Despite this, qualitative approaches are gaining favour, particularly with the increasing focus upon the personal experiences of people in receipt of health and social care. Indeed, it is now often suggested that qualitative approaches, such as ethnography, have equal value in the development of evidence and in understanding the complex and multifaceted nature of human existence within a health and social care context (Charmaz and Olesen, 1997; Newton et. al., 2000; Savage, 2000; Bloor, 2001).

One important reason for using ethnography within health and social care contexts is to deepen our understanding of the factors influencing professional and clinical practice. Much of what we do in our everyday lives and the meanings behind our actions are implicit and tacit and, as such, not open to immediate interpretation or discovery. As Herbert (2000: 553) suggests, 'The tissue of social life is not always observable. The meanings of objects and events are often revealed through practices, reactions, cursory comments and facial expressions'. This is no less true of professionals and clinicians within health and social care settings. The need to understand the rules, values and beliefs informing the behaviour of health and social care professionals is of particular importance as their actions have significant implications for individuals using their services.

The value of ethnographic research in developing this deeper understanding of healthcare practice is highlighted in studies by Smith et al. (2003) and Gabbay and le May (2004) where the implicit, personal and 'internalised tacit' mechanisms informing actions had a significant influence on how anaesthetists gained expert knowledge and how clinicians (doctors and nurses) derived their healthcare decision-making. Indeed, in Gabbay and le May's research, these factors had a greater influence than the standard routes advocated towards evidence-based practice, such as evidence-based guidelines.

Beyond this, ethnography can help us to understand the experiences of those who use health and social care services and the perceptions, beliefs and cultures informing their access to services. This is especially the case when researching groups whose needs have traditionally been hard to ascertain – such as people with dementia whose language ability may be impaired (Kontos, 2004, 2005; McColgan, 2005); children, where research has traditionally interpreted their actions with adult-centred frames of reference (Mayall, 2000; Edmond, 2005); and ethnic groups, who may be difficult to access using conventional survey methods (Harper, 2000). It is also very relevant when topics are of a sensitive nature – such as substance misuse (Borgois, 1998) and sexual practice and identity, including HIV and AIDs (Herdt, 2001).

Additionally, ethnography generates rich qualitative data which can supplement and offer depth to evaluations of policy directives and their impact upon those people they are designed to affect. For example, Newton et al. (2000) successfully used ethnography to add rich and meaningful data to an evaluation of deinstitutionalisation policies and practices for people with long-term mental illness. Within this context, ethnography can also be used to identify risk conditions, probing areas where measurement is problematic and there is a need to get at the implicit and tacit issues influencing risk, including sensitive issues such as errors in drug administration (Dixon-Woods, 2003: 326–7).

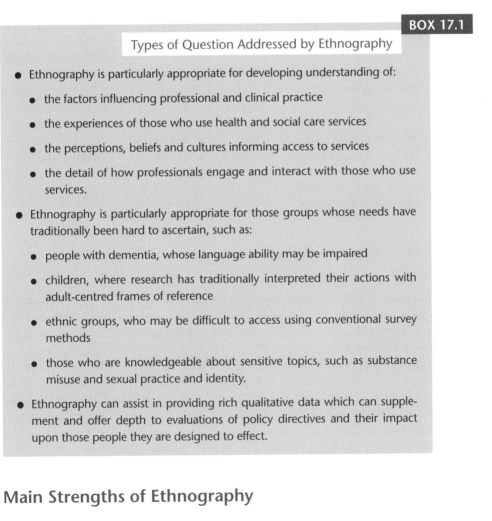

BOX 17.1

Types of Question Addressed by Ethnography

- Ethnography is particularly appropriate for developing understanding of:

  - the factors influencing professional and clinical practice

  - the experiences of those who use health and social care services

  - the perceptions, beliefs and cultures informing access to services

  - the detail of how professionals engage and interact with those who use services.

- Ethnography is particularly appropriate for those groups whose needs have traditionally been hard to ascertain, such as:

  - people with dementia, whose language ability may be impaired

  - children, where research has traditionally interpreted their actions with adult-centred frames of reference

  - ethnic groups, who may be difficult to access using conventional survey methods

  - those who are knowledgeable about sensitive topics, such as substance misuse and sexual practice and identity.

- Ethnography can assist in providing rich qualitative data which can supplement and offer depth to evaluations of policy directives and their impact upon those people they are designed to effect.

Main Strengths of Ethnography

Some of the key strengths of ethnography are highlighted in the previous section and include the ability to: understand the implicit and tacit aspects of culture informing our everyday lives; access the views and experiences of groups who have previously been hard to engage; and provide rich data which can assist in the evaluation of policy and practice within health and social care. Further strengths are, however, worthy of mention.

First, ethnography is able to provide 'thick description'.[1] Some research methodologies achieve only 'thin description', 'a bare report of the "facts" independent of intentions or circumstances' (Brewer, 2000: 39). Thin description may not suffice in determining the answers to the research questions being studied, such as whether people with dementia can express a sense of selfhood when their experience of dementia is severe and they have all but lost language ability (Kontos, 2004). Thick description, in contrast, provides a detailed discussion of the social processes and the context in which they occur, whilst also describing in depth the circumstances in which the description was produced (Brewer, 2000).[2]

Another strength of ethnography is that it is not limited to one epistemological or theoretical orientation and is thus a versatile methodology. This does not mean that it is acceptable for a researcher to produce a text without a theoretical orientation, or indeed to be anything other than explicit about that orientation. Rather, this lack of alignment creates flexibility for researchers to draw upon a range of epistemological positions, including critical theory; symbolic interactionism; phenomenology; feminism; and constructionism. As Robertson and Boyle (1984) indicate, the epistemology on which an ethnography is based is determined by the researcher. It is additionally influenced by their epistemological and ontological values (Mackenzie, 1994).

Main Weaknesses of Ethnography

Ethnography has been criticised for its non-standardised data collection techniques, subjectivity and reliance on interpretation (Spradley, 1980; Mackenzie, 1994; Carspecken 1995; Brewer; 2000). Because of this, it has been suggested that ethnography is not subject to replication and is therefore not scientific (Hammersley, 1998; Brewer, 2000; Herbert, 2000). Although all research is subject to interpretive practices, this critique requires ethnographers to be explicit and transparent about the processes and theories informing their research in order that others can judge the credibility of their results and conclusions (Hammersley, 1998; Brewer, 2000; Herbert, 2000). Furthermore, it needs researchers to be reflexive and transparent about their role in the research and the impact and effects of their presence upon it.

A second suggested limitation is that ethnography studies small samples or groups of people and the findings cannot therefore be considered generalisable. However, ethnography deliberately sacrifices breadth for depth in order to achieve a richness of data (Hammersley, 1998). Furthermore, if the research is rigorous and transparent in the selection and description of the sample and the context, then the reader can judge for themselves if the research can be applied more widely (Brewer, 2000; Herbert, 2000). Nonetheless, Savage (2000) suggests that poor generalisability is a potential reason for the lack of funding for ethnographic research within healthcare.

Third, ethnography involves time-consuming and lengthy fieldwork (Murphy, 2005). Even if data collection is limited to interviews (see below), the nature of the ethnographic interview is different from, and requires a longer term commitment to the participants than, a single interview (Spradley, 1979). This commitment of time is essential if meaningful data are to be collected, but this inevitably has implications in terms of increased costs and research time (Dixon-Woods, 2003).

MAIN STRENGTHS AND WEAKNESSES
... OF ETHNOGRAPHY

Strengths

Ethnographic research enables:

- 'Thick description' – that is, detailed discussion of the social processes and the context and circumstances in which they occur in order to achieve a rich understanding of the actions, beliefs, constructions and meanings associated with the group being studied.

- Probing of areas where measurement is problematic and there is a need to get at the implicit and tacit issues.

- Access to groups which tend to be hard to engage.

Weaknesses

Ethnography is criticised for:

- Its subjectivity and reliance on interpretation.

- The use of small samples or groups of people which mean that findings cannot be considered generalisable.

- Being time-consuming and thus costly to undertake.

Conducting an Ethnography

Planning

Key stages in planning an ethnography are: developing the research focus and the questions arising from this focus; selecting and accessing the setting to be studied; identifying ethical issues arising from the study and addressing any concerns (including securing ethical approval); clarifying the theoretical framework that will inform the study; and planning the financial and human resource factors influencing its completion (see also Chapter 2). Particular aspects of these stages warrant further consideration.

Developing the research question(s)

It is necessary to develop clear and focused research questions which are nevertheless open to change as the study progresses. Hammersley and Atkinson (1995) refer to an approach developed by Malinowski, entitled 'foreshadowed problems'. The researcher is encouraged to utilise a range of sources – including theory, experience of social situations and other analytical frameworks – to assist in the development of questions, while recognising that these questions are likely to require further consideration and development as the research progresses (Hammersley and Atkinson, 1995: 24–36).

Selecting the setting and negotiating access

Selection of the research setting and negotiating access are challenging issues in ethnographic research (Edmond, 2005). In particular, the researcher needs to reflect on sampling and consider whether the chosen setting reflects common issues relevant to other similar settings and/or whether it has specific characteristics that warrant further study. Negotiating access is an ongoing process in which the researcher must be vigilant about the impact of the research on the participants (Edmond, 2005).

Research ethics

Ethical issues are very important in ethnography because of the lengthy, in-depth nature of the fieldwork and the vulnerability of the groups and sensitivity of the topics often being studied. Most obviously, consideration should be given to the protection of participants' identity (Murphy and Dingwall, 2001) and ways of managing the development and ending of relationships built up over long periods of time.

Researcher reflexivity

The researcher must also reflect carefully on the values, beliefs and personal perspectives that might influence their research (Carspecken, 1995). Rachel (1996) indicates that the challenge for the ethnographer is to become part of the world being studied whilst simultaneously remaining separate enough to study and attempt to understand the wider social, historical and political context within which the setting exists (and the influence that they as researchers have on the setting being studied):

Fieldwork

The fieldwork phase of an ethnographic study is lengthy and involves considerable commitment on the part of the researcher. Fieldwork involves the collection of data through three specific methods: participant observation; interviews; and documentation.

Participant Observation

Within participant observation, the roles played by the researcher constitute a continuum from participant, participant-as-observer, observer-as-participant, and observer (see also Chapter 16). The nature of the role adopted will depend on a variety of factors, though the most common role is participant-as-observer. In all cases, however, the key task of the researcher is to make a detailed written record of the 'what, where, when, how and why' of events occurring in the field. To this end, Carspecken (1995) stresses the importance of 'low inference recording', whereby the researcher makes notes which detail the actions and language of the participants without reference to their own perceptions. The researcher's reflexive responses to the research are added subsequently.

Interviews

Ethnographic interviews differ from other forms of qualitative interviewing in a number of ways. First, they are conducted in the context of an existing relationship with a researcher who has usually also been observing the setting (Spradley, 1979; Hammersley and Atkinson, 1995). Second, they are more likely to be unstructured than other one-to-one interviews (see, for example, Chapter 14). And third, they are frequently carried out with the same individuals on a number of occasions over a period of time. In ethnographies, interviews commonly focus on narratives and oral histories which enable the participants to reveal their lives by creating autobiographical accounts of themselves and their social context (Brewer, 2000). According to Harper (1998), the 'funnel approach' – whereby a broad opening question is funnelled into a branching system of alternatives – is a particularly useful technique. Although some ethnographic studies involve interviews without any other form of data collection, they are still considered ethnographic because of the nature and style of the interview process which is likened to having extended 'natural conversations' (Burgess, 1984).

Documentation

The collection of documents – ranging from official records through to lay accounts of everyday life – has traditionally constituted part of ethnographic work and was widely used in the Chicago School (Hammersley and Atkinson, 1995). Documents can form valuable sources of data about the construction of everyday life and about the workings of organisations. Hammersley and Atkinson (1995: 168) nevertheless caution that documents must be 'treated as social products: they must be examined, not relied on uncritically as a research resource'.

Analysis

Ethnography analysis 'can be defined as the process of bringing order to the data, organising what is there into patterns, categories and descriptive units and looking for relationships between them' (Brewer, 2000: 188). Analysis is informed by two key aspects: the specific purpose of the research and the epistemology underpinning the research. As already argued, ethnography can draw upon many different epistemological positions, some of which have their own analytical frameworks, such as phenomenology.

Common methods of analysis include grounded theory (Strauss and Corbin, 1998), analytical induction, (Katz, 2001) and systems analysis (Carspecken, 1995). While differences exist in each type, all approaches emphasise the need for structure and a systematic approach (Brewer, 2000). This structure includes the assertion that analysis should be inductive, that is it should attempt to follow as closely as possible the results arising from the participants and the setting, placing these in the social, political and historical context in which they exist.

Analysis should begin alongside the data collection, with the researcher reading and re-reading notes and transcripts to familiarise themselves with all the material collected. This will enable initial relationships, perspectives and themes to emerge and these can be noted down tentatively. To facilitate the analysis process, the data should be organised into manageable units – usually with the assistance of a computer software package such as NVivo or Ethnograph (Hammersley and Atkinson, 1995; Brewer, 2000). From this, it should be possible to produce a description of the context of the research and a detailed account of the key events or behaviours being studied (Hammersley and Atkinson, 1995; Brewer, 2000). A typology or theory relating to the context, which utilises examples from the data to support the conclusions drawn, can then be developed (Hammersley and Atkinson, 1995). The various 'voices' that are involved in the research – including that of the researcher – should all be represented when the study is written up (Brewer, 2000: 124).

An Example of Ethnography

Background

'Voices from Southside Chicago: Healthcare Experiences of Elderly African-American Women' was a University of Chicago study conducted in three Southside Chicago hospitals and funded by the Chicago Community Trust and the National Institute of Aging (Kaplan and Harper, 1996; Harper et al., 1998). The starting point of the ethnographic component was that emergency rooms are not necessarily appropriate entry points for older people into hospital medical care and may reflect failures in primary, community and home health-care. To explore this, Harper and Kaplan examined hospital 'admission events' in elderly women's lives, including possible breakdowns in both formal primary and preventative healthcare and the informal care-giving structure provided by family, neighbours and friends.

The study drew on Chicago's African-American population, a strongly residentially segregated group comprising 95% of people living in the South- and Westsides of Chicago. The ethnographic research took place in Southside residential areas dominated by gangs and drug dealers. Those living there have poor socio-economic and health status indicators, including high mortality rates; low median incomes; high levels of poverty and receipt of public aid; and high homicide rates. Several of the community areas have a higher than average population aged over 65 years, with nearly half of these older individuals living alone. The communities thus include a high percentage of vulnerable elderly people.

As previously discussed, ethnographic research can allow voices that normally go unheard to speak. Consistent with this, the study sought to present a complete voice that would tell its story intact and also interpret those stories. Using a framework from the British tradition of qualitative feminist research (McIntyre, 1985; Finch, 1986; Stacey, 1992), mirrored by a smaller North American group (Romalis, 1985), the research aimed to make older African-American women's own perceptions of their needs central to relevant policy debates.

Methodology

Sixty-three life histories and/or ethnographic stories were collected by two researchers from older women visiting the emergency rooms of three Chicago hospitals, with some further conversations taking place following admittance to one of the hospitals. The women all lived in the surrounding communities, which had the highest rates of social deprivation, disease and mortality in the city. The interviews focused on narratives, life history and oral history, creating autobiographical accounts which revealed not only the lives of the individual women but also the social contexts in which those lives existed. The method used was the 'funnel interview' (Harper, 1998). Here a broad opening question is employed allowing a free narrative to develop. This is then funnelled into a branching system of alternatives devised by the interviewer to ensure that the narrative, while still free, is guided within the framework.[3] The main gatekeeper for the study was the director of the emergency room (ER) of one of the three hospitals, who provided a valuable entry to the research setting and was used in the analysis as a control to maintain reliability of interpretation. The researchers were fully integrated into the ERs, wore white hospital coats and were identified as being associated with the medical staff. This was for their own protection in a dangerous study environment, but also to engender an atmosphere of neutrality and trust from the women.

Potential participants were identified at triage on entry to the ER. The researcher identified herself and asked permission to accompany them during their visit. The researcher then became a companion to the women – staying all day and night if necessary and returning for multiple visits if a woman was admitted. In one case, the researcher remained with the woman until her death. In addition to extended open interviews and conversations, the researchers undertook participant observation within the ERs, collecting detailed fieldnotes of the 'what, where, when, how and why' of the ER setting and attended (with permission) medical interviews and examinations. In this way, an understanding of the values and beliefs informing the behaviour of health and social care professionals was gathered. Open interviews and conversations were also held with family members and visitors. Additionally, contextual material was collected from hospital records. Confidentiality, anonymity and ethics were kept at the forefront of the study.

Findings and impact

The study allowed the voices of older African-American women living in Chicago to inform policy debates that would have a direct impact on their lives. Findings focused on the stress of multigenerational care and the problems older black women living in those communities had in accessing healthcare. It was evident that little attention had hitherto been given to the tremendous stresses experienced by older women who still headed multigenerational households, particularly those situated in extreme environmental conditions, including abandoned and deteriorating housing and overcrowding. The daily stresses of dwelling in substandard conditions compounded the severe psychological and emotional strains of managing children (including adult children) damaged by crime and drug and alcohol abuse.

The women's stories showed how these problems were compounded by fear and social isolation which prevented them from accessing parts of the community. For example, although elderly African-American women generally qualified for Medicare and/or public aid, many were unaware of their rights to this support. Transport costs and the perceived barriers to receiving free transport tokens militated against taking up the broad range of care scattered across the community. Meanwhile, the lack of access to telephones in the home caused problems when they tried to find out clinic hours and schedule follow-up appointments. Lack of dissemination of information about primary and preventative healthcare was a further barrier to meeting their needs. Indeed, the women found the complexities of gaining knowledge about possible healthcare and associated services particularly daunting.

The study also revealed the need for greater recognition in healthcare planning of the diverse health needs and healthcare perceptions of this group of people. A lack of autonomy, fatalism and dependency ran through their stories. Their accounts revealed a lack of access to high-quality primary care, but also showed how the diversity and scatter of agencies created confusion and necessitated time-consuming travel around the city. Ultimately, both the extended family and the older woman were treated for specific social and health problems, rather than holistically.

Further Reading

Brewer, J.D. (2000) *Ethnography* **(Buckingham: Open University Press).**

This text can help students understand how to carry out ethnography and will enable them to develop an understanding of the many different issues that need to be considered in order to achieve a competent end result. Using examples throughout, the author considers the strengths and weaknesses of the methodology and guides the reader through the key theoretical and practical steps involved.

Hammersley, M. and Atkinson, P. (1995) *Ethnography: Principles in Practice*, **2nd edn (London: Routledge).**

This book offers a systematic account of ethnographic principles and practice. The authors state that their aim is to steer a course between a practical 'how to' text and one which grapples with the theoretical underpinnings of ethnography. Although the book is certainly to be valued for its comprehensive coverage, it is probably not ideal for the complete novice. Indeed, readers are advised to have a general grasp of social research and some of its epistemological and ontological underpinnings in order to understand the first few chapters.

Murphy, E. and Dingwall, R. (2001) 'The ethics of ethnography'. In Atkinson, P., Coffey, A., Delamont, S., Lofland, J. and Lofland, L. (eds), *Handbook of Ethnography* **(London: Sage Publications).**

In this chapter, Murphy and Dingwall provide a very useful and comprehensive account of the key ethical issues involved in conducting ethnographic research. In so doing, they enable the researcher to consider the many moral challenges that they will need to address in order to negotiate ethical approval, conduct their fieldwork and successfully analyse and present their results.

Spradley, J.P. (1979) *The Ethnographic Interview* (Belmont, CA: Wadsworth Thomson Learning) and Spradley, J.P. (1980) *Participant Observation* (New York: Holt, Rinehart and Winston).

These two texts offer comprehensive guides to developing, carrying out and analysing ethnographic interviews and participant observation. They are written in accessible styles and, despite being targeted at anthropologists, can be recommended to the novice health and social care researcher.

 # References

Bloor, M. (2001) 'The ethnography of health and medicine'. In Atkinson, P., Coffey, A., Delamont, S., Lofland, J. and Lofland, L. (eds), *Handbook of Ethnography* (London: Sage Publications), pp. 177–87.

Borgois, P. (1998) 'The moral economies of homeless heroin addicts: Confronting ethnography, HIV risk, and everyday violence in San Francisco shooting encampments', *Substance Use Misuse*, **33**, 2323–51.

Brewer, J.D. (2000) *Ethnography* (Buckingham: Open University Press).

Burgess, R. (1984) *In the Field* (London: Routledge).

Carspecken, P. (1995) *Critical Ethnography in Educational Research: A Theoretical and Practical Guide* (New York: Routledge).

Charmaz, K. and Olesen, V. (1997) 'Ethnographic research in medical sociology: Its foci and distinctive contributions', *Sociological Methods Research*, **25**, 452–94.

Deegan, M.J. (2001) 'The Chicago School of Ethnography'. In Atkinson, P., Coffey, A., Delamont, S., Lofland, J. and Lofland, L. (eds), *Handbook of Ethnography* (London: Sage Publications), pp. 11–25.

Denzin, N.K. (1989) *Interpretive Interactionism* (Newbury Park, CA: Sage).

Dixon-Woods, M. (2003) 'What can ethnography do for quality and safety in health care?' *Quality and Safety in Health Care*, **12**, 326–7.

Edmond, R. (2005) 'Ethnographic research methods with children and young people'. In Greene, S. and Hogan, D. (eds), *Researching Children's Experience: Approaches and Methods* (London: Sage Publications) pp. 123–40.

Finch, J. (1986) *Research and Policy* (London: Falmer).

Gabbay, G. and le May, A. (2004) 'Evidence-based guidelines or collectively constructed mindlines? Ethnographic study of knowledge management in primary care', *British Medical Journal*, **329**, 1013–7.

Goffman, E. (1961) *Asylums: Essays on the Social Situation of Mental Patients and Other Inmates* (Garden City, NY: Anchor Books).

Goffman, E. (1963) *Stigma: Notes on the Management of Spoiled Identity* (Englewood Cliffs, NJ: Prentice Hall).

Hammersley, M. (1998) *Reading Ethnographic Research*, 2nd edn (Harlow: Longman).

Hammersley, M. and Atkinson, P. (1995) *Ethnography: Principles in Practice*, 2nd edn (London: Routledge).

Harper, S. (1998) *The Health and Social Welfare of an African-American Elderly Population: Research in Chicago's Emergency Room*, WP298 (Oxford: Centre on Population Ageing).

Harper, S. (2000) 'Five voices from southside Chicago: Healthcare experiences of elderly African-American women'. In Dark, J., Ledwith, S. and Woods, R. (eds), *Women and the City: Visibility and Voice in Urban Space* (Basingstoke: Palgrave – now Palgrave Macmillan), pp. 19–34.

Harper, S. and Vlachantoni, A. (2005) *A Job for Late Life? Work and Retirement Aspirations of Older Self-employed Women in the UK*, Working Paper (Oxford: Oxford Institute of Ageing).

Harper, S., Walter, J. and Kaplan, L. (1998) *Underuse of Primary Care and Overuse of Emergency Care: Chicago's African-American Population,* WP498 (Oxford: Centre on Population Ageing).

Harper, S., Leeson, G., Aboderin, I. and Ruicheva, I. (2004) *Grandmother Care,* Report to the Nuffield Foundation (Oxford: Oxford Institute of Ageing).

Herbert, S. (2000) 'For ethnography', *Progress in Human Geography,* **24**, 550–68.

Herdt, G. (2001) 'Stigma and the ethnographic study of HIV: Problems and prospects', *Aids and Behaviour,* **5**, 141–9.

Jordan, S. and Yeomans, D. (1995) 'Critical ethnography: Problems in contemporary theory and practice', *British Journal of Sociology of Education,* **16**, 389–408.

Kaplan, L. and Harper, S. (1996) *Emergency Room Use by Chicago's African-American Population.* Conference Paper. Washington, DC: Gerontological Society of America, November.

Katz, J. (2001) 'Analytic Induction'. In Smelser, N.J. and Baltes, P.B. (eds), *International Encyclopedia of the Social and Behavioral Sciences,* http://www.sscnet.ucla.edu/soc/faculty/katz/pubs/Analytic_Induction.pdf (accessed 6 December, 2007).

Kontos, P.C. (2004) 'Ethnographic reflections on selfhood, embodiment and Alzheimer's disease', *Ageing and Society,* **24**, 829–49.

Kontos, P.C. (2005) 'Embodied selfhood in Alzheimer's disease: Rethinking person-centred care', *Dementia,* **4**, 553–70.

Laing, R.D. (1960) *The Divided Self: An Existential Study in Sanity and Madness* (Harmondsworth: Penguin).

MacDonald, S. (2001) 'British Social Anthropology'. In Atkinson, P., Coffey, A., Delamont, S., Lofland, J. and Lofland, L. (eds), *Handbook of Ethnography* (London: Sage Publications), pp. 60–79.

Mackenzie, A. (1994) 'Evaluating ethnography: Considerations for analysis', *Journal of Advanced Nursing,* **19**, 774–81.

Malinowski, B.K. (1922) *Argonauts of the Western Pacific: An Account of Native Enterprise and Adventure in the Archipelagoes of Melanesian New Guinea* (London: George Routledge and Sons).

Mayall, B. (2000) 'Conversations with children: Generational issues'. In Christensen, P. and James, A. (eds), *Research with Children: Perspectives and Practices* (London: Falmer Press).

McColgan, G. (2005) 'A place to sit: Resistance strategies used to create privacy and home by people with dementia', *Journal of Contemporary Ethnography,* **34**, 410–33.

McIntyre, S. (1985) 'Gynaecologist/women interaction'. In Ungerson, C. (ed.), *Women and Social Policy* (London: Macmillan – now Palgrave Macmillan), pp. 175–84.

Murphy, E. and Dingwall, R. (2001) 'The ethics of ethnography'. In Atkinson, P., Coffey, A., Delamont, S., Lofland, J. and Lofland, L. (eds), *Handbook of Ethnography* (London: Sage Publications), pp. 339–51.

Murphy, F. (2005) 'Preparing for the field: Developing competence as an ethnographic field worker', *Nursing Research,* **12**, 52–60.

Newton, L., Rosen, A., Tennant, C., Hobbs, C., Lapsley, H.M. and Tribe, K. (2000) 'Deinstitutionalisation for long-term mental illness: An ethnographic study', *Australian and New Zealand Journal of Psychiatry,* **34**, 484–90.

Pring, J.T. (1995) *Pocket Oxford Greek Dictionary* (Oxford: Oxford University Press).

Rachel, J. (1996) 'Ethnography: Practical implementation'. In Richardson, J.T.E. (ed.), *Handbook of Qualitative Research Methods for Psychology and the Social Sciences* (Leicester: British Psychological Society), pp. 113–24.

Robertson, M.H.B. and Boyle, J.S. (1984) 'Ethnography: Contributions to nursing research', *Journal of Advanced Nursing,* **9**, 3–49.

Romalis, S. (1985) 'Struggle between providers and recipients'. In Lewin, E. and Olsen, V. (eds), *Women, Health and Healing* (London: Tavistock), pp. 174–208.

Savage, J. (2000) 'Ethnography and health care', *British Medical Journal,* **321**, 1400–2.

Smith, A., Goodwin, D., Mort, M. and Pope, C. (2003) 'Expertise in practice: An ethnographic study exploring acquisition and use of knowledge in anaesthesia', *British Journal of Anaesthesia,* **91**, 319–28.

Spradley, J.P. (1979) *The Ethnographic Interview* (New York: Holt, Rinehart and Winston).

Spradley, J.P. (1980) *Participant Observation* (New York: Holt, Rinehart and Winston).

Stacey, M. (1992) *Regulating British Medicine* (New York: Wiley).

Strauss, A. and Corbin, J. (1998) *Basics of Qualitative Research: Techniques and Procedures for Developing Grounded Theory*, 2nd edn (Thousand Oaks, CA: Sage).

Tedlock, B. (2000) 'Ethnography and ethnographic representation'. In Denzin, N.K. and Lincoln, Y.S. (eds), *Handbook of Qualitative Research*, 2nd edn (Thousand Oaks, CA: Sage), pp. 455–71.

Toren, C. (1996) 'Ethnography: A theoretical background'. In Richardson, J.T.E. (ed.) *Handbook of Qualitative Research Methods for Psychology and the Social Sciences* (Leicester: British Psychological Society), pp. 102–12.

Notes

1 According to Denzin (1989: 83) thick description, 'presents detail, context, emotion and the web of social relationships. Thick description invokes emotionality, and self-feelings. It establishes the significance of an experience or the sequence of events. In thick description, the voices, feelings, actions and meanings of interacting individuals are heard'.

2 It should, however, be recognised that this thick description cannot be a complete description of the context being studied, as interpretations can and do differ and are dependent on the observer and their theoretical orientation (Brewer, 2000: 43).

3 This combination of narrative and semi-structured questions has been used successfully in a range of research by Harper (Harper et al., 2004; Harper and Vlachantoni, 2005).

Critical Incident Technique 18

HELEN AVEYARD AND JOANNE NEALE

Introduction

The critical incident technique (CIT) is a systematic, inductive, predominantly qualitative research method which is sometimes referred to as the critical event technique or critical incident analysis. The CIT involves collecting descriptions of events and behaviours – known as critical incidents – that will help to explain or understand a particular topic, most commonly an area of practice. A critical incident can be a minor or major event or behaviour. However, it should comprise a clearly demarcated scene which directly affects (either positively or negatively) the issue being researched.

Information on critical incidents can be collected in a variety of ways, such as by direct observation, one-to-one interviews, focus groups, formal records, and self-report questionnaires. The kinds of critical incidents described tend to be extreme or unusual behaviours and events, since these are the easiest to identify and are thought to shed most light on research problems. Once collated, the critical incident data are sorted, grouped and analysed – usually using some form of textual, content or thematic analysis. They are then reported primarily with the intention of solving practical problems or improving practice.

Historical Context

The CIT is a relatively new research approach that was initially developed and described by Flanagan (1954). Flanagan's work was conducted as part of the Aviation Psychology Program of the US Army Air Forces in the Second World War. The Second World War had generated an urgent need to identify and describe the components of successful and less successful bombing missions in order to strengthen pilot performance and air defence mechanisms. Accordingly, Flanagan asked pilots and their instructors to record incidents which they perceived as either effective or ineffective in bombing missions. This information, Flanagan argued, would provide a focused approach to the observation and analysis of pilot action which would be preferable to vague generalised statements about behaviour.

From his analyses, Flanagan was able to determine the required criteria for a successful bombing task. In the process of this, he also defined the terms 'incident' and 'critical incident'. An 'incident', he argued, was *any observable human activity that is sufficiently complete in itself to permit inferences and predictions to be made about the person performing the act'* (p. 327). That is, the observer should be able to infer from the incident why someone behaved as they did and the likely implications of this. Meanwhile, for an incident to become 'critical', it *'must occur in a situation where the purpose or the intent of the act seems fairly clear to the observer and where its consequences are sufficiently definite to leave little doubt concerning its effects'* (p. 327). That is, the observer should be fairly certain about the impact of the incident on the topic of inquiry.

Since a critical incident is effectively a stand-alone event or behaviour which can be interpreted by an observer without additional information, the success of the technique depends on the ability of the observer to identify critical incidents accurately. In view of this, Flanagan (1954) emphasised that those collecting critical incident data should be aware of the exact purpose of the activity being examined, the specific judgements they have to make about whether incidents fit the criteria for being 'critical' for the purposes of the study, and whether all relevant factors necessary to provide a full understanding of the incident have been described.

In practice, Flanagan's bombing missions were particularly suited to the CIT. This was because the components of a successful bombing mission were largely self-evident, with success or failure being immediately apparent. In addition, those observing and identifying critical incidents tended to be pilot instructors who were well qualified to judge what was critical and what was not. Despite this, some of Flanagan's early work involved the identification of critical incidents by pilots-in-training and, in these cases, accounts of the successes and failures of bombing missions might have been compromised by the relative inexperience of the observers.

Flanagan (1954) acknowledged that the application of the technique he had defined would probably not be appropriate in all settings. Indeed, he recognised that in contexts other than bombing missions it may be less easy to identify critical incidents which provide a valid insight into the situation or event under study. Thus, he argued that the CIT should be regarded as a flexible set of principles to be *'modified and adapted to meet the specific situation at hand'* (p. 335). As advised by Flanagan, the method has now been adapted and used in a variety of ways within a variety of disciplines, including management, human resources, education, marketing, the service industry, and health and social care.

Current Use

Within market research, Bitner et al. (1990) used the CIT to identify the particular events that caused customers to distinguish between very satisfactory and very unsatisfactory service encounters. To this end, they collected information on 700 incidents (approximately half satisfactory and half unsatisfactory) from customers of airlines, hotels and restaurants. Categorisation of the incidents led Bitner et al. to conclude that the CIT was a useful method for assessing customer satisfaction/dissatisfaction and that it could potentially be used by managers in other service sector industries. Following this endorsement, the use of the CIT within service and market research increased sharply.

The CIT has also been used in management. For example, a study of the workplace by Liefooghe and Olafsson (1999) invited focus group participants to identify incidents from their own experience which they considered to be bullying. Participants were asked questions about these incidents to ensure that full details were obtained. The focus group discussion then explored how bullying was interpreted by the different involved parties. Liefooghe and Olafsson did not state how many bullying incidents were reported and did not comment specifically on the effectiveness of the use of focus groups for the collection of critical incident data. However, the method clearly enabled the researchers to access information that the participants themselves identified as significant.

Educational research has likewise taken advantage of the CIT. Following concern that deputy-head teachers were often left alone in charge of potentially serious situations, Kerry (2005) used the method to explore the role of the deputy head in primary schools. Twenty-two newly appointed deputy heads were asked to record critical incidents about their experiences on a pre-designed proforma. They were then invited to answer specific questions about the incidents they had reported and asked to match each incident with one of 15 job roles identified during their induction training. The study showed that only eight of the 15 job roles featured in the critical incidents reported. The significance of the duties undertaken by deputy heads and the importance of their role in sustaining the effectiveness and public image of the school were, however, revealed.

Within the field of health and social care, researchers have used the CIT to investigate aspects of clinical practice, nursing education and nursing care quality (Bailey, 1956; Benner, 1984; Pryce-Jones, 1992; Grant et al., 1996). For example, Keegan et al. (2001) used the method to study relatives' views of different types of care service received within the last year of a patient's life. To this end, they interviewed 155 relatives of patients who had died during a 12-month period. For ethical reasons, these relatives were not interviewed until at least 10 months after the relative's death and the authors commented that the verifiability of the incidents was thus difficult to establish. Nonetheless, examples of good and poor care were successfully collected and the findings showed that relatives considered all aspects of care to be significant towards the end of life – although the attitudinal and dignity-preserving aspects were particularly important. The authors concluded that the approaches adopted in hospice care should be adapted and applied in the acute hospital setting.

Health-related research has additionally shown how the CIT can be developed and modified to suit the needs of a particular study. Thus, Griffiths et al. (2001) used an adaptation of the CIT in interviews conducted within the general practice setting to explore the reasons for hospital admission for asthma in a multicultural population. The adaptation had previously been described by Bradley (1992) and involved systematically recording anecdotal events described in general practice. However, unlike Bradley, Griffiths et al. did not ask their participants to give specific examples of critical incidents in the interviews. Rather, they used an interview guide to steer participants through a number of key topics, such as experience of admission, coping with asthma and causes of exacerbation. Information on critical events arose spontaneously during the course of the interviews and this enabled the researchers to identify specific reasons for admission to hospital rather than vague generalisations.

A study of nursing care by Norman et al. (1992), meanwhile, found that patients were often unable to identify 'critical incidents' relating to good and bad nursing because the incidents they identified were not clearly demarcated events that stood alone for independent analysis – in other words, they did not fulfil Flanagan's criteria as critical incidents. Norman et al. found that participants did not necessarily distinguish between what happened on a certain occasion and what often happened. That is, patient experiences did not stand out as independent events but merged into one general overall recollection. Furthermore, Norman et al. felt that repeated happenings were potentially more significant than one-off incidents, an argument which they related to the complex nature of human–human interaction:

> Human beings are complex creatures with varied histories and memories who create and recreate meaning within the social situation they experience. The implication of this is that incidents cannot be abstracted from the chronological temporal flow of human experience. The meanings of critical observed happenings which are located within incidents are not created anew but are the product of previously created meanings which are carried forwards from previous incidents. As such, human beings will inevitably describe one incident in the light of related incidents and the meaning of observable events is of crucial importance. (Norman et al., 1992: 599)

Accordingly, Norman et al. suggested that it might be more appropriate to collect accounts of 'critical happenings' rather than critical incidents in some health and social care contexts. These critical happenings, they argued, were likely to be revealed by a critical incident but did not require a full critical incident in order to be recorded. In their later work, Redfern and Norman (1999) deliberately adopted the term 'critical happenings' to identify the main events that were significant to patients' and nurses' perceptions of nursing care quality. Nurses and patients were asked to describe incidents that they had observed or experienced which they considered to be indicators of high- or low-quality nursing. The interview transcripts were then read to identify 'critical happenings' and a 'quality indicator' was derived from each happening. These 'quality indicators' were subsequently classified into sub-categories which were ranked according to how many respondents identified quality indicators in each category.

BOX 18.1

Types of Question Addressed by the Critical Incident Technique

- What particular events cause customers to distinguish between very satisfactory and very unsatisfactory services? (Bitner et al., 1990)

- How can bullying be identified and explained? (Liefooghe and Olafsson, 1999)

- What is the role of deputy-head teachers in primary schools? (Kerry, 2005)

- What are the positive and negative components of palliative care from the perspective of relatives? (Keegan et al., 2001)

- What are the reasons for hospital admission for asthma in a multicultural population? (Griffiths et al., 2001)

- What are indicators of nursing care quality from the perspective of patients and nurses? (Norman et al, 1992; Redfern and Norman, 1999)

Main Strengths of the Critical Incident Technique

A key strength of the CIT is its objectivity. This is because the data collected are reports of actual events that have happened rather than very generalised statements about what people 'tend to do' or what people say they 'would be likely to do' in a particular situation. This avoids the criticism – often levelled at the qualitative interview (see Chapter 14) – that there is a wide gap between what people say they do and what really happens. Furthermore, detailed accounts of critical incidents can function as objective observations of practice, even if the particular behaviours or events are not directly observed. So, the CIT effectively permits observational data to be collected without the intrusion that occurs with direct observation (see Chapter 16) and, as a result, information can be gathered on areas of practice that might otherwise remain hidden.

A further strength of the CIT is its flexibility. As already indicated, the way critical incident data are collected can be adapted to suit the needs of the study and those who participate in it. For example, data can be gathered by direct observation of practice or formal records. These methods might be most appropriate if those involved have difficulty identifying or articulating critical incidents, perhaps because of their limited technical knowledge or because they are unwell. Critical incidents can also be collected on a report form or questionnaire at the time of, or soon after, the incident occurring. The advantage of this is that information on many incidents can be collected relatively easily and economically. Additionally, critical incident data can be collected via in-depth interviews or focus groups. Using these approaches, the interviewer is able to guide participants to ensure that relevant incidents are recounted. Equally, they can probe for further details if necessary.

When participants self-report critical incidents (either in written or verbal format), the CIT has the added advantage that it is the participants themselves who nominate salient events. This ensures that the incidents recorded and analysed are those which those involved in the events and behaviours – rather than the researchers – deem important and meaningful. In healthcare, this can be particularly useful in enabling clinicians better to understand their roles and the impact of their actions; the feelings, emotions and reactions of their patients; and the complex dimensions of patient–professional interactions.

Finally, the CIT is particularly suited to obtaining information on occasional or rare events that tend to be overlooked by other research methods. Occasional or rare events – such as deaths, missed diagnoses, prescribing errors, and accidents – can have very serious implications for patient well-being and safety. Yet, the causes of these events can be difficult to understand. The CIT offers an opportunity to explore how and why very occasional or rare events occur and can also take account of positive events and behaviours that may have prevented negative outcomes.

Main Weaknesses of the Critical Incident Technique

An important weakness of the CIT is that it is highly dependent on the appropriate identification of incidents which directly affect the topic of inquiry. As suggested previously, identifying incidents that have a direct impact on the success or failure of a bombing mission is not overly difficult since outcomes in terms of bombing targets are fairly easy to measure objectively. Identifying incidents that directly affect other outcomes – such as an improvement or deterioration in a patient's level of anxiety about their illness or their desire for one particular form of treatment rather than another – is likely to prove more difficult. In health and social care, this can be complicated by the subjective nature of many research topics – particularly when these relate to human experiences, feelings and emotions.

A further weakness of the CIT is that events and behaviours need to be remembered accurately and reported in detail. Success in achieving this will depend on how long ago events occurred, the recall ability of participants, and the extent to which discrete events or behaviours can be easily identified. Those who are very unwell or who have poor cognitive functioning may find it difficult to participate meaningfully. Meanwhile, distant and more mundane incidents are more likely to be forgotten than recent and unusual incidents. It is also possible that participants will under-report or even omit to report events and behaviours that reflect badly on themselves – especially if they have acted illegally or immorally.

Although the flexibility and adaptability of the CIT constitute important strengths of the approach, they can also be perceived as weaknesses. As already discussed, information on critical incidents can be collected in a wide range of ways – through direct observation, records, self-report proforma, interviews and so on. Butterfield et al. (2005) have commented that the diversity of approaches to using the CIT has now problematically blurred the boundaries around what constitutes the method and what does not. Indeed, Redfern and Norman's (1999) use of the technique to collect 'critical happenings', rather than critical incidents, illustrates this point neatly. If discrete critical incidents are not discernible and critical happenings have to be collected, it could be argued that the study does not fall into the remit of the CIT.

MAIN STRENGTHS AND WEAKNESSES
... OF THE CRITICAL INCIDENT TECHNIQUE

Strengths

- A key strength of the CIT is its objectivity. This is because the data collected are reports of actual events that happened rather than very generalised statements about what people 'tend to do' or what people say they 'would be likely to do' in a particular situation.

- The CIT enables observations of practice to occur without the intrusion that inevitably accompanies direct observation – so, information can be collected about areas of practice that might otherwise remain hidden.

- The CIT is a flexible method as the collection of data can be adapted to suit the needs of the study and those who participate in it.

- Within the CIT, it tends to be the participants themselves who nominate salient events. This ensures that the incidents recorded and analysed are those which those involved in the events and behaviours – rather than the researchers – deem meaningful.

- The CIT is particularly suited to obtaining information about occasional or rare events that tend to be overlooked by other research methods.

Weaknesses

- The identification of incidents which directly affect subjective outcomes – such as those relating to human experiences, feelings and emotions – is not an easy task.

- Participants may not be able to remember or report critical incidents in adequate detail.

- Participants may under-report or even omit to report events and behaviours that reflect badly on themselves – especially if they have acted illegally or immorally.

- In recent years, the CIT has been adapted and changed to the point where the boundaries around what constitutes a CIT study and what does not have now blurred.

Conducting a Critical Incident Study

As explained previously, there is no one set approach to undertaking the CIT. Data can be gathered through a variety of structured or unstructured methods. Consequently, those who encounter research papers where the technique has been used are urged to scrutinise the methods for details about the particular approach taken. Meanwhile, those who use the CIT must be able to justify why it – rather than any other method – has been chosen and provide a clear and transparent account of the processes followed so that the quality of their study can be accurately assessed. In this regard, Flanagan (1954) identified five steps to be followed when undertaking a CIT study and these are briefly outlined below.

In the **first stage** of the CIT, the researcher is required to give a clear statement of what is being investigated – that is, the general aim of the study. This will involve defining a research question or a particular problem. As already discussed, the CIT is particularly suited to researching aspects of practice and suitable research questions are often those seeking to identify factors underpinning good or poor practice.

The **second stage** of the CIT involves specifying the criteria to be used in deciding which incidents should be included in the research. These criteria need to be established at the start of the study in the same way that those reviewing literature (Chapters 4 and 5) set inclusion and exclusion criteria for the literature they seek. This process helps to ensure that there is a clear strategy for identifying critical incidents and that only data on incidents relevant to the research topic are collected. For example, in research to develop a measurement of engagement between HIV/AIDS patients and nurses, incidents were only selected if they described the circumstances surrounding a nursing care event; presented a description of the interaction which occurred between the patient and a specific nurse; and clearly described the behavioural outcomes that occurred as a result of the care-giving event (Kemppainen et al., 1999).

The **third stage** of the CIT is where the data are collected. The researcher should adopt the most appropriate method of gathering the information on critical incidents that meet the criteria specified in stage 2. This will often depend on who is best placed to identify and record this material – an independent observer or individuals who were actually involved in the incidents. Once this has been decided, detailed accounts of each incident need to be collected. According to Kemppainen (2000), this requires a description of the situation that led to the incident (to help understand why certain actions were or were not taken); the actions and behaviours of the main person or people involved in the incident (to clarify who exactly did what and when); and the outcome of the incident (to enable inferences about the behaviour and its impact on the research question or problem to be made).

Although the size of a CIT study is determined by the number of critical incidents reported (rather than the number of individuals collecting or reporting the incidents), there is no such thing as an ideal number of critical incidents.

Rather, Flanagan argued that incidents should be collected until redundancy or 'saturation' in the data appears – that is, until no new information arises from the most recently collected critical incidents. Specifically, Flanagan (1954) argued that if few new insights were developed from the last 100 incidents collected, then saturation had been achieved. However, in practice, valuable studies have been conducted on a much smaller scale than this.

When interviews are used to collect data from individuals who have been involved in critical incidents, it is sensible to include a heterogeneous group of participants since this will facilitate the collection of diverse and exhaustive descriptions (Weisgerber et al., 1990, cited in Kemppainen, 2000). Participants must also be encouraged to provide clear, thorough and accurate descriptions of events and behaviours. For this, the researcher needs to probe participants for as much detail as possible about every incident. They should also seek to conduct the interviews as soon as possible after the time of the events being reported as this will help to improve recall. Meanwhile, to prevent essential aspects of data being forgotten or lost, it is advisable that interviews are audio recorded and fully transcribed.

Analysis of the critical incident data collected occurs in the **fourth stage** of the research process. Although Flanagan (1954) argued that the critical incident was the main unit of analysis, Redfern and Norman (1999) claimed that 'critical happenings', as revealed by critical incidents, are central. Irrespective of this difference of opinion, information on critical incidents is generally analysed through an inductive process. To this end, incidents are sorted and grouped into categories. This enables patterns and differences in the frequency of similar incidents to be seen and overarching themes to be identified. In other words, types of textual, content and thematic analyses are employed to classify the data and give it an overall structure.

In the final **fifth stage**, the data are interpreted. It is important to remember that those who participate in CIT interviews are only asked to describe events and behaviour. As Bitner at al. (1990) noted, it is the researcher who takes responsibility for abstraction and inference. In the interpretation of the data, the main findings should be explored and compared with the results of other research, possible explanations for the findings need to be suggested and tested, and improvements in practices and systems should be recommended.

To date, there has been little formal evaluation of the CIT – particularly in terms of the methodological strengths and weakness of its many diverse applications. Reflecting on this, Butterfield et al. (2005) have recommended a number of strategies to promote the credibility of the technique. Some of these – providing a clear articulation of what constitutes a critical incident for the purposes of the study, accuracy in the collection of incidents, and the continued collection of critical incidents until data saturation has been reached – have already been discussed. Other strategies to promote credibility include 'member checking' (returning the initial classification of critical incidents to the participants for confirmation), asking an independent judge to classify critical incidents into the researcher's categories (a high level of agreement between the independent judge and the researcher indicating the robustness of the categories), and calculating the number of participants contributing critical incidents to a category (where more than 25% of participants contributing to a category is considered significant).

An Example of a Critical Incident Study

A study which incorporated many of Butterfield's recommendations is 'Patients' experiences of support while waiting for cardiac surgery: A critical incident technique analysis'. This was published in the *European Journal of Cardiovascular Nursing* in 2004 and involved the collection and analysis of 223 critical incidents. The authors were Bodil Ivarsson, Sylvia Larsson and Trygve Sjöberg, who were based in the Department of Cardiothoracic Surgery at the University Hospital of Lund and the Department of Nursing at Lund University, Sweden. The research was supported by grants from the Swedish Heart Lung Foundation, Lund University Hospital, Southern Sweden Nurses' home and Swenurse.

The aim of the Ivarsson et al. study was to describe patients' experiences of support in the form of important events during the waiting period for cardiac surgery. The authors justified their topic by reference to evidence that waiting for a heart operation can be a long and traumatic period, with patients experiencing high levels of stress and anxiety, particularly when they have been told that they might die without surgery. Ethical approval was received from the Ethics Committee of the Medical Faculty of Lund University and permission to select informants was given by the directors of the participating units. Twenty-six individuals – with diverse socio-demographic characteristics and patient experiences – who were on the waiting list for elective bypass or valve surgery at a cardiothoracic surgical clinic were then chosen to participate.

The 26 individuals were contacted by letter and informed that their participation would be voluntary and confidential. They were also asked to provide written consent. Data were collected by a semi-structured interview guide, which had previously been piloted and amended slightly. The guide allowed the patients to describe in their own words events that were related to the support they had experienced whilst waiting for heart surgery. Each interview lasted between 10 and 38 minutes, was tape-recorded and transcribed verbatim. The transcripts were reviewed and descriptions of 223 critical incidents – events described by the patients as positive or negative in relation to their experience of support – were identified.

The 223 identified incidents were abstracted from the interview text, given labels, and grouped into 19 sub-categories of behaviour. These 19 sub-categories of behaviour were then further grouped into six categories:

- Patient found strength

- Life and way of living of patient had changed

● Patient was given attention

● Patient took part in care

● Patient was dissatisfied with the organisation of the healthcare system

● Social network was not supported.

The above categories were grouped under two main headings – internal factors and external factors. Because the last five interviews generated no new sub-categories, the researchers concluded that data saturation had been reached. Meanwhile, to enhance credibility of their analyses, all incidents were identified and classified independently by two researchers (who disagreed about only one incident).

Analyses showed how internal and external factors influenced patients' coping strategies. Moreover, both primary and secondary care staff required a better understanding of patients' needs prior to cardiac surgery so that they could offer them appropriate information and support. The authors concluded that their findings could be used to develop an intervention programme to improve the situation of heart surgery patients and their next of kin. This, they suggested, might include a nurse-led pre-admission clinic with a telephone information function, a 24-hour internet-based support system, and an evidence-based multiprofessional manual to ensure consensus and standardisation.

Further Reading

Butterfield, L.D., Borgen, W.A., Norman, E., Maglio, A. and Magilo, A.T. (2005) 'Fifty years of the critical incident technique', *Qualitative Research*, 5, 475–97.

This article provides a comprehensive account of the origins and development of the CIT, including a useful commentary offering suggestions on how to achieve credibility when using the approach.

Flanagan, J.C. (1954) 'The critical incident technique', *Psychological Bulletin*, 51, 327–58.

This is the original text in which Flanagan outlines the use of CIT for exploring human behaviour.

Ivarsson, B., Larsson, S. and Sjöberg, T. (2004) 'Patients' experiences of support while waiting for cardiac surgery: A critical incident technique analysis', *European Journal of Cardiovascular Nursing*, 3, 183–91.

This article offers a detailed description of how the CIT has been applied within a nursing context.

Norman, I., Redfern, S.J., Tomalin, D.A. and Oliver, S. (1992) 'Developing Flanagan's critical incident technique to elicit indicators of high and low quality nursing care from patients and their nurses', *Journal of Advanced Nursing*, 17, 590–600.

This interesting paper introduces the concept of 'critical happenings' rather than 'critical incidents' as the basic unit of analysis within the CIT.

References

Bailey, T.J. (1956) 'The critical incident technique in identifying behavioural criteria of professional nursing effectiveness', *Nursing Research*, **5**, 52–64.

Benner, P. (1984) *From Novice to Expert* (Menlo Park, CA: Addison-Wesley).

Bitner, M., Booms, B. and Tetreault, M. (1990) 'The service encounter: Diagnosing favourable and unfavourable incidents', *Journal of Marketing*, **54**, 71–84.

Bradley, C.P. (1992) 'Turning anecdotes into data: The critical incident technique', *Family Practice*, **9**, 98–103.

Butterfield, L.D., Borgen, W.A., Norman, E., Maglio, A. and Magilo, A.T. (2005) 'Fifty years of the critical incident technique', *Qualitative Research*, **5**, 475–97.

Flanagan, J.C. (1954) 'The critical incident technique', *Psychological Bulletin*, **51**, 327–58.

Grant, N.K., Reimer, M. and Bannatyne, J. (1996) 'Indicators of quality in long-term care facilities', *International Journal of Nursing Studies*, **33**, 469–78.

Griffiths, C., Kaur, G., Gantley, M., Feder, G., Hillier, G., Goddard, J. and Packe, G. (2001) 'Influences on hospital admission for asthma in south Asian and white adults: Qualitative interview study', *British Medical Journal*, **323**, 962.

Ivarsson, B., Larsson, S. and Sjöberg, T. (2004) 'Patients' experiences of support while waiting for cardiac surgery: A critical incident technique analysis', *European Journal of Cardiovascular Nursing*, **3**, 183–91.

Keegan, O., McGee, H., Hogan, M., Kunin, H., O'Brien, S. and O'Siorain, L. (2001) 'Relatives' views of health care in the last year of life', *International Journal of Palliative Nursing*, **7**, 449–56.

Kemppainen, J.K. (2000) 'The critical incident technique and nursing care quality research', *Journal of Advanced Nursing*, **32**, 1264–71.

Kemppainen, J.K., O'Brien, L., Williams, H., Evans, L., Newman-Weiner, K. and Holzemer, W. (1999) 'Quantifying patient engagement with nurses: A validation of a scale with AIDS patients', *Outcomes Management for Nursing Practice*, **3**, 167–74.

Kerry, T. (2005) 'Critical incidents in the working lives of a group of primary deputy heads', *Improving Schools*, **8**, 79–91.

Liefooghe, A. and Olafsson, R. (1999) '"Scientists" and "amateurs": Mapping the bullying domain', *International Journal of Manpower*, **20**, 39–49.

Norman, I., Redfern, S.J., Tomalin, D.A. and Oliver, S. (1992) 'Developing Flanagan's critical incident technique to elicit indicators of high and low quality nursing care from patients and their nurses', *Journal of Advanced Nursing*, **17**, 590–600.

Pryce-Jones, M. (1992) 'Assessing the quality of discharge procedures for elderly people', *Health Services Management*, **88**, 23–6.

Redfern, S. and Norman, I. (1999) 'Quality of nursing care perceived by patients and their nurses: An application of critical incident technique, Part 1', *Journal of Clinical Nursing*, **8**, 407–21.

Weisgerber, R.A., Levine, R. and DuBois, P. (1990) *Research to Identify Critical Factors Contributing to Entry and Advancement in Science, Mathematics, and Engineering Fields by Disabled Persons: Final Report* (Palo Alto, CA: American Institute for Research).

Part 5

Bringing it all Together

Mixed Methods Research: Quantity Plus Quality

ROBERT WALKER

19

Introduction

Had this book been published 40 years ago, it probably would not have been organised into sections on quantitative, qualitative and desk-based research. Desk-based research was then associated with the humanities, with scholarship; it was what philosophers and historians did. Quantitative methods, still often known as 'statistics', were the rapidly advancing social research frontier reliant on hand counts, Kalamazoo cards[1] and, if fortunate, computers that filled half a building but took three days to generate a cross-tabulation. Social science had come of age; theories were being evolved and tested quantitatively with survey data. Outside of marketing, qualitative research was usually called ethnography and was largely the preserve of anthropologists.

How things have changed in social science. In Britain, qualitative methodology has long been in the ascendancy, especially in sociology, health services research, education and, perhaps too, in social policy and geography. Only economics, psychology and demography sustain a quantitative core. Moreover, for much of this period there has been a tendency in academe to separate qualitative and quantitative research, with specialist journals and segregated methods of teaching. The time has come to end this separatist tendency and the intention in this chapter is to explain how. But first it is necessary to review the origins of the quantitative–qualitative divide.

Competing Paradigms

It is possible to interpret the advance of qualitative research in terms of a paradigm shift (Morgan, 2007). In the 1960s and 1970s, much of social science was seeking to ape the approach of the natural sciences in prioritising formal theory, deductive reasoning, hypothesis generation and empirical testing based on careful measurement. Because experiments were difficult to construct in the social sciences, *post hoc* statistical control was used as a substitute. However, a number of scholars, notably Guba and Lincoln (1989), became frustrated at, among other things, the apparent inability of social science to grapple with the complexity and intentionality of people's lives. Normal social science, or rather a caricature of it, was labelled 'positivism' and an alternative, variously termed 'naturalistic enquiry', 'constructivism' or 'interpretivism', was presented in opposition and juxtaposition to it.

This critique was primarily conducted in metaphysical terms. It sought to demonstrate that the nature of reality determined what could be known and circumscribed the methodology that should be used. Ontology (the nature of existence) and epistemology (what it is possible to know) were prioritised above decisions about methodology (ways of finding out). If reality was, as constructivists would argue, what people perceived or defined reality to be, then it could only be accessed through interaction and empathy with individual research subjects, and this, in turn, could only be achieved by using the techniques of qualitative research (Guba and Lincoln, 1989; Shadish, 1995). Positivism, and with it quantitative social science, was toppled from its position as the dominant (albeit often aspirational) paradigm and relegated, as illustrated by the structure of this volume, to just one of a number of ways of studying the social world.

Some argue that the time is ripe for another paradigm shift, to mixed methods research. However, before considering this possibility, two further observations are in order. First, the overthrow of positivism was effectively a political act. A prevailing paradigm determines by whom research agendas will be set, which research questions will be asked and what projects funded, what jobs opportunities will become available and which skills and aptitudes will be rewarded (see also Chapter 1). Challenging positivism therefore meant confronting the status quo and the vested interests within academic power structures. The success of this challenge warrants study in its own right, but one important factor was the growth of emancipatory politics based on race and ethnicity, gender and sexuality. These political movements readily associated positivism with the powers of oppression and rejoiced in the liberation offered by qualitative methodology; the latter at last giving voice to the oppressed and so being morally superior to quantitative research.

The second observation concerns the oppositional basis of the paradigm shift away from positivism. Kuhn (1962) anticipated that when one scientific paradigm succeeded another, the change would be triggered by an increasing number of inexplicable anomalies that could only be resolved by the new paradigm that would then generate fresh areas of enquiry. However, because positivism was replaced on grounds of ontology and epistemology, the anomalies were avoided rather than resolved. Constructivists, who were newly in the ascendant, addressed different kinds of question in different ways; positivist quantitative research continued but generated incommensurable kinds of knowledge. There was little scope for dialogue; each side argued that the questions asked by the other were either trivial or impossible to answer given the nature of reality and the research tools in use.

A Different Paradigm

Reality has differed somewhat from the rhetoric. Hidden in a footnote to Guba and Lincoln's contribution to the *Handbook of Qualitative Research* is the acknowledgement that 'workaday scientists rarely have either the time or the inclination to assess what they do in philosophical terms' (1994: 117). In truth, the choice of method is not usually predetermined by ontological considerations. Moreover, while quantitative research may have fallen out of favour in academe, it has become the foundation of evidence-based policy and practice. Qualitative researchers, ethnographers especially, frequently use survey evidence, while the design of surveys is often preceded by qualitative piloting and, less frequently, quantitative analysis is informed by parallel qualitative findings. Likewise, for a couple of decades, large-scale policy evaluations in Britain have often embraced a mixture of quantitative and qualitative methods (Cabinet Office, 2004).

This practice of mixed methods, driven by the dictum 'whatever works', obviously sits uncomfortably within the strictures of a paradigm that limits the possibility of constructive dialogue across the methodological divide by declaring that only one method is appropriate. In fact, this dilemma has seldom proved an obstacle for people who practise mixed methods research: for them, the approach has been productive, generating knowledge, research funds or both (Bryman, 2007). However, several authors have sought to address the problem from a range of philosophical perspectives: realism (Pawson and Tilley, 1997); pragmatism (Powell, 2002, 2003; Johnson and Onwuegbuzie, 2006; Morgan, 2007); and systems theory (Barnes et al., 2003; Walker 2007). Perhaps the most elegant solution is that proposed by Morgan (2007) based on pragmatism. Pragmatism sidesteps ontology by arguing that all that is known about reality is known through human experience of it. It therefore offers an epistemological basis for what scientists do; namely seek to solve problems identified through their experience. Their success in solving problems justifies their activity and the method, or combination of methods, used.

Table 19.1 compares qualitative and quantitative approaches with the pragmatic perspective that legitimates the use of mixed methods on the grounds of their contribution to solving problems. Qualitative research is associated with inductive reasoning (that is, building theory from data) and quantitative with deduction (that is, testing theory with data). However, pure deductive and inductive reasoning are comparatively rare in social science, a reality reflected in pragmatism's reliance on abduction, an iterative process in which hypotheses are derived from observation and subsequently tested against data. Similarly, the double dichotomy that associates quantitative research with objectivity and qualitative research with subjectivity, though a useful didactic device, oversimplifies the research process. Pragmatism acknowledges this and that the researcher typically moves between different objective and subjective reference points, engaging in dialogue with research subjects, research peers and consumers of research. Finally, pragmatism seeks a compromise between the context-specific nature of qualitative research and the automatically assumed generalisability of quantitative research. Knowledge acquired in one setting is often applied in another. Pragmatism insists that the basis for making such transfers is clearly articulated and justified.

Table 19.1 Alternative paradigms

	Qualitative approach	Quantitative approach	Pragmatic approach (mixed methods)
Ontology	Reality is individualistic and relative	A real (absolute) existence	No assumption about reality
Connection of theory and data	Induction	Deduction	Abduction
Relationship to research process	Subjectivity	Objectivity	Intersubjectivity
Inference from data	Context	Generality	Transferability

Source: Adapted from Morgan (2007)

What is Mixed Methods Research?

It may seem odd to have used so many words establishing the legitimacy of mixed methods research before actually defining what it is. However, in one respect the meaning of mixed methods research is self-evident: different techniques or approaches used within a single study. Also, the maxim that 'you recognise it when you see it' holds good. Nevertheless, there is still considerable debate about what counts as mixed methods research (Johnson et al., 2007). The editorial to the first issue of the *Journal of Mixed Methods Research* (*JMMR*, 2007) recognises a series of different types of mixed method studies but all are characterised by a combination of quantitative and qualitative approaches (Table 19.2). In other words, mixing one-to-one interviews (Chapter 14) and focus groups (Chapter 15) or a survey (Chapter 9) and a randomised controlled trial (Chapter 11) do not count. This distinction is emphasised in the working definition of mixed methods research proposed by the journal:

> Research in which the investigator collects and analyzes data, integrates the findings, and draws inferences using both qualitative and quantitative approaches or methods in a single study or a program of inquiry. (*JMMR*, 2007: 4)

This is a useful definition that will be adopted here. However, its limitations should be noted. As is evident from Table 19.2, the definition reflects a binary view of research methodology. This denies the possibility of other kinds of research that are neither quantitative nor qualitative. Where, for example, does desk-based research fit and the systematic review of qualitative research? It also precludes a true fusion of methodologies that is arguably evident in, for example, attempts to use qualitative methods to *measure* policy outcomes (Thornton and

Corden, 2002) or in computational economics, an academic analogue to playing The Sims computer game on a PC or PlayStation2 (Tesfatsion, 2005).

Table 19.2 Types of mixed methods research identified by the *Journal of Mixed Methods Research*

Designs are 'mixed' because they utilise quantitative and qualitative approaches in one or more of the following ways:

● Two types of research questions (with qualitative and quantitative approaches)
● The manner in which the research questions are developed (participatory vs. pre-planned)
● Two types of sampling procedures (for example probability and purposive)
● Two types of data collection procedures (for example focus groups and surveys)
● Two types of data (for example numerical and textual)
● Two types of data analysis (statistical and thematic)
● Two types of conclusions (emic and etic[1] representations, 'objective' and 'subjective', and so on).

1 An 'emic' account is a culturally specific description given in terms meaningful to the respondent or actor. An 'etic' account is supposedly culturally neutral and is provided by an observer.

Source: Adapted from *JMMR* (2007)

Although the *JMMR* definition prioritises integration, this can differ in timing and degree (Figure 19.1). Johnson et al. (2007) identify research designs from the purely qualitative to the purely quantitative. At the midpoint, equal status is assigned to the two perspectives. Between the midpoint and the extremes lie a large number of possible permutations. These range from those in which quantitative methodology dominates and qualitative methods play a subsidiary role, perhaps in aiding survey design or in interpreting statistical relationships, to designs that are inherently qualitative but use quantitative research in a supportive role, with survey or socio-economic data perhaps being used to situate a case study. It is, at least, arguable that as mixed methods research has become more accepted, there has been a migration in the density of projects from the extremes to the more challenging, and potentially more creative, midpoint.

Figure 19.1 includes a second discriminating dimension, project time. The argument is that the balance of quantitative and qualitative research may change over the duration of a project. In the classic development of a quantitative survey, qualitative research may only dominate in the design phase when focus groups and in-depth interviews are used to explore concepts and to develop terminology and question wording. In studies of the effectiveness of health interventions, quantitative methods may feature at the beginning, establishing baseline data, and at the end when these are compared with outcomes to establish impact. Qualitative fieldwork may predominate in the intervening period with a focus on implementation, and at the analysis stage when attention turns to explaining or accounting for the policy outcomes observed. However, particularly with midpoint designs that balance qualitative and quantitative perspectives and prioritise integration, the linear conception of project time, from design through to dissemination, may disintegrate as analysis leads to, for example, redesign.

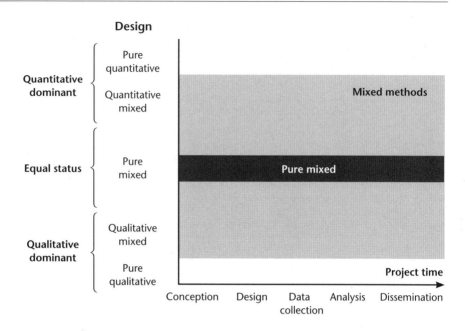

Figure 19.1 Types of mixed methods research

Source: Adapted from Johnson et al. (2007)

What should by now be apparent is that mixed methods research is characterised by its diversity. There is no fixed formula for what mixed methods research is or how it should be done.

Uses of Mixed Methods Research

Pragmatism legitimates the mixing of qualitative and quantitative methods to the extent that they solve research problems better than either approach employed in isolation. What then is the added value that results from mixed method research? At heart, this is an empirical question that cannot yet be answered since systematic comparison of the different methods is rare. However, it is possible to document the justification for mixed methods research offered by its proponents.

Table 19.3 lists both the rationale that exponents give for using multi-method research and the ways in which it is actually used in practice, as assessed by Alan Bryman (2006). The table is based on 232 articles published between 1994 and 2003 that were listed in the Social Science Citation Index (SSCI) and identified by a search of 'relevant key words or phrases such as "quantitative" and "qualitative", or "multi(-)method", or "mixed method", or "triangulation" [that] appeared in the title, key words or abstract' (Bryman, 2006: 100). The analysis covers sociology, social psychology, human, social and cultural geography, management and organisational behaviour and media and cultural studies. Because the SSCI is restricted to 'scholarly' journals, it unfortunately excludes the important and creative applied work undertaken for government and business that is not written up for academic consumption.

In Table 19.3 Bryman's detailed analysis is nested within a broader fivefold conceptual framework of mixed methods research suggested by Greene et al. (1989). Greene et al.'s first rationale or justification for combining methods is '*development*'; that is, using results from one method to inform or develop another. Examples include qualitative piloting during survey development, employing a survey sample to identify or recruit respondents with specific characteristics for in-depth interview, and fieldwork to establish the quality of service delivery in a policy experiment.[2] In studies using mixed methods with the aim of development, the individual methods are not necessarily accorded equal status and the ontological and epistemological bases of the dominate methodology may be retained.

Table 19.3 Uses of mixed methods research

	Percentage of studies			
	Rationale		Practice	
	Primary	All given[1]	Primary	All identified[1]
1 Development	10.3		8.6	
Instrument development		7.8		9.1
Sampling		13.4		18.5
2 Initiation	0.4		1.3	
Confirm and discover		3.9		6.5
3 Triangulation	7.8		12.5	
Triangulation – Validity and precision		12.5		34.5
Diversity of views (perspective)		11.2		15.1
4 Expansion	25.4		31.5	
Completeness		13.0		28.9
Utility		0.9		0.9
5 Complementarity	28.9		44.8	
Different things				
Different research questions		5.6		4.3
Process		2.2		2.6
Strengthening				
Offset		3.0		1.7
Enhancement		31.5		52.2
Credibility		0.9		2.2
Interpretation				
Diversity of view (ascribing meaning)[2]		X		X
Illustration		1.7		22.8
Explanation		5.6		13.8
Context		3.4		4.3
Unexpected results		0.0		0.9
Other/unclear		3.4	1.3	6.1
Not stated	27.2	26.7		0.4

1 Percentages do not add to 100 per cent because more than one rationale/use was coded.
2 Included in 'Diversity of views (perspective)' above.

Source: Adapted from Bryman (2006)

'*Initiation*', Greene et al.'s second justification for mixed methods, directly embraces the epistemological conflicts between quantitative and qualitative methodologies. Initiation seeks to reformulate questions or reinterpret findings defined within one tradition by reference to insights from the other. It, therefore, exploits the contradiction and paradox arising from different perspectives. Initiation is rarely used, either in practice or as an explicit rationale for mixed methods, but one example, cited by Greene et al. (1989), is Maxwell et al.'s (1986) evaluation of Medical Care Evaluation Committees in physicians' education. This employed ethnography within an experimental framework. The researchers anticipated that participation in the committees by physicians would directly increase the latter's knowledge and, hence, performance. However, the ethnography revealed that confidence, which was increased by participation, was a crucial mediating variable.

'*Triangulation*', adding methods to corroborate findings, is a much more frequently cited rationale for using mixed methods in the literature. Although it was not often given as the main justification in the studies reviewed by Bryman, a third or more of the studies revealed that researchers used triangulation in practice. Campbell and Fiske (1959) are credited with the introduction of the term but Denzin (1970) popularised four kinds of triangulation: data; investigator; theory; and methodological. Inherent in these writers' account of triangulation is the positivistic notion that there is some objective truth which is imperfectly revealed by each method; the greater the overlap in findings, the greater their validity is presumed to be (Golafshani, 2003). However, triangulation need not trap the researcher within a positivistic framework. Within other methodologies, difference may be perceived as the product of varying methods identifying disparate aspects of reality or, even, offering glimpses of different realities perceived by different (kinds of) people.

Triangulation interpreted in this wider, less positivistic, way connects with '*Expansion*' and '*Complementarity*', two further justifications for mixed methods research that both stress its 'added value'. Expansion refers to the ability to increase the range and breadth of an enquiry, to approach completeness and, thereby, to add understanding and, important for practitioners, practical, real-world utility to research findings (Walker and Duncan, 2007). Complementarity highlights the combining of research methods throughout the life of a project to achieve such completeness. Almost two-thirds of the studies reviewed by Bryman cited expansion and complementarity as reasons why mixed methods were used, and over three-quarters of the studies were judged to have exploited these characteristics in the design of projects and/or in analysis.

Complementarity means that different kinds of research question – for example, 'How many?' and 'How come?' – can be addressed empirically within the same project; for instance, quantitative techniques might be used to map structures and qualitative ones to explore process. Complementarity can also facilitate interpretation in a number of ways. Examples include: adding quantitative context to ethnographic findings; using qualitative evidence to illustrate a statistical relationship or to help to explain it; and 'revisiting' an unanticipated result, perhaps investigating it with follow-up in-depth interviews. Interpretation can be further facilitated by carrying through into the interpretation the views of different actors – including researchers from contrasting traditions (Bryman merged this aspect of complementarity within a category labelled 'diversity of views'; it is reported under 'triangulation' in Table 19.3 above). Finally, complementarity may enhance the reliability or trustworthiness of research. The limitations of one method may, on occasion, be offset by the strengths of another. Understanding may be enhanced if different methods add to the levels of resolution considered or add tiers of meaning. Credibility can be increased if different methods generate consistent results or if they provide detailed understanding of discrepancies.

The reasons for mixed method research are therefore legion and the fact that a quarter of the authors in Bryman's 2006 study did not even bother to justify their use of mixed method designs suggests that they may be operating within a paradigm in which the use of mixed methods is self-evident. There can be dangers in this as is discussed towards the end of the chapter.

An Example of a Mixed Methods Study

While authors of other chapters have chosen to shop-front recent research, the example reported here dates from 1990–2 and demonstrates, among other things, that multi-method research is not as new as some advocates of a multi-method paradigm would suggest (Figure 19.2). Although not a study of health or social care, it concerns the process of identifying and responding to need. Conducted under contract from the then UK Department of Health and Social

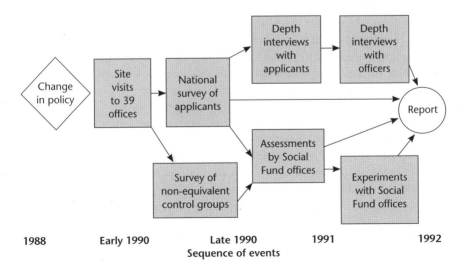

Figure 19.2 Social Fund evaluation

Source: Adapted from Walker, R. (2000) 'Welfare policy: Tendering for evidence'. In Davies, H., Nutley, S. and Smith, P. (eds) *Evidence and Public Policy* (Bristol: Policy Press) pp. 141–66

Security, the study is a post facto evaluation of the Social Fund, a national system of largely discretionary loans and grants intended to meet the one-off financial needs of people living on social assistance (Huby and Dix, 1992). Payments are made from a fixed budget allocated to local offices and were generally only available to people already receiving a social assistance benefit (called Income Support).

The style of the evaluation was pluralistic, examining the effectiveness of the policy with respect to the various, and sometimes divergent, objectives of different policy actors (Smith and Cantley, 1985). Prospective evaluation was considered to be impractical since the policy was already in place. The evaluation sought to determine the extent to which the Social Fund was targeted on people who were most in need, an objective that was complicated by the discretionary, budget-driven nature of the scheme. Only Social Fund officers using discretion could determine whether a person was eligible, but even their discretion was fettered by budgetary constraints.

The core of the project was a survey interview with a clustered, stratified national random sample comprising four non-equivalent comparison groups:

1 Successful applicants to the Social Fund

2 Applicants who had been refused a Social Fund award

3 Income Support recipients who had not applied to the Social Fund (to establish how far need was going unmet) and

4 Housing Benefit recipients who, while ineligible for Social Fund payments, were included as proxies for low-income families generally.

The sample, stratified by geography, was clustered in the areas served by 39 benefit offices. Site visits of two to three days' duration had previously been made to each of the areas and this had involved observation of office procedures and in-depth interviews with office staff and welfare rights workers (Walker et al., 1992). The aim of the visits was to understand how the scheme was variously administered and how staff used discretion to determine individual need (see Figure 19.3).

Insights into the way decisions were made, together with an understanding of claimants' experiences as mediated through welfare rights advisers, were used to inform the content and structure of the survey interview schedules. In total, 1,724 structured home interviews were undertaken to collect information on incomes, perceived needs, 'objective' needs and budgeting strategies. Social Fund officers, seconded to the research team, revisited applicants to conduct need assessments with reference to the priorities and budgetary constraints of the appropriate local office in which they were temporarily based. These assessments, which were purely for research purposes, provided a basis for judging how many people would have been successful had they made an application to the Social Fund and, hence, a measure of unmet need.

Thirty-one of the survey respondents who had applied to the Social Fund were re-interviewed in depth to gain greater insight into how needs were

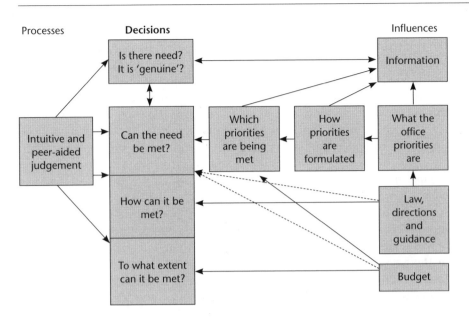

Figure 19.3 How Social Fund officers made decisions

Source: Adapted from Walker et al. (1991)

perceived and identified by people on low incomes and to explore how the decision to claim was made. Twenty-seven of these respondents gave consent to the officer who dealt with their last application being interviewed, and subsequently 26 interviews were undertaken with staff to investigate how the claims had been dealt with. Finally, laboratory experiments were conducted in which specimen applications, developed to replicate needs scenarios based on 'objective' information gathered in the survey, were 'processed' by Social Fund officers under different budgetary constraints.

The study showed that it was impossible to predict which applicants would be awarded payments from the Social Fund on the basis of either objective or self-assessed measures of need. Officers varied noticeably in their interpretation of the regulations and reached very different decisions on the basis of the same facts. The 'laboratory work' suggested that budgetary constraints were likely to have reduced the percentage of successful applications by 31 per cent. Clearly, the Social Fund did not target help to those in greatest need as was intended. On the other hand, it did successfully cap expenditure on exceptional needs, which no previous scheme had done. The Social Fund scheme continues with only minor modifications.

Making Multi-method Research Happen

The Social Fund evaluation illustrates mixed methods being used to develop the survey questionnaire; to triangulate the perspectives of applicants, staff and welfare rights advisers, sometimes concerning the same event; and to expand the study to investigate process as well as outcomes. Arguably, it even demonstrates the less common use of mixed methods research to facilitate initiation; that is, to explore paradox. So, while the Social Fund regulations were couched in positivistic terms based on the idea of objective need, the practice of discretion was more amenable to a constructivist analysis. However, the major rationale for using mixed methods was complementarity: it would have been impossible to understand need assessment without observing applicant interviews, to measure policy outcomes without survey data from comparison groups, or to assess the impact of budgetary constraints without experimental data. Likewise, the analysis was enriched by the ability to refer to multiple sources to understand why the Social Fund did not address need rather than merely being able to state the extent of mismatch between need and delivery.

Many factors can, of course, conspire to frustrate integration within mixed methods research. Drawing upon interviews with 20 UK social scientists, Bryman (2007: 12) notes, for example, the methodological preferences that lead some researchers 'to emphasise one set of findings' over another and the skill specialisms in teams that impede integration. Beneath these particular barriers lie the narrow methodological training of most researchers, the methods-bound perspectives of the academic disciplines and the sheer range of skills required. Such factors militate against the lone researcher utilising multiple methods; instead privileging multi-disciplinary teams. Nonetheless, effective team working depends on easy communication, openness, trust, time, good management and supportive structures that are often missing from universities and shotgun research collaborations created in response to financial opportunities (Walker and Wiseman, 2006). The Social Fund evaluation benefited from a closely knit team of researchers, each trained in more than one discipline, who had previously experimented with different methodologies.

Bryman also points to other barriers, such as one set of data being intrinsically more interesting than another, the structure of research projects that make integration difficult, and the deleterious consequences for integration of survey analysis being quicker than qualitative. These are effectively design problems that can often be offset at the planning stage. For example, research questions can be broken down into their constituent elements, and details of how each will be informed by various components of the research specified. Equally, a Gantt[3] chart, or its equivalent, can be used to ensure that reporting sequences are optimised (and made robust to unanticipated eventualities), so permitting each component maximally to inform, or be informed by, the others (see also Chapter 2). The fact that integration can also be restricted by external factors, notably limited time horizons, is more problematic.

Other barriers to integration identified by Bryman reflect uncertainties about the nature of evidence and of truth itself: the different demands made by different audiences; the gate-keeping role of methodologically narrow-minded publishers; and the need to bridge ontological divides. Bryman notes how different audiences and editorial boards expect different kinds of evidence and different kinds of evidence may be required on varying occasions. For example, Walker and Duncan (2007) opine that government ministers may be persuaded of a policy by qualitative research, since this is similar in form (although, of course, not necessarily in content) to the accounts that they are used to hearing from constituents, but would generally require quantitative evidence to defend it. However, if the rationale for mixed method designs is as compelling as documented above, the added value of integrated mixed method research may quell resistance to it. Freshwater (2007: 139) has warned of the danger of mixed methods research moving away from providing explanations of the world from a particular perspective to 'becoming a narrative with a legitimising function', namely that of justifying itself. If this is to be avoided, it is probably necessary to progress beyond the combination of methods, the 'sets of findings' referred to by Bryman (2007), towards full integration.

For Moran-Ellis et al. (2006: 50), integration means the assembly of different entities in research in which the 'material differences' of the 'separate entities are not erased, but work synergistically to produce a whole that is greater than the sum of its parts'. They identify several types or degrees of integration including *Separate Methods, Integrated Analysis'*, in which a common analytic method, quantitative or qualitative, formal or informal, is applied to data generated by different methods, and *'Separate Methods, Separate Analysis, Theoretical Integration'* in which the findings of separately conducted analyses are only integrated through theoretical interpretation. The former approach can necessitate questionable transformations to harmonise data types or the explicit or unacknowledged oversight of material differences in data or epistemology. The latter strategy, though common in literature review, may be as difficult to justify as it is fruitfully to achieve. They, therefore, applaud the attempts by Pawson (1995) and Coxon (2005) to integrate methods at the outset of research and to retain that integration throughout analysis and interpretation. To achieve this successfully, returns one to the importance of design and to the foresight and planning that are required to generate circumstances in which imagination and creativity can extract added value from mixed methods research. The added value would be judged, pragmatically, in terms of whether mixed methods research provides better answers to research questions.

Quantity and Quality

Mixed methods research is not new. What is new is a growing confidence that it has much to offer beyond what quantitative research and qualitative research have delivered individually, and that the different ontologies and epistemologies can be accommodated intellectually. It is too early to say whether a mixed methods paradigm underpinned by pragmatism will become dominant in the way that positivism, and to a lesser extent, constructivism once were. However, the quantitative–qualitative dichotomy is too limiting to be sustainable in a world crying out for knowledge, answers and solutions.

Mixed method research is to other research what binocular vision is to monocular sight; it adds depth, relief and field. However, while mixed methods research can be effective, this does not mean that it is always influential. Plans to reform the Social Fund on the basis of the evaluation were discarded following a change of government. Moreover, while mixed methods research carries over the strengths of its constituent methodologies, it also acquires the weaknesses, only some of which can be offset through the use of complementary methods. Furthermore, it is not only necessary to accommodate to the complexity of design, fieldwork and analysis that is typically demanded by mixed methods research, but also to accept discrepancies in findings. There is a need to accommodate to the increased uncertainty that is likely to accompany the richness of understanding arising from multiple perspectives.

But while multi-method research may be difficult, it is certainly not impossible and its potential is enormous. A final barrier to integrating methods identified by Bryman (2007) was the supposed lack of exemplars. It is possible that Bryman's respondents reached this conclusion because they were looking in the wrong place, to academic social science. Within applied social science, in government, business and commerce, mixed methods research is commonplace if not the norm. These sectors have not tripped up over ontology but have successfully employed the pragmatic maxim that 'what works, works; quantity and quality'. While not all such research is excellent, enough is sufficiently good to provide models from which to learn.

Acknowledgement

This chapter benefits much from insight and stimulus provided by Professor Alan Bryman who, nevertheless, cannot be held responsible for any deficiencies.

References

Barnes, M., Matka, E. and Sullivan, H. (2003) 'Evidence, understanding and complexity: Evaluation in non-linear systems', *Evaluation*, **9**, 265–84.

Bryman, A. (2006) 'Integrating quantitative and qualitative research: How is it done?' *Qualitative Research*, **6**, 97–113.

Bryman, A. (2007) 'Barriers to integrating quantitative and qualitative research', *Journal of Mixed Methods Research*, **1**, 8–22.

Cabinet Office (2004) *'Trying It Out' Review of the Effectiveness of Government Pilots* (London: Cabinet Office).

Campbell, D. and Fiske, D. (1959) 'Convergent and discriminant validation by the multitrait-multimethod matrix', *Psychological Bulletin*, **56**, 81–105.

Collins, K., Onwuegbuzie, A. and Sutton, I. (2006) 'A model incorporating the rationale and purpose for conducting mixed methods research in special education and beyond', *Learning Disabilities: A Contemporary Journal*, **4**, 67–100.

Coxon, T. (2005) 'Integrating qualitative and quantitative data: What does the user need?', *FQS (Forum: Qualitative Social Research)*, **6**, URL: http://www.qualitativeresearch.net/fqs/fqs-eng.htm.

Denzin, N. (1970) 'Strategies of multiple triangulation'. In Denzin, N. (ed.), *The Research Act* (New York: McGraw Hill), pp. 297–331.

Freshwater, D. (2007) 'Reading mixed methods research: Contexts for criticism', *Journal of Mixed Methods Research*, **1**, 134–46.

Golafshani, N. (2003) 'Understanding reliability and validity in qualitative research', *The Qualitative Report*, **8**, 597–607.

Greene, J., Caracelli, V. and Graham, W. (1989) 'Towards a conceptual framework of mixed method evaluation designs', *Educational Evaluation and Policy Analysis*, **11**, 255–74.

Guba, E. and Lincoln, Y. (1989) *Fourth Generation Evaluation* (Newbury Park, CA: Sage).

Guba, E. and Lincoln, Y. (1994) 'Competing paradigms in qualitative research'. In Denzin, N. and Lincoln, Y. (eds), *Handbook of Qualitative Research* (Thousand Oaks, CA: Sage), pp. 105–77.

Huby, M. and Dix, G. (1992) *Evaluating the Social Fund*. Department of Social Security Research Report 9 (London: HMSO).

JMMR (2007) 'The new era of mixed methods', *Journal of Mixed Methods Research*, **1**, 3–7.

Johnson, B. and Onwuegbuzie, A. (2006) 'Mixed methods research: A research paradigm whose time has come', *Educational Researcher*, **33**, 14–26.

Johnson, R.B., Onwuegbuzie, A. and Turner, L. (2007) 'Toward a definition of mixed methods research', *Journal of Mixed Methods Research*, **1**, 112–33.

Kuhn, T. (1962) *The Structure of Scientific Revolutions*, 3rd edn (Chicago, IL: University of Chicago Press).

Maxwell, J., Bashook, P. and Sandlow, C.J. (1986) 'Combining ethnographic and experimental methods in educational evaluation.' In Fetterman, D. and Pitman, M. (eds), *Educational Evaluation: Ethnography in Theory, Practice, and Politics* (Beverly Hills, CA: Sage), pp. 121–43.

Moran-Ellis, J., Alexander, V., Cronin, A., Dickinson, M., Fielding, J., Sleney, J. and Thomas, H. (2006) 'Triangulation and integration: Processes, claims and implications', *Qualitative Research*, **6**, 45–59.

Morgan, D. (2007) 'Paradigms lost and pragmatism regained: Methodological implications of combining qualitative and quantitative methods', *Journal of Mixed Methods Research*, **1**, 48–76.

Pawson, R. (1995) 'Quality and quantity, agency and structure, mechanism and context, dons and cons', *BMS, Bulletin de Methodologie Sociologique*, **47**, 5–48.

Pawson, R. and Tilley, N. (1997) *Realistic Evaluation* (London: Sage).

Powell, T. (2002) 'The philosophy of strategy', *Strategic Management Journal*, **23**, 873–80.

Powell T. (2003) 'Strategy without ontology', *Strategic Management Journal*, **24**, 285–91.

Shadish, W. (1995) 'Philosophy of science and the quantitative–qualitative debates: Thirteen common errors', *Evaluation and Program Planning*, **18**, 62–75.

Smith, G. and Cantley, C. (1985) 'Policy evaluation: The use of varied data in a study of a psychogeriatric service'. In Walker, R. (ed.) *Applied Qualitative Research* (Aldershot: Gower), pp. 156–74.

Tesfatsion, L. (2005) 'Agent-based computational economics: A constructive approach to economic theory'. In Judd, K. and Tesfatsion, L. (eds), *Handbook of Computational Economics, Volume 2: Agent-Based Computational Economics* (North Holland: Elsevier/Handbooks in Economics Series).

Thornton, P. and Corden, A. (2002) *Evaluating the Impact of Access to Work: A Case Study Approach*. Research and Development Report WAE138 (Sheffield: Claimant Unemployment and Disadvantage Analysis Division, Department for Work and Pensions).

Walker, R. (2007) 'Entropy and the evaluation of labour market interventions', *Evaluation*, **13**, 193–219.

Walker, R. and Duncan, S. (2007) 'Knowing what works: Policy evaluation in central government'. In Bochel, H. and Duncan, S. (eds) *Professional Policy Making for the Twenty First Century* (Bristol: Policy Press).

Walker, R. and Wiseman, M. (2006) 'Managing evaluations'. In Shaw, I., Greene, J. and Mark, M. (eds) *Handbook of Policy Evaluation* (London: Sage), pp. 360–83.

Walker, R., Dix, G. and Huby, M. (1991) 'How Social Fund officers make decisions'. In Carter, P., Jeffs, T. and Smith, M. (eds), *Social Work and Social Welfare Yearbook 3* (Milton Keynes: Open University Press).

Walker, R., Dix, G. and Huby, M. (1992) *Working the Social Fund* (London: HMSO).

Notes

1 Punch cards in which alphanumerical characters were represented as patterns of holes that enabled mechanical sorting. They were named after the town where they were invented, Kalamazoo in Michigan, USA.

2 Collins et al. (2006) label each of these three examples: 'instrument fidelity'; 'participant enrichment' and 'treatment integrity' respectively.

3 A Gantt chart is a horizontal bar chart that depicts activities as blocks arrayed over time such that the left- and right-hand ends of each block correspond to the beginning and end date of an activity. Time management software such as Microsoft Project generates them as visual displays.

Dissemination

20

JOANNE NEALE

Introduction

As earlier chapters of this book have revealed, there are many ways of answering research questions, testing out hypotheses and exploring new areas of enquiry. In order to conduct a successful study, the researcher must first have some basic understanding of the issue to be investigated and sufficient methodological knowledge to be able to select the most appropriate techniques of data collection and analysis to address the problem. Thereafter, it is often necessary to review and revise previous decisions and plans as unforeseen problems emerge and opportunities arise.

The mechanics of conducting a study can be so complex and all-consuming that it is easy to see why researchers, and particularly novice researchers, do not always pay close attention to how they can best disseminate the outputs of their research. As the dissertation deadline looms, funding for the Ph.D. studentship ends or the delivery date of that commissioned report draws near, individuals commonly focus on producing the minimum written requirements for their institution or funder. Once those deadlines have passed, it is tempting to heave a sigh of relief and turn off the computer. To prevent this from happening, dissemination needs to be seen as a fundamental part of the research process. Accordingly, it needs to be written into the research timetable and, whenever possible, costed into funding applications (see Chapter 2).

What is Dissemination?

Dissemination is essentially the process of sharing information and knowledge with the largest audience possible in order to improve the accessibility of research findings (Saywell et al., 2007). This can be achieved through the production of diverse research outputs, such as dissertations, theses, research reports, books and book chapters, academic journal articles, professional journal articles, the mass media, leaflets, the internet and presentations. Different types of research output tend to have different audiences and tend to be suited to different types of message. As a result, the findings from any given study will usually be disseminated best by using a range of techniques and by producing a variety of outputs (ibid.).

Dissemination can, of course, be both a lone activity and a collaborative venture. Research conducted in teams usually produces multi-authored outputs and these are likely to benefit from the bringing together of researchers' different perspectives, experiences and knowledge. Joint dissemination can also generate new ideas, increase the number of potential outputs from a project, and offer team members opportunities for mutual support (Woods, 1999; Williams, 2002). Simply being part of a research team does not, however, guarantee authorship of an output. This rather has to be earned by fulfilling three basic criteria:

● Having generated at least part of the intellectual content of an output (for example, by designing the study or collecting or analysing the data

● Participation in writing, critically reviewing or revising the output

● Being able to defend publicly all the intellectual content of the output (Huth, 1990: 44).

Why Disseminate?

But why should the busy researcher, already coping with the day-to-day stresses of undertaking a study and meeting a final deadline, commit themselves to additional work? This question has many potential answers. Some might argue that dissemination is a moral obligation, particularly if the research has been publicly funded. In other words, other academics, professionals and the general public have 'a right' to access any new information produced. Good dissemination can also increase the impact of the study and enhance the likelihood that it will positively affect policy or practice. Equally, dissemination can promote the profile of the researcher/s and their institution/s which, in turn, might attract further research funding. Beyond this, preparing the findings of a study for wider consumption can help researchers to clarify their thinking. And last but not least, seeing one's name in print or presenting to an appreciative audience can, of course, be both rewarding and enjoyable.

Some General Guidelines for Successful Dissemination

Later sections of this chapter will review particular types of dissemination in more detail. Prior to this, some general guidelines on how to share research findings are suggested. Planning and early groundwork are certainly two useful starting points. These include selecting aspects of the data that will be of most interest and relevance to particular audiences and identifying the most appropriate type of research output (journal article, book, newspaper and so on) for a specific finding. Where more than one researcher is involved, the planning stage should also involve making decisions about who will be responsible for particular aspects of dissemination and the ordering of authors' names on outputs. Indeed, early discussions about such matters can prevent unhelpful misunderstandings and disputes later down the line.

Good planning equally means allowing sufficient time to complete the various stages of preparing materials for dissemination. Once the analyses are finalised, this will still involve reading, thinking, note-taking, preparing a plan or outline of the proposed output, drafting, redrafting, compiling a reference list, clearing any copyright permissions, checking and polishing. The first full draft of any output should always be put to one side for a while before being critically reviewed and revised. Although this review process can be undertaken by the researcher themselves, it is often helpful to invite a colleague or peer to make considered and constructive comments. These activities cannot, however, be undertaken well if the first full draft is not ready until the night before a deadline.

Clarity is a further fundamental principle of effective dissemination. There is little point in preparing a presentation or writing up findings for publication if the key messages being conveyed are vague, confused or overly complex. This further underlines the importance of knowing the needs of the audience being targeted. For example, the examiner of a Ph.D. will want and expect a higher level of technical and methodological detail than the reader of a newspaper or magazine article. All users of research will, meanwhile, appreciate materials that are clearly presented, logically ordered and easy to navigate. They will also expect outputs to contain accurate, up-to-date information and to tell a complete story. It should not be necessary to refer to another document or source in order to understand the one immediately to hand.

One strategy that can help to ensure that dissemination proceeds smoothly is to adopt a relatively structured approach to working on each research output. This might mean blocking out regular periods of time for dissemination activities, just as though they were fixed appointments in a diary. It might also mean breaking the preparation of research outputs down into smaller, more manageable tasks (Burnard, 1996). So, rather than thinking of producing a full Ph.D. thesis or book, it can be easier to identify chapters and, within chapters, sections and sub-sections of text. The IMRAD (introduction, methods, results and discussion) format can be helpful to this end since it encourages aspects of dissemination to be treated as discrete entities. Researchers can then set realistic and achievable targets for each period of dissemination work they undertake.

While the importance of reading the related literature must be emphasised, it is not necessary to be the world-leading expert in a field before dissemination can begin. Being able to talk coherently and with authority about one's findings is generally a good sign that it is time to start sharing information more widely. Those who are still uncertain about whether or not they are ready to disseminate from their study may wish to ask themselves the following five questions:

1. What are the main messages I want to convey from my data?

2. Who will be interested in these messages?

3. How do my findings add to the existing literature?

4. What are the strengths and weaknesses of my research?

5. What are the implications of my findings for policy and/or practice?

(See also Woods, 1999, p. 83 for a similar discussion). Once these questions can be answered, dissemination can almost certainly begin.

Dissertations and Theses

The student dissertation or thesis is probably the first substantial piece of research dissemination that most individuals ever undertake. Generally speaking, dissertations are written by final year undergraduates and Masters students as part of the requirements of their degree. In the UK, undergraduate dissertations are commonly about 10,000 words and Masters student dissertations about 20,000 words, although Master of Philosophy dissertations can be up to 60,000 words. Theses are submitted by doctoral students (Ph.D. or D.Phil.) as the final formal report of their research and tend to be between 80,000 and 100,000 words in length (Burnard, 1996).[1]

Allison and Race (2004) argue that students should always be conscious of the intended audience and purposes of academic dissertations and theses. That is, they are likely to be read by only two or three individuals (usually the external and internal examiners). Moreover, they have very specific purposes. These are to assess the student's ability to identify a problem, analyse the problem, carry out appropriate literature and other searches, develop a research design, select or devise appropriate data-collecting instruments, implement the design in practice, collate and analyse data using appropriate techniques, deduce conclusions, and write up and present a report in accordance with established practices (Alison and Race, 2004: 13).

Most academic institutions provide their students with guidelines or regulations regarding the length, structure and format of their dissertation or thesis (Levin, 2005). This is often accompanied by clear information on handing in arrangements and the marking criteria for assessment. This formalised approach tends to result in the production of fairly standardised documents containing a title page, abstract, acknowledgements, introduction, literature review, aims and methods section, findings, discussion, conclusions, references and appendices (where the appendices might contain material that is relevant but not essential to the reader's comprehension, such as questionnaires, interview schedules, or detailed tables and charts) (Burnard, 1996).

Despite this broad uniformity of style, dissertations and theses in practice vary widely in their content and quality. As with any form of research output, a logical structure and clear progressive argument will help to distinguish a strong dissertation or thesis from a mediocre or poor one. Equally, good writing skills can make a significant difference to the final product. For instance, it is always advisable to write as concisely as possible, using short sentences and paragraphs and avoiding complex punctuation (Burnard, 1996). Paragraphs should generally contain only one idea or theme and linking statements should provide continuity from one paragraph to the next (Williams, 2002).

For all researchers, but especially the dissertation or thesis writer, it can be helpful to divide the writing process into stages. Haynes (2001: 111) usefully identifies two: the compositional and the secretarial. In the compositional stage, the writer concentrates on producing words, getting the subject matter in order and covering all the ground. In the secretarial stage, the focus turns to presentation. That is, ensuring that the layout is clear, the punctuation, grammar and spelling are accurate, and the references are correct and in a consistent format. The secretarial stage can also be a good time to make sure that the writing style is concise and flows in a rhythmical way when read aloud.

Research Reports

Of the many forms of dissemination, the research report is perhaps the closest in form and structure to the university dissertation or thesis. The main audience of a research report is usually the research funder, such as a government department, public body or private company. The latter will often have commissioned a piece of research in order to gain insights into a particular issue that concerns them or to answer a specific question that is crucial to their organisation (see also Chapter 1). Where the findings are relevant to others – perhaps to other academics or to the general public – reports may be published like books or uploaded to websites where they can be accessed and downloaded by anyone interested in their content.

Just as it is not sensible to begin writing a dissertation before checking any relevant university guidelines, so one should not begin to write a report before clarifying with the funder the intended audience, any terms of references, formatting requirements, length, and submission deadline. Ascertaining this information should help to determine the tone and style of writing, but also the best way of organising and presenting the material. More general tips for preparing research reports are to ensure that the binding and paper are sturdy enough to withstand heavy use and the margins are wide enough to allow all text, tables and diagrams to be viewed with ease. In addition, a good contents list should enable the reader to turn easily to the information that most interests them (Emden and Easteal, 1993).

Books and Book Chapters

Very broadly speaking, academic books fall into two main categories: monographs and textbooks. Monographs are based on original research, often Ph.D. theses. In contrast, textbooks provide an authoritative summary of existing research and the state of knowledge in any given field. Like all published output, academic books can be single authored or multi-authored and should always be clearly written and logically organised. Crucially, however, they must also have a market and sell. Academic book publishing is a competitive business and those who wish to write in this form must demonstrate to potential publishers that they are a sound investment. This means researching the market, identifying other competitor publications, and specifying the context in which the book they want to write would be used (Haynes, 2001).

Authoring a book has many advantages over other forms of publication. For example, it allows the researcher to write about their subject at length, permits a high level of freedom of expression, reaches a wider audience than most other forms of academic writing, and – assuming it is done well – enhances status amongst students and peers. It is, however, a lengthy undertaking and requires a degree of time commitment that other research outputs do not tend to demand. Writing a book chapter is a considerably less ambitious undertaking than writing a sole-authored book, but the success or otherwise of the final product lies beyond the control of any single contributor. One all too frequent problem is that the publication of an edited book is delayed by one or two slow chapter writers or even a slow editor.

Academic Journals

According to Weiner (1998), academic journals provide up-to-date thinking and current research at the cutting edge in a particular discipline. Academic journals tend to be published under the aegis of professional bodies or subject associations and have a national and international readership (Allison and Race, 2004). Most have editorial boards and use expert referees to determine whether or not any submission received is of a sufficiently high standard to be published. It is largely because of this peer review process and their focus on publishing the most recent original research that papers appearing in academic journals are generally considered to be of the highest quality and the most prestigious.

One reason why journals contain the most recent research in any given field is that they are published on a regular basis (usually weekly, monthly, bi-monthly or quarterly). They are also able to publish papers that are too short, too ephemeral, or too obscure for books because their readership and thus their commercial success are not dependent on any single article (Burnard, 1996). The format of papers appearing in academic journals is, meanwhile, diverse and includes research papers, literature reviews, case studies, brief reports, opinion pieces, clinical notes, examples of best practice and letters to the editor.

Those seeking to publish in an academic journal should begin by identifying an appropriate journal for the message they want to convey and the audience they want to target. This is often best achieved by physically scanning recent issues of journals that seem promising and reading any recent papers related to one's own research. Academic journals invariably provide information in each issue and on their web page regarding their scope and readership. They also usually provide clear guidelines on the types of papers accepted, maximum length, layout, formatting of tables and illustrations, the use of footnotes and referencing system (Allison and Race, 2004). Researchers can additionally send editors a short abstract of their proposed paper and ask whether a full submission would be welcome.

According to Day (1996), editors of academic journals value papers that are logically structured, have a sharp focus, produce conclusions that address the aims identified at the outset, and are written in a concise and economical style. They will also be looking for work of a very high academic standard. Researchers are commonly under pressure to publish in their field's leading journals and this is a laudable goal. Despite this, an honest appraisal of one's own intended paper can sometimes indicate that it is unlikely to meet the very high standards of publication required or that the message would be better targeted at a non-specialist audience. In this case, submission to a less prestigious peer-reviewed journal or a decision to prepare the findings in a different format for a professional or lay audience might prove wiser (Thyer, 1994).

Professional Journals

Whilst the traditional academic journal is underpinned by original research and tends to have a relatively small and specialised audience, the professional journal is more concerned with practice and experience and generally has a much larger audience (Murray, 2005). Good examples of professional journals from the health and social care field include *Nursing Times*, *Community Care* and *Mental Health Today*. Since professional journals tend not to be peer-reviewed, they are sometimes seen as having a lower status than academic journals. However, it is better to see them as offering an alternative, rather than an inferior, form of dissemination. This is because they serve a different purpose and reach a different audience from highly academic publications.

When a research project produces knowledge that is likely to be of direct relevance to those practising in the health and social care world, it is always sensible to consider writing something for a professional journal. Nonetheless, it is important to remember that the style and format of any such piece will need to be fairly informal and even journalistic. Short sentences written in the active voice are usually best. Again, good preparation is to read a number of recent issues of the intended publication and contact the editor to discuss the content, tone and style before actually starting. Many professional publications have writers' guidelines similar to academic journals. Some will willingly send their in-house writers to interview researchers and then write up the article themselves. Others will accept academics' submissions but want to edit any unsuitable prose into their own house style.

The Mass Media

Historically, writing for or presenting directly to the mass media have not been priority activities for university researchers. However, this is beginning to change and increasing numbers of academics (sometimes referred to as 'media dons') are now routinely engaging with television, radio and the local and national press. Reasons for not working with journalists can include fear of losing control of one's own research findings, concern about having aspects of one's work misrepresented or slanted for popular appeal, and finding it too difficult – or inappropriate – to present very complex subjects in simple sound bites (particularly where this can result in context and qualification being lost).

More positively, reasons why researchers might work with the media include raising awareness of a particular research topic, helping to educate the public, opportunities for increasing the profile of one's discipline in the public eye, encouraging others – especially children – to take up a scientific career, engendering public support for science, generating extra money for one's field, and having a forum for expressing a personal opinion (Williams, 2002; Day and Gastel, 2006). It can, of course, also provide a little additional personal income and be personally satisfying.

An important key to disseminating research findings through the mass media is to remember that members of the public are not experts in any particular field and nor will they necessarily have an interest in the findings of a specific study. In consequence, it is essential to consider what the interests of the audience in question are likely to be and how best to engage them. This can be facilitated by providing real-life examples, using simple analogies, avoiding technical terms, and repeating the most salient points (Day and Gastel, 2006). If an interview with a reporter is involved, the researcher should be clear in advance about the most important messages they want to present and know how to convey these in simple and concise language. In addition, written materials can be given to reporters to foster accuracy and promote the efficient use of interview time (ibid.).

Leaflets

The production of leaflets is a particularly effective method of disseminating the most important findings of a study to patients and service users, to those who might have participated in the research, or to a lay audience who might be interested in the topic. For instance, leaflets can easily be distributed at sites where the research occurred or where those who might be affected by the research findings congregate. In the health and social care field, this might include doctors' surgeries, hospitals, social services departments and voluntary sector agencies.

A good leaflet should be eye-catching and sensibly set out, using easily understood headings and subheadings. The title will tell the reader about the research topic and encourage them to read on. The language used should appeal to the audience being targeted and the key messages must be clearly signposted. The use of bullet points, text boxes and the creative use of font sizes can be helpful for this purpose – although it is worth noting that upper case letters, italics and underlining can make text difficult to read. The first paragraph should ideally provide a general introduction and tell the reader what they will learn by reading on. Subsequent paragraphs should be short and precise, each making a separate point. The leaflet should then end in a friendly way, with details of who conducted the study and how or where to obtain further information (Cambridge ESOL, 2007).

Web Pages

Paper-based research outputs tend to have one important characteristic in common. That is, they are linear in structure. In other words, the reader will usually begin with the introduction and end with the conclusion, although they may of course dip into and out of sections if they are seeking particular information. In contrast, web pages are designed to be interactive and therefore commonly present their content in a nonlinear format. Thus, there is no expectation that the reader will access information in any particular order or have any knowledge from a previous web page when opening up a new one (Bonime and Pohlmann, 1997). Today, universities and research centres routinely have web pages that provide an overview of their research, profiles of their researchers and details of their research publications.

Dorner (2002: 25) helpfully explains some of the respective benefits of paper and web-based research outputs. Paper outputs, she argues, are suited to retaining the reader's attention over a long period of time. They generally offer reliable information, standardised display, clear readable typography and good image reproduction. They also look and feel good. In contrast, web pages are better for quick navigation and accessing up-to-date information, for example recent research findings. Display can be personalised and they are excellent for searching, combining media forms (visuals, audio, animation and text), and providing layers of detail through hyperlinks.[2] Web pages additionally offer good accessibility to those with disabilities.

A number of specific features are, however, required for effective web design. For instance, each page should communicate who owns the site and when the information on it was originally created and last updated. There should likewise be a link back to an appropriate home page and meaningful headings, subheadings and hyperlinks to facilitate navigation. Essentially, each web page must tell the user where they are, where they have been and where they can go (Nielson, 2000). It should also offer self-contained information so that understanding is not too dependent on what precedes or follows it (Bonime and Pohlmann, 1997; Maciuba-Koppel, 2002).

Because screen resolutions vary and can be tiring on the eyes, writing for the web should be particularly concise. Web pages should ideally be less than three hundred words and written in short paragraphs and sentences that are easy to scan and digest (Dorner, 2002; Maciuba-Koppel, 2002). Fonts should be checked for on-screen readability, but also print quality (Dorner, 2002). In general, the best web writing tends to be informal and direct, written in the present or present perfect tense. It should use active rather than passive verbs and first person rather than third person subjects. The overall tone is upbeat and positive, illustrating the immediacy and interactive nature of online information (ibid.).

Oral Presentations

Oral presentations can take the form of informal talks to fellow students or colleagues, but also national and international presentations to experts in a research field. Those making verbal presentations are generally asked to speak for a predetermined period of time, though seldom for longer than one hour and often for as short as ten minutes. In addition to providing an opportunity for showcasing polished research, oral presentations can offer a valuable forum for testing out thoughts on work in progress and for receiving critical feedback. Having to articulate key elements of one's research (sometimes in a very limited amount of time and to a lay audience) can be an excellent means of crystallising ideas and increasing clarity of expression.

Day and Gastel (2006) argue that oral presentations are generally best arranged in the same order as a written paper. That is, beginning with a statement of the problem and ending by suggesting a solution. The middle will cover methods and key results. Nonetheless, it is not advisable to provide an extensive review of the literature or too much detail on the study design and analyses. The audience for an oral presentation will generally be more diverse than the readership of a scientific paper, and so the presentation of too much technical information may cause them to lose interest or become confused. Likewise, too many ideas presented too quickly can obscure the key messages that one is trying to convey (Davis, 1997; Day and Gastel, 2006).

Visual aids, particularly PowerPoint slides, are increasingly the norm when presenting research at seminars or conferences. Visual aids can help to reinforce salient points, compensate for language barriers and bring research findings alive. If used badly, however, they can obstruct effective communication by diverting the audience's attention away from the speaker's words. Good visual aids should be well-organised and coordinate closely with what is being spoken. They should also be legible and easy to understand. As a rule, bullet points are easier to read than paragraphs of text and graphs are clearer than tables. Importantly, slides should not be cluttered with too many words, colours, or images (Davis, 1997; Day and Gastel, 2006).

When giving an oral presentation, speakers need to be conscious of their own physical presence and body language. A good presenter will speak slowly and clearly, make eye contact with the audience and convey enthusiasm for their topic. They will not fiddle with the microphone, put their hands in their pockets, mumble into their notes, or overrun beyond their allotted time. During their talk, they will use short pauses to allow the audience to reflect on key issues and they will be ready to deviate from their prepared material if the audience's attention or understanding seems to be straying (Davis, 1997). As with any other form of dissemination, knowing the audience and advanced preparation, including constructive self-criticism or feedback from a colleague, will help to ensure a successful delivery.

Poster Presentations

Poster presentations are based on visual information – written text, tables, graphs and illustrations – supplemented by the author's spoken explanation. The poster is usually on display for several hours at a conference or meeting and the authors will be present during part of that time to discuss the content with viewers (Davis, 1997). Poster displays were first used in the US in the mid-1970s when conference organisers found that they could not accommodate everyone who wanted to present verbally (Maugh, 1974). At that time, the opportunity to present a poster was commonly offered as a second best option for those who were not invited to speak. Today, the poster presentation has come to be seen as a valued form of dissemination in its own right.

An important advantage of a poster display over an oral presentation is that there is greater opportunity for one-to-one interaction between the author and the audience. Questions can be asked and answered more easily and information, including contact details, exchanged (Davis, 1997). The poster display thus provides a good opportunity for networking and for receiving feedback and comment (Day and Gastel, 2006). It can also be better than an oral presentation for showing the results of a complex study or for conveying multiple findings (ibid.).

Before beginning work on a display, it is again important to clarify the intended audience and any requirements of the organisers – particularly the height and width of space available. It is also essential that material is presented in a coherent and orderly fashion (such as the IMRAD format) and is clearly legible (Davis, 1997). The poster should be aesthetically pleasing with an interesting, descriptive title to help capture the reader's interest. Short paragraphs, written in simple language without too much technical jargon, will then help to retain the audience's attention. Although bullet points and lists are more appropriate than large chunks of text, pre-prepared handouts with additional detail can be used to satisfy those who want to know more (Davis, 1997; Day and Gastel, 2006).

Conclusions

Dissemination is a fundamental part of the research process. There is very little point in undertaking any scientific study if the findings are not shared with an audience, or better still many audiences. Some forms of dissemination (particularly dissertations, theses and reports) are non-negotiable requirements of undertaking a project. Other forms are not compulsory and this leaves the researcher with decisions to be made about how much dissemination to undertake, to whom and in what form. In a world of finite resources and competing priorities, these decisions should be made carefully.

Preparing findings for publication or presentation is hard work and requires the researcher to open themselves up to external criticism. There will likely be setbacks, including rejection letters from editors and unappreciative audiences, along the way. Consequently, perseverance, a willingness to learn and a relatively thick skin are required. As argued in Chapter 1, the findings of any research project are but a drop in a much larger ocean of uncertainty. Nonetheless, they can add to an existing body of knowledge or may begin to chip away at a prevailing set of beliefs and methods of practice. A successful dissemination strategy will help to ensure that a study's findings have maximum impact. Beyond this, good dissemination can raise the profile of a researcher and their institution and be personally very rewarding. Yet, to ensure that these benefits are achieved, it is necessary to do one's homework. This means identifying key messages, researching the best audiences and thinking through the pros and cons of different types of research output. It is wrong to assume that the leading journal in the field is the only place to publish. In reality, different aspects of one's data will be suited to different dissemination forms. The goal is to capitalise on all of the alternatives by being aware of the many options that exist and making sensible and informed choices.

References

Allison, B. and Race, P. (2004) *The Student's Guide to Preparing Dissertations and Theses,* 2nd edn (London: RoutledgeFarmer).

Bonime, A. and Pohlmann, K.C. (1997) *Writing for New Media* (New York: John Wiley and Sons).

Burnard, P. (1996) *Writing for Health Professionals: A Manual for Writers,* 2nd edn (London: Chapman and Hall).

Cambridge ESOL (English for Speakers of Other Languages) (2007) *Skills for Life: Writing Levels 1 and 2 – Leaflets and Information Sheets* (http://www.cambridgeesol.org/teach/SfL/Levels_1_and_2_Writing/About%20the%20paper/Leaflets/leaflets.htm) (accessed 1 January, 2008).

Davis, M. (1997) *Scientific Papers and Presentations* (San Diego, CA: Academic Press).

Day, A. (1996) *How to Get Research Published in Journals* (Aldershot: Gower).

Day, R.A. and Gastel, B. (2006) *How to Write and Publish a Scientific Paper,* 6th edn (Cambridge: Cambridge University Press).

Dorner, J. (2002) *Writing for the Internet* (Oxford: Oxford University Press).

Emden, J.V. and Easteal, J. (1993) *Report Writing,* 2nd edn (Maidenhead: McGraw-Hill Book Company).

Haynes, A. (2001) *Writing Successful Textbooks* (London: A & C Black Ltd).

Huth, E.J. (1990) *How to Write and Publish Papers in the Medical Sciences,* 2nd edn (Baltimore, MD: Williams and Wilkins).

Levin, P. (2005) *Excellent Dissertations!* (Maidenhead: Open University Press).

Maciuba-Koppel, D. (2002) *The Webwriter's Guide: Tips and Tools.* (Amsterdam: Focal Press).

Maugh, T.H. (1974) 'Poster sessions: A new look at scientific meetings', *Science,* **184**, 1361.

Murray, R. (2005) *Writing for Academic Journals* (Maidenhead: Open University Press).

Nielson, J. (2000) *Designing Web Usability: The Practice of Simplicity* (Indianapolis, IN: New Riders Publishing).

Saywell, D., Cotton, A. and Woodfield, J. (2007) *Spreading the Word: Disseminating Research Findings,* Synthesis note (http://www.lboro.ac.uk/departments/cv/wedc/publications/snstw/snstw.pdf) (accessed 1 January, 2008).

Thyer, B.A. (1994) *Successful Publishing in Scholarly Journals* (Thousand Oaks, CA: Sage Publications).

Weiner, G. (1998) *Getting Published: An Account of Writing, Refereeing and Editing Practices (1996–8),* final report to the ESRC (Image) Education-line, 26 August.

Williams, D. (2002) *Writing Skills in Practice: A Practical Guide for Health Professionals* (London: Jessica Kingsley Publishers).

Woods, P. (1999) *Successful Writing for Qualitative Researchers* (London: RoutledgeFalmer).

Notes

1   Although they might be less than this in the natural sciences.
2   Hyperlinks are direct links to another section in the same document or to another document that may be on another website.

Index

A letter *n* and a number following a page number refers to a note number on that particular page.